Y0-ABY-957

PROSTATIC CANCER

Gerald P. Murphy, M.D., Editor

PSG Publishing Company, Inc.
Littleton, Massachusetts

Library of Congress Cataloging in Publication Data

Main entry under title:

Prostatic cancer.

Includes index.
1. Prostate gland—Cancer. I. Murphy, Gerald Patrick.
[DNLM: 1. Prostatic neoplasms. WJ752 P966]
RC280.P7P76 616.9'94'63 78-55284
ISBN 0-88416-190-0

Printed in the United States of America.

International Standard Book Number: 0-88416-190-0

Library of Congress Catalog Card Number: 78-55284

CONTRIBUTORS

Malcolm A. Bagshaw, M.D.
Professor and Chairman
Department of Radiology
Stanford University School of Medicine
Stanford, California

Pierluigi E. Bigazzi, M.D.
Associate Professor of Pathology
University of Connecticut School of Medicine
Farmington, Connecticut

T. Ming Chu, Ph.D.
Professor and Director, Diagnostic Immunology Research and Biochemistry
Roswell Park Memorial Institute
Buffalo, New York

Donald S. Coffey, Ph.D.
Professor of Pharmacology and Experimental Therapeutics
Professor of Urology
Professor of Oncology
Johns Hopkins University School of Medicine
Baltimore, Maryland

Virginia Ernster, Ph.D.
Assistant Research Epidemiologist
University of California Medical Center, San Francisco
San Francisco, California

John F. Gaeta, M.D.
Associate Professor of Pathology
State University of New York at Buffalo School of Medicine
Buffalo, New York

William A. Gardner, Jr., M.D.
Chief of Laboratory Service
Veterans Administration Hospital
Professor of Pathology
Vanderbilt University School of Medicine
Nashville, Tennessee

Ruben F. Gittes, M.D.
Professor of Urological Surgery
Harvard Medical School
Urologist-in-Chief
Peter Bent Brigham Hospital
Boston, Massachusetts

John T. Isaacs, Ph.D.
Postdoctoral Fellow
Department of Pharmacology and Experimental Therapeutics
Johns Hopkins University School of Medicine
Baltimore, Maryland

James P. Karr, Ph.D.
Deputy Director for Scientific Affairs
National Prostatic Cancer Project
Roswell Park Memorial Institute
Buffalo, New York

Mani Menon, M.D.
William Wallace Scott Fellow in Urology
Johns Hopkins University School of Medicine
Baltimore, Maryland

Donald J. Merchant, Ph.D.
Professor and Chairman
Department of Microbiology and Immunology
Eastern Virginia Medical School
Norfolk, Virginia

Arnold Mittelman, M.D.
Program Director
Surgical Oncology, Colon-Rectal Service
Roswell Park Memorial Institute
Buffalo, New York

Gerald P. Murphy, M.D., D.Sc.
Project Director
National Prostatic Cancer Project
Roswell Park Memorial Institute
Buffalo, New York

Jeffery Pollen, M.D.
Assistant Research Surgeon
Division of Urology
University of California, San Diego, School of Medicine
San Diego, California

Avery A. Sandberg, M.D.
Chief, Medicine C Department
Roswell Park Memorial Institute
Buffalo, New York

Joseph D. Schmidt, M.D.
Professor of Surgery
Head, Division of Urology
University of California, San Diego, School of Medicine
San Diego, California

Zew Wajsman, M.D.
Cancer Research Clinican II
Department of Experimental Surgery
Roswell Park Memorial Institute
Buffalo, New York

Patrick C. Walsh, M.D.
Professor and Director
Department of Urology
Johns Hopkins University School of Medicine
Baltimore, Maryland

Robert M. Weisman, Ph.D.
Department of Oncology
Johns Hopkins University School of Medicine
Baltimore, Maryland

Warren Winkelstein, M.D., M.P.H.
Professor of Epidemiology
Dean, School of Public Health
University of California, Berkeley
Berkeley, California

Robert F. Zeigel, Ph.D.
Associate Cancer Research Scientist
Associate Professor of Microbiology
Roswell Park Memorial Institute
Buffalo, New York

CONTENTS

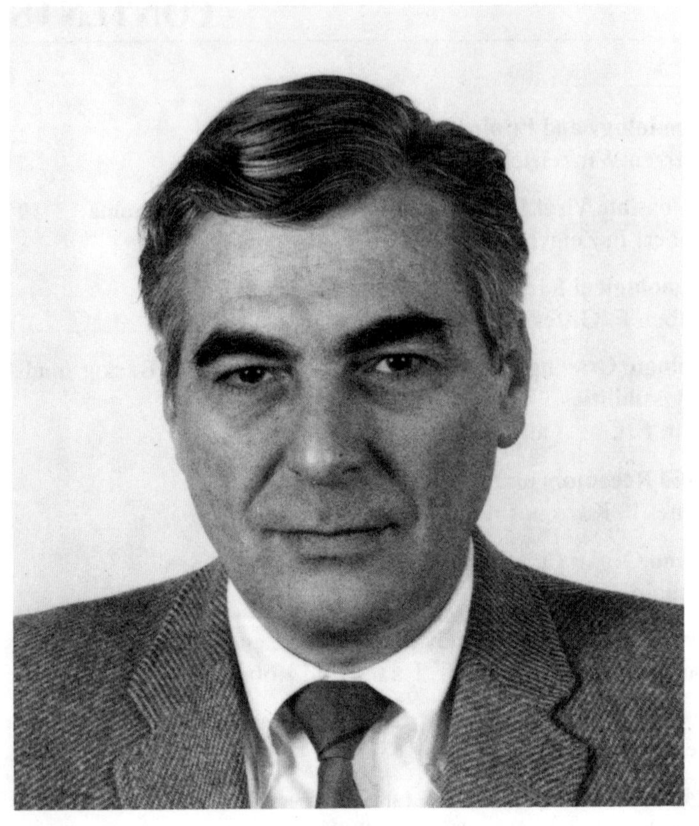

JACK SAROFF, PH.D.
ASSISTANT DIRECTOR
NATIONAL PROSTATIC CANCER PROJECT
1972–1977

INTRODUCTION

The management of prostate cancer in all its forms in man has undergone a substantial adjustment in our thinking within this decade. Reasons for this include the evolution of treatment, the application of new scientific concepts, and further progress in all fields of medicine. However, specifically, in terms of hormonal factors, the accuracy of diagnosis, the determination of the extent of disease, and the application of multimodal therapy, have resulted in initial changes in the approach to the management of cancer as we know it.

The authors contributing to this book are individuals involved with the day-to-day progress in all aspects of this field. At various times many of them have served effectively and worked with, or have been involved in, the National Prostatic Cancer Project, a program supported by the National Institutes of Health. Throughout all of our endeavors Dr Jack Saroff has assisted us, both in the preparation of this book and in many of the concepts that will be expressed. His recent and untimely death has deprived us not only of a good friend and colleague but of one who has made substantial contributions to the management of prostate cancer. Thus, by common consent, we dedicate this book to him.

Gerald P. Murphy, M.D., D.Sc.
Director
National Prostatic Cancer Project

Buffalo, New York
February 6, 1978

Epidemiology and Etiology

1

Warren Winkelstein, Jr.,
and Virginia L. Ernster

Cancer of the prostate is a disease of unknown etiology. Several reviews of the epidemiologic aspects of this neoplasm have been published.[1-4] It is primarily a disease of older men; mortality rates increase markedly with age after about the fiftieth year. This malignancy occurs with strikingly different frequencies in various regions of the world, across racial groups, and over different time periods. In the United States today, it accounts for 10% of cancer mortality in males and ranks second in overall cancer incidence among men.[5-6] In this chapter the etiologic hypotheses and inferences that can be derived from our knowledge of the epidemiology of prostatic cancer will be discussed.

Epidemiology, the study of disease distribution in human populations and the factors which affect it, has been useful in eliciting some of the associations of particular cancers, viz, smoking and lung cancer, ionizing radiation and leukemia, and occupational exposure to aniline dyes and bladder cancer. Whereas the laboratory investigator can usually specify exact experimental conditions, epidemiologists must study human populations in their environment, with all their biologic, behavioral, and environmental variables. Variation in disease is often based on such characteristics as age, marital status, sexual practices, occupational exposures, and diet, all of which "naturally" differ among populations. Any demographic or biologic characteristic, social practice, or environmental exposure found to increase the chances of developing a disease is known as a *risk factor*; conversely, any practice or exposure which lowers those chances is thought to be *protective.*

Etiology—the cause of a disease—does not derive solely from epidemiologic studies. Usually, however, hypotheses initiated in clinical or laboratory settings must be tested using epidemiologic methods. For example, the association of cigarette smoking and lung cancer, first suggested on the basis of clinical observations, was strengthened considerably through case-control studies. Evidence of the carcinogenicity of diethylstilbestrol (DES) in mice reported over two decades ago has been cited as a parallel study to that linking vaginal adenocarcinoma in young women to DES. In any instance, valid etiologic inferences must be consistent with the epidemiologic evidence, that is, they must fit the distribution of purported risk factors and disease in the population.

EPIDEMIOLOGY

The validity of inferences derived from epidemiologic studies depends on the accuracy with which the observations are made. This applies both to the independent variables postulated to affect the occurrence of the disease (ie, risk factors) as well as to the identification of cases of the disease under study. With respect to prostatic cancer, the latter issue is particularly troublesome.

For most cancers, disease is manifested by clinical signs and symptoms prior to death. Thus, epidemiologic studies can be designed for representative sampling. However, for prostatic carcinoma, a substantial but undetermined proportion of the disease is latent and only incidentally discovered at autopsy or when surgical intervention is undertaken for other reasons. Thus, samples of clinically diagnosed cases may not be completely representative of all men at risk of developing the disease. Moreover, the possibility that men with latent cancer will be included in control groups in epidemiologic studies is substantially greater for prostatic than for other cancers. This bias would, however, have the effect of diminishing true differences between cases and controls rather than artificially demonstrating differences which do not exist.

The problem created by the occurrence of latent prostatic cancer has an indeterminate effect on the interpretation of descriptive statistics such as mortality and incidence rates over time, and comparisons between groups with different medical care systems and case-recording mechanisms. At the present time, we know of no way out of this dilemma and would question comparative statistics drawn from countries that vary considerably in their medical-screening and case-reporting facilities. On the other hand, where the levels of medical diagnosis and care are high and where statistics are gathered according to standardized and rigorous procedures, we expect the latency bias to be minimized.

Descriptive Statistics: Mortality and Incidence

Age-Specific Mortality and Incidence by Race The most useful indicators of the extent of disease occurrence in a population are mortality rates (ie, deaths per unit population per year) and incidence rates (ie, *new* cases per unit population per year). While prevalence (all existing cases per unit population at a *particular* point in time) is a practical measure for the purpose of planning for health and medical care services, it is not useful for developing etiologic hypotheses and inferences. The epidemiologist would even prefer not to use mortality rates because case fatality (ie, deaths per 100 cases during a particular time period) varies greatly among different cancers and, indeed, for the same cancer at different places and at different times. Nevertheless, mortality statistics are often the only data available. For the United States, complete mortality statistics have been collected on a nationwide basis since the 1930s. An excellent representative estimate of cancer incidence is available from the Third National Cancer Survey (1969–1971), and an ongoing network of cancer registries now exists across the country (Surveillance, Epidemiology and End Results—SEER—program of the National Cancer Institute).

In Figure 1, age-specific prostatic cancer mortality and incidence rates for whites and blacks are shown for the United States in 1970. Prostatic cancer is relatively rare under the age of 50, after which time it rises more rapidly with age than any other cancer. Both mortality and incidence increase at an almost constant exponential rate, indicated by the nearly straight line of the curves shown in Figure 1. Although it is tempting to interpret the difference between incidence and mortality as a measure of severity or survivorship, the reader is cautioned that many other factors may be operative, including differential risks by age of dying of other causes as well as the fact that deaths at one age may not be referent to the same individuals who are incident cases at that age.

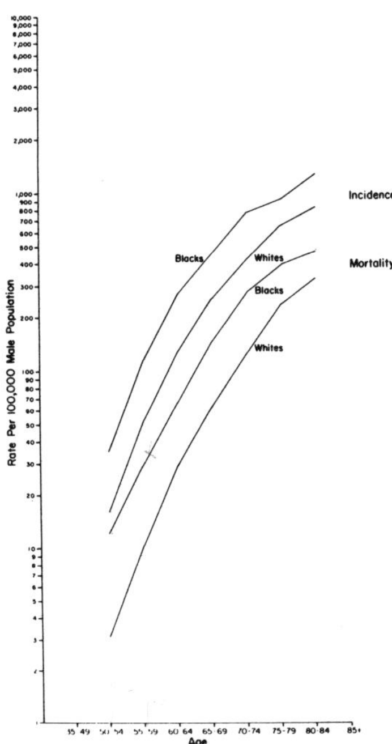

Figure 1. Age-specific prostatic cancer mortality and incidence rates per 100,000 males, whites and blacks, United States, 1970 (Cutler and Young, 1975[6]).

The most striking aspect of the epidemiology of prostatic cancer in the United States is the racial difference in occurrence. Age-adjusted rates among blacks are approximately 65% higher than among whites.[6] However, black rates have not always exceeded those of whites, a phenomenon discussed below.

Time Trends (Age-Adjusted) As shown in Figure 2, age-adjusted prostatic cancer death rates for all males in the United States have been relatively stable since 1940. In the decade 1930 to 1940 there was an increase of approximately 40%. This could well be explained by improvements in mortality reporting and changes in the international coding procedures according to which causes of death are ascribed. However, the overall mortality picture generally reflects the white experience. When nonwhites are considered separately, a somewhat different pattern emerges, with a steady increase in age-adjusted rates apparent from 1930 on. This has resulted in a shifting of the positions of the two racial groups relative to one another. Until 1945, at all ages combined, whites had higher death rates than nonwhites. However, as early as 1930, prostatic cancer mortality among young men was higher in nonwhites than whites. With time, successively older age groups followed this pattern. By 1965 nonwhite rates for all age groups through age 85 had exceeded comparable white rates.

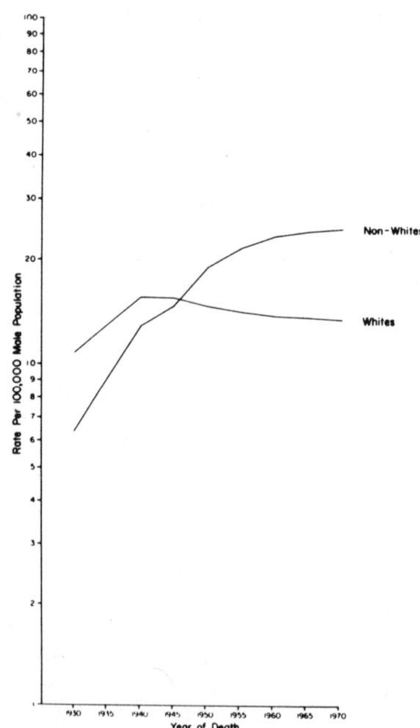

Figure 2. Age-adjusted mortality rates for prostatic cancer per 100,000 males, 1930–1970, by race (United States Public Health Service, *Vital Statistics of the United States.* (Mortality Series 1935–1970.)

Additional insight into time trends can sometimes be provided by an analysis of age-specific rates calculated for birth cohorts. Thus one views the mortality experience at each age of a given generation as opposed to a cross-sectional analysis which examines the experience of several generations simultaneously. When this was done for prostatic cancer, it appeared that the nonwhite birth cohorts of 1896 to 1900 experienced relatively higher rates at almost all ages as compared with both earlier and later cohorts (see Table 1).[7] In fact Table 1 suggests a general decline in mortality at each age for which data are available for birth cohorts following 1896 to 1900. Of course, prostatic cancer occurs more frequently in the older age groups, and data are not yet available for the complete lifespan of the 1896 to 1900 cohort or for subsequent cohorts. Thus it will be of interest to monitor such rates in the future. If trends observed in younger men persist, one can anticipate that mortality from prostatic cancer in blacks will stabilize and possibly even begin to decline in the not too distant future.

Table 1. Prostatic Cancer Mortality Rates Per 100,000 By Cohort for U.S. Nonwhite Males Born 1861–1920 (sources same as Figure 2)

	Birth Cohorts											
Age	1861–1865	1866–1870	1871–1875	1876–1880	1881–1885	1886–1890	1891–1895	1896–1900	1901–1905	1906–1910	1910–1915	1916–1920
40–44						1.10	2.02	1.65	2.15	1.61	1.26	2.68
45–49					3.48	4.76	6.55	7.23	4.71	4.66	2.73	2.43
50–54				5.41	11.35	15.95	15.65	23.35	16.34	15.82	13.39	12.03
55–59			18.78	22.40	32.08	41.41	39.05	44.44	30.85	32.43	29.90	
60–64		23.98	45.90	50.19	60.42	77.72	84.21	81.35	77.39	68.21		
65–69	35.12	60.24	72.26	74.05	97.25	141.06	147.39	177.09	149.00			
70–74	66.50	90.10	125.96	148.03	168.49	224.73	235.89	276.70				
75–79	151.36	129.82	219.20	234.44	299.59	304.24	399.90					
80–84	155.56	299.06	380.56	371.54	359.15	471.30						

A similar cohort analysis of mortality for whites in the United States revealed no such generational pattern, a finding consistent with the fact that cross-sectional rates for whites have shown very little change in the past five decades.

Geographic Variation: International and National The study of geographic differences in disease occurrence provides an opportunity to identify genetic or environmental factors which may be of etiologic importance. Such comparisons, however, suffer due to variations in diagnosis, differences in case fatality rates, and inaccuracy and incompleteness of records. While an exhaustive compendium of international incidence statistics has been compiled it is our feeling that incidence data for most countries have not yet reached the point where they can be used for comparative purposes.[8] Recognizing that international mortality data require cautious interpretation, we have nonetheless reached the following conclusions based on an examination of the most frequently consulted sources of international mortality statistics.[9,10]

For those nations for which statistics are available, it appears that the developed nations of Western Europe, North America, and Australia/New Zealand generally have the highest age-adjusted rates. The range of differences between them is quite small and could easily be accounted for by random variation. A second group of countries with intermediate rates can be identified in eastern and southern Europe. Included in this group are several countries in Latin America. Again, variation between these countries is not remarkable. Finally, there is a third group characterized by extremely low rates, comprised of countries in eastern Asia. Japan is perhaps the most interesting and important of these, since its vital statistics system is thought to be of a particularly high caliber. Furthermore, the presence of substantial numbers of Japanese migrants to the United States, where overall mortality rates are relatively high, provides an opportunity to study the issue of genetic vs environmental etiology. Unfortunately, mortality statistics are unavailable for most countries of the world, including many nations in Africa, South and Central Asia, the Near East, and much of Latin America.

Within the United States published data concerning geographic variations of prostatic cancer mortality are inconsistent. When age-adjusted mortality rates for white males by state for the pericensal period 1959 to 1961 were examined, it appeared that rates in the three northern New England states and most of the northern tier states west of the Mississippi to the Pacific Coast were from 1½ to 2 times higher when compared with most of the southern tier states east of Arizona and Utah.[11] A rather different pattern is evident in the recently published *Atlas of Cancer Mortality,* which provides age-adjusted mortality rates for white males by county for the 20-year period 1950–1969.[12] Maps in the *Atlas* show that a number of counties in the upper midwest states of Minnesota and Iowa had an apparent excess of prostatic cancer mortality, and scattered high-rate counties were found in the Rocky Mountain plateau area, Texas, the southeastern states, and in the upper mid-Atlantic and central New England areas.[12]

Incidence data are not available for most of the United States, but an examination of the nine areas included in the Third National Cancer Survey shows no clear-cut regional patterns despite a range of rates from a low of 37 per 100,000 males in Pittsburgh to a high of 54 per 100,000 in Minneapolis-St. Paul.[6]

From the foregoing it appears that no obvious regional pattern for prostatic cancer exists in the United States. It may well be that individual counties identified in the recent *Atlas* will be found to have particular environmental characteristics which lead to increased risk of the disease, but this has not as yet been investigated.

Analytic Epidemiology: Environmental Factors

Nature (Genetic vs Nurture): Migrant Studies The marked racial and international differences in prostatic cancer statistics might be explained on either a genetic or an environmental basis. Migrant studies are particularly useful for making this distinction if the assumption can be made that migrants are genetically representative of the native populations from which they come. If genetic mechanisms are responsible for disease occurrence, then one would expect rates in the host country to be quite similar to those in the country of origin. Alternately, if environmental factors are dominant, one would expect migrants to assume rates experienced in the host country.

The extensive migrant populations in the United States have been studied for many cancers. With respect to prostatic cancer, the migration experience of the Japanese is particularly relevant. Most of the Japanese migration to the United States came from a limited geographic area around Hiroshima, suggesting a homogeneous genetic makeup among the migrants. Within the United States migrants settled in two distinct areas, namely, Hawaii and California. In Table 2, recent mortality rates are shown for Japanese in Japan, Hawaii, and California. These data reveal a clear difference between the low rates in Japan and the much higher rates in Hawaii and California.

Table 2. Average Annual Prostatic Cancer Mortality by Age for Japanese in Japan, Hawaii, and California

	Japan (1970)*		Hawaii (1968–1972)†		Calif. (1969–1973)‡	
Age	Population	Deaths/ 100,000	Population	Deaths/ 100,000	Population	Deaths/ 100,000
55–64	3,798,000	3.2	9,638	4.2	817	—
65–74	2,361,000	14.7	5,203	24.8	550	36.4
75+	862,000	43.8	2,826	184.0	409	195.6

* World Health Organization 1973.
† L. Kolonel (unpublished data).
‡ Bragg and Austin (unpublished data).

Since large-scale migration has not occurred for many years, one may infer that rates among Japanese-Americans will increasingly reflect the influence of members of the second and subsequent generations. In 1970 the age-adjusted incidence rate for prostatic cancer among Japanese in the five San Francisco Bay Area counties participating in the Third National Cancer Survey was 6.3 (S.E. ± 3.1) per 100,000, and by 1975 this figure had already climbed to 49.6 (S.E. ± 23) per 100,000 according to K. Bragg and D. F. Austin (personal communication, 15 July 1977). Of course, these rates are based on very small numbers and must be interpreted cautiously. Nevertheless, all of these observations taken together suggest that environmental factors predominate in determining risk of prostate cancer.

Further support for the environmental hypothesis comes from the observation that the prevalence of latent prostatic carcinoma is the same in autopsy series among Japanese in Japan and in Hawaii.[13] This suggests that an environmental factor(s) precipitates the change from latent to clinical disease.

An examination of mortality rates among migrants to the United States from European countries generally reveals no such definitive change in the direction of host-country rates as revealed for Japanese. No doubt this is due in part to the fact already indicated that rates in those countries from which the bulk of European migration occurred are much closer to those in the United States as a whole, probably reflecting greater similarities in life style.

Environmental Factors In this section, urban/rural comparisons of prostatic cancer rates, and possible associations of the disease with measures of air pollution, occupation, and smoking behavior, will be discussed.

When 1950 age-adjusted incidence rates were compared for urban and rural areas of New York, Connecticut, and Iowa, areas which had good registries at the time, a small excess of about 10% was observed in urban areas.[1] However, when age-adjusted mortality rates between urban and rural counties of the entire United States for the period 1950 to 1969 were examined, no difference was observed.[14] Elsewhere, a case-control study of prostatic cancer patients and other hospitalized men found a higher proportion of cases to be residents of small towns.[15] Given these rather contradictory results, it is not possible to conclude that there is any appreciable difference between urban and rural areas in the occurrence of prostatic cancer.

The lack of an association between prostatic cancer and urbanization seems inconsistent with findings elsewhere of an association between suspended-particulate air pollution and mortality from this disease as observed in two community-wide studies of air pollution effects in the United States.[16,17] Both of these studies controlled for differences in social class. However, the possibility that the association might be explained by other unaccounted-for covariables cannot be assessed.

Based on previous suggestions in the literature, the authors of one of the air pollution studies hypothesized a possible carcinogenic effect from airborn cadmium particles.[16] Animal studies had shown cadmium to be a carcinogen capable of inducing testicular tumors in rats.[18] An excess of prostatic cancer mortality had also been reported based on uncontrolled observations among cadmium workers.[19,20] Later, a careful retrospective case-control study, using a lifetime cadmium exposure index based on dietary, smoking, and occupational histories, found no significant differences.[21] Another retrospective case-control study examined general occupational differences between cases and controls and also found no differences, although the study groups were drawn from a very homogeneous socioeconomic population.[22] Our own comparisons of occupations for deaths due to prostatic cancer and matched controls revealed that cases were more likely to have belonged to certain occupational groups, including compositors/typesetters, painters, and shipfitters.[23] Elsewhere, a cohort study of workers in a cadmium smelter demonstrated an excess of observed over expected prostatic cancer deaths in those men whose cadmium exposure had begun at least 20 years prior to death.[24] Finally, in a cohort of 6,000 rubber workers, excess deaths from prostatic cancer were observed in several job categories, one of which involved cadmium exposure.[25] These studies can hardly be considered definitive of occupational hazards for prostatic cancer, and more work along these lines is to be encouraged.

The prostate is among the major cancer sites for which an association with smoking has not been demonstrated despite a number of studies addressed to this question.[26] This lack of an association was most recently confirmed in an examination of smoking history among cancer patients included in the Third National Cancer Survey.[27]

Behavioral Factors In attempting to explain the marked racial differential in prostatic cancer occurrence, one must consider the possibility that it might be accounted for by factors associated with socioeconomic status (SES). It is possible that some social factors independent of racial differences might be associated with the etiology of prostatic cancer. Numerous studies have examined this question; most of them predated the dramatic black/white reversal in prostatic cancer rates, and few had similar results. Moreover, the studies that did include racial groups other than whites pooled "nonwhite" races together and also predated the dramatic black/white reversal in prostatic cancer rates. These studies have been reviewed recently and analyzed further, using both mortality and incidence data separately for whites and blacks from Alameda County, California, for the five-year pericensal period 1968 to 1972.[28] No SES gradient in prostatic cancer rates was observed for either whites or blacks, and black excess risk for the disease held up within age-specific comparisons for every socioeconomic level studied. As indicated earlier, the black/white difference in prostatic cancer is of recent origin, so that failure to explain it on the basis of SES should not necessarily be interpreted as supporting a genetic hypothesis.

Religion has proved to be a useful characteristic to measure in many epidemiologic studies since it is frequently a good indicator of sexual practices, fertility, dietary habits, smoking, alcohol use, and circumcision. Religion has been a study variable in several prostatic cancer studies. Investigations in New York City have indicated that Jews have a slightly lower risk for the disease.[29-31] It was thought that circumcision might be protective. However, a later study failed to demonstrate a difference in circumcision status between cases of prostatic cancer and controls.[32] The author suggested that reports of lower risk among Jews might well be explained by the fact that a large proportion of New York's Jewish population of immigrants were from low-risk eastern European countries. Two of the earlier studies, however, controlled for nativity and found that both American-born and foreign-born Jews were at low risk, although the latter had slightly lower rates.[29,30] Findings of religious differences in risk for the disease among blacks have not been reported.

National mortality data for the pericensal period 1959 to 1961 revealed a gradient from the lowest risk of death from prostatic cancer for single men, increasing for married, widowed, and divorced men, respectively.[11] An excess risk among married men suggests the possibility of a positive association between fertility and prostatic cancer. Various studies have examined this and it does appear that married men with children have a moderately increased risk of developing the disease compared both with single men and married men with no children.[15,33,22] However, the studies on which this conclusion is based show small differences in actual risk and do not represent the majority of cases. In addition, a case-control study involving several hundred men with prostatic cancer showed no relationship between the disease and marital status, age at first marriage, or number of children.[32]

Studies of sexual practices of individuals with cancers of sexual sites have been particularly fruitful with respect to the establishment of hypotheses regarding the causation of cervical cancer. Only a few such studies have been reported to date for prostate cancer. Two retrospective case-control studies have shown cases to have an excess in past history of venereal disease, number of sexual partners, and frequency of coitus.[34,35] Reports have also appeared from two additional studies in progress. In one, the previous observations are supported.[36] More frequently than controls, cases report a history of association with prostitutes, prior venereal disease, genital infections in the spouse, and earlier age at first intercourse. In the other study, cases had later initiation and earlier cessation of sexual activity. These findings were interpreted by the author to indicate greater sexual repression throughout the lifespan.[37]

Thus, although the bulk of the evidence from these case-control studies suggests that sexual activity or associated factors increase risk for prostatic cancer, at least one study contradicts this conclusion. Furthermore, one of the completed studies included only 39 cases, another had a high nonresponse rate for the questions related to sexual practices, and the data from the remaining two are preliminary.[34-37]

The geographic variation and changes in incidence among migrants raises the question of the possible influence of diet on the cancer. There are several ways that dietary behavior could be influential: ingestion of carcinogenic agents, malnutrition with consequent interference with normal metabolism, and changes in plasma lipids resulting in alteration of hormone transport to the target organs. Although several investigators have suggested the attractiveness of a dietary etiology in the case of hormone-dependent cancers such as prostate, these mechanisms have not yet been studied.[38-40]

Biologic Factors It has frequently been assumed that demonstrations of familial aggregation are strongly supportive of genetic factors in the etiology of disease, but they can alternately bolster hyotheses related to common environmental exposure. None of the studies of familial clustering in prostate cancer has attempted to untangle these influences, although admittedly the task would be a difficult one from the standpoint of study design. Two studies were conducted prior to 1960, one in the predominately Mormon population of Utah and the other in Milan, Italy.[41,42] Both found a more frequent family history of prostatic cancer in cases than controls, although in the Utah study at least, this was true only for brothers and not fathers of the propositi. In both studies the frequency of concordance (the occurrence of prostatic cancer in both a case and a relative) was low, about 5% or less. In three case-control studies primarily concerned with sexual factors, an excess of familial prostatic cancer was observed among cases.[34-36] Two of the study populations were very small in number, however.

Benign prostatic hypertrophy (BPH) has been seriously considered as a possible precursor of carcinoma of the prostate. Its high prevalence particularly in the older age groups which are most susceptible to prostate cancer, makes its evaluation as a risk factor problematic from the viewpoint of study design. It is difficult to constitute a comparison group without BPH for the purpose of investigation. Thus it is not surprising that two carefully designed and executed historical prospective studies came to opposite conclusions. The study which showed no increased risk for development of prostatic cancer among men with benign prostatic hypertrophy included cases operated on or biopsied for BPH. By excising latent disease or reducing the amount of potential substrate tissue, the probability of subsequent cancer might have been artificially reduced.[43] The other study included men diagnosed as having benign prostatic hypertrophy after referral to a major cancer research center because of suspicion of cancer. Since both benign hyperplasia and cancer produce enlargement of the prostate, any missed cancer diagnosis would have biased the case group in this study toward increased incidence.[44] Although the relationship of benign prostatic hypertrophy to cancer of the prostate is unknown, the issue remains important. In the study which claimed an association, the excess risk was substantial and the investigators estimated that 43% of prostatic cancer might be attributable to prior benign disease. They suggested a "randomized clinical trial of prostatectomy in symptom-free patients with benign prostatic hypertrophy . . . ," a recommendation which, aside from its ethical and practical problems, should only be undertaken after more definitive epidemiologic study.

It has been suggested that hormonal factors may be involved in the etiology of the disease because of the possible relationship between fertility and prostatic cancer. Evidence in support of this hyothesis includes the fact that androgens are needed for normal prostatic development and the observation that eunuchs have atrophic prostates and apparently do not develop prostatic cancer.[45] Autopsy studies have shown the frequency of occult prostatic carcinoma in men dying of nonprostatic disease to be lower in men with evidence of hepatic cirrhosis.[46,47] This condition is associated with diminished clearance and elevated blood levels of endogenous estrogens. Moreover, the growth of many prostatic carcinomas is retarded by estrogen therapy and by orchiectomy. In another controlled study of prostatic cancer, lowered excretion of androsterone and a higher proportion of estrogen as estrone and estradiol were reported.[48] However, we are not aware of any studies which have reported differences in hormonal levels and excretion patterns between whites and blacks with respect to prostatic cancer risk, and no clear differences between hormone levels of Japanese and Caucasian Americans have been demonstrated.[32] Indirect measures of hormonal activity have also been studied. Somatotype, gynandromorphy, androgyny, baldness, and pilosity in early life were not linked with prostate cancer in a historic case-control study.[43]

Whether or not hormones are causally associated with prostatic cancer must be determined by prospective investigation because there is no way to distinguish the sequence of hormonal changes and cancer in a retrospective study where the subjects are discovered after the onset of disease.

Based on associations between herpes simplex virus-II (HSV-2) and cervical cancer observed in case-control studies, it has been hypothesized that a transmissable agent might also be involved in the etiology of prostatic cancer. Limited microbiologic investigations have been undertaken. Although serologic studies have suffered from small numbers and inadequate controls, no associations have been revealed for HSV-2 or simian virus (SV-40).[49] Virologic evidence is also meager. Some investigators have reported isolation of cytomegalo-virus (CMV) from semen and HSV from prostatic fluid but others have failed in similar efforts.[50-53] Other relevant research has examined prostatic cancer tissue by electron-microscopy and identified herpes-like particles; reverse transcriptase activity in prostatic cancer tissue has been reported but not confirmed; and viral transformation of tissue cultures of human prostatic gland has not been demonstrated.[54-57]

An interesting association has been demonstrated between secular trends in the incidence of gonorrhea in Denmark and the occurrence of prostatic cancer in that country 40 years later. This has led to the hypothesis that treatment of gonorrheal infections in the prechemotherapy era may have been implicated in the etiology of the disease. The authors predict a future decline in prostatic cancer as affected cohorts die out.[58]

ETIOLOGY

Several classes of etiologic agents are now recognized as being carcinogenic or cocarcinogenic. Thus, we recognize extrinsic agents (chemical, physical, and viral), and intrinsic agents (genetic and hormonal). The effects of these agents are undoubtedly influenced by host and environmental factors such as age, sex, occupational experience, geographic location, and social milieu. Some of the risk factors identified in epidemiologic studies of prostatic cancer suggest etiologic hypotheses consistent with the foregoing classes of agents. However, in most cases the evidence from various studies is contradictory and, as stated earlier, the etiology of prostatic cancer remains unknown. Some hypotheses are discussed below.

Genetic Hypotheses

The relatively high occurrence of prostatic cancer among American blacks compared with whites and the relatively low occurrence among Asians, suggest a genetic mechanism in the etiology of prostatic cancer. However, the recent marked changes in rates among blacks and migrant Asians argue against a primary role for genetic factors. Nevertheless, combined action of genetic and environmental factors could very well exist. A paradigm is the supposed etiology of xeroderma pigmentosum in which persons heterozygous and homozygous for the gene are predisposed to the development of cancer only when exposure to a specific agent has occurred, in this case ultraviolet radiation.[59] Such a model illustrates how a population genetically predisposed to cancer might demonstrate increased incidence only in the presence of concomitant environmental carcinogens. Using such a model, the differing rates observed in white, black, and Asian Americans would be attributable to differing combinations of gene frequency and exposure to environmental carcinogens across these groups and over a period of time. The consistent finding from five separate small case-control studies that men with prostatic cancer report a more frequent family history of the disease than do controls also supports the possibility of at least a genetically influenced susceptibility. While it seems unlikely that genetic mechanisms account for a very substantial proportion of cases, the frequency of latent carcinoma might well mask a much stronger familial aggregation than that already observed. It bears repeating, however, that familial aggregation can also result from common environmental exposure among family members.

Hormonal Hypotheses

Perhaps the etiologic mechanism with the most epidemiologic support relates to the hormone dependency of prostatic cancer. To reiterate, the disease does not occur among eunuchs, it shows a modest relationship with fertility, its occurrency is lower than expected in men with elevated blood levels of endogenous estrogens (cirrhotics), and cases are characterized by lowered excretion of androsterone and altered proportions of estrogens compared with controls. A role for hormones is further supported by the demonstrated effectiveness of hormone treatments in the ablation of some prostatic tumors. The picture is confused, however, by the conflicting results of several case-control studies that have attempted to assess the role of benign prostatic hypertrophy as a precursor for prostatic cancer and others designed to evaluate factors related to sexual activity.

Infectious Hypotheses

The possibility that prostatic cancer could be etiologically analogous to cervical cancer has led to the hypothesis of venereal transmission of an infectious agent. As indicated previously, the results of studies of sexual activity have been somewhat inconsistent, some indicating that many partners and a history of venereal disease are risk factors for prostatic cancer, whereas at least one study has shown the opposite, finding that repression of sexual activity was more characteristic of men with prostatic cancer than controls. Serologic and virologic studies of suspected viral carcinogens in prostatic fluid have also yielded inconsistent results. Furthermore, if venereal mechanisms are important etiologically and are presumed to involve transmission in early adulthood, one might expect an earlier peak in disease occurrence since most known oncogenic agents appear to have incubation or latency periods of 15 to 30 years.

Chemical Hypotheses

Several studies of prostatic cancer and particular occupations have led to the specific hyothesis that exposure to cadmium and its compounds increases risk for the disease. This possibility is also supported by two independent community studies of the effects of particulate air pollution on disease occurrence that showed a positive association for prostatic cancer. On the other hand, the lack of any difference in occurrence between urban and rural areas and across socioeconomic groups, as well as an absence of any association with smoking, argues against a chemical etiology.

SUMMARY

The rather meager and contradictory epidemiologic information about prostatic cancer has not led to the formulation of a coherent etiologic explanation for the disease. While something is known of the distributional characteristics of prostate cancer—particularly its age-dependence, its racial and geographic differences in occurrence, and its time trends—the reasons for these have not been satisfactorily explained. Perhaps the most productive direction that research could take would be to concentrate study on the relatively rare cases of prostate cancer in young men. Etiologic agents might be identified more easily in this population because causally significant events might be easier to recall in the young. In addition, environmental or other exposures may have been more intense (higher dose) in cases of early onset, and age-matched controls would be less likely to have occult prostatic cancer. Needless to say, such research should include white and black populations.

REFERENCES

1. King, H., Diamond, E., and Lilienfeld, A. M. Some epidemiological aspects of cancer of the prostate. *J Chronic Dis.* 16:117-53, 1963.

2. Higgins, I.T.T. The epidemiology of cancer of the prostate. *J Chronic Dis.* 28:343-8, 1974.

3. Owen, W. L. Cancer of the prostate: a literature review. *J Chronic Dis.* 29:89-114, 1976.

4. Hutchison, G. B. Epidemiology of prostatic cancer. *Semin Oncol.* 3:151-9, 1976.

5. Silverberg, E. Cancer Statistics, 1977. *CA.* 27:26-41, 1977.

6. Cutler, S. J., and Young, J. L. Jr., eds. *Third National Cancer Survey: Incidence Data.* Washington: National Cancer Institute, Monograph 41, March 1975.

7. Ernster, V. L., Selvin, S., and Winkelstein, W. Jr. Cohort mortality for prostatic cancer among US nonwhites. *Science.* 200:1165-6, 1978.

8. Doll, R., Muir, C., and Waterhouse, J.A.H., eds. *UICC Cancer Incidence in Five Continents,* Vol. 2. New York: Springer-Verlag, 1970.

9. *World Health Statistics Annual 1970.* Geneva, World Health Organization, 1973.

10. Segi, M., Kurihara, M., and Matsuyama, T. *Cancer mortality for selected sites in 24 countries, No. 5 (1964–1965).* Sendai, Japan: Department of Public Health, Tohoku University of Medicine, 1969.

11. Lilienfeld, A., Levin, M. L., and Kessler, I. I. *Cancer in the United States.* Cambridge: Harvard University Press, 1972.

12. Mason, T. J., McKay, F. W., Hoover, R. et al. *Atlas of Cancer Mortality for U.S. Counties: 1950–1969.* Washington: United States Department of Health, Education, and Welfare; Public Health Service, 1975.

13. Akazaki, K., and Stemmermann, G. N. Comparative study of latent carcinoma of the prostate among Japanese in Japan and Hawaii. *J Natl Cancer Inst.* 50:1137-44, 1973.

14. Hoover, R., Mason, T. J., McKay, F. W. et al. Geographic patterns of cancer mortality in the United States. Edited by Joseph F. Fraumeni. In *Persons at High Risk of Cancer.* New York: Academic Press, 1975, pp 343-60.

15. Armenian, H. K., Lilienfeld, A. M., Diamond, E. L. et al. Epidemiologic characteristics of patients with prostatic neoplasms. *Am J Epidemiol.* 102:47-54, 1975.

16. Winkelstein, W. Jr., and Kantor, S. Prostatic cancer: relationship to suspended particulate air pollution. *Am J Public Health.* 59:1134-38, 1969.

17. Hagstrom, R. M., Sprague, H. A., and Landau, E. Mortality from cancer in relation to air pollution. *Arch Environ Health.* 15:237-48, 1967.

18. Malcolm, D. Potential carcinogenic effect of cadmium in animals and man. *Ann Occup Hyg.* 15:33-6, 1972.

19. Kipling, M. C., and Waterhouse, J. A. II. Cadmium and prostatic carcinoma. *Lancet* 1:730-1, 1967.

20. Potts, C. L. Cadmium proteinuria–the health of battery workers exposed to cadmium oxide dust. *Ann Occup Hyg.* 8:55-61, 1965.

21. Kolonel, L. N. *An epidemiological investigation of cadmium carcinogenesis.* Doctoral thesis, University of California, Berkeley, 1972.

22. Greenwald, P., Damon, A., Kirmss, V. et al. Physical and demographic features of men before developing cancer of the prostate. *J Natl Cancer Inst.* 53:341-6, 1974a.

23. Ernster, V. L., Selvin, S., Brown, S. M. et al. *Occupation and Prostatic Cancer.* Presented at the Tenth Annual Meeting of the Society for Epidemiologic Research, Seattle, June 15–17, 1977.

24. Lemen, R. A., Lee, J. S., Wagoner, J. K. et al. Cancer mortality among cadmium production workers, *Ann NY Acad Sci.* 271:273-9, 1976.

25. McMichael, A. J., Spirtas, R., Gamble, J. F. et al. Mortality among rubber workers: relationship to specific jobs. *J Occup Med.* 18:178-85, 1976.

26. Hammond, E. C. Tobacco. Edited by Joseph F. Fraumeni. In *Persons at High Risk of Cancer.* New York: Academic Press, 1975, pp 131-8.

27. Williams, R. R., and Horm, J. W. Association of cancer sites with tobacco and alcohol consumption and socioeconomic status of patients: interview study from the Third National Cancer Survey. *J Natl Cancer Inst.* 58:525-47, 1977.

28. Ernster, V. L., Selvin, S., Sacks, S. T. et al. Prostatic cancer: mortality and incidence rates by race and social class. *Am J Epidemiol.* 107:311-20, 1978.

29. Newill, V. Distribution of cancer mortality among ethnic subgroups of the white population of New York City, 1953–1958. *J Natl Cancer Inst.* 26:405-17, 1961.

30. MacMahon, B. The ethnic distribution of cancer mortality in New York City, 1955. *Acta Unio Intern Contra Cancrum.* 16:1716-24, 1960.

31. Seidman, H. Cancer death rates by site and sex for religious and socioeconomic groups in New York City. *Environ Res.* 3:234-50, 1970.

32. Wynder, E. L., Mabuchi, K., and Whitmore, W. Epidemiology of cancer of the prostate. *Cancer.* 28:344-60, 1971.

33. Lancaster, H. O. The mortality in Australia from cancers peculiar to the male. *Med J Aust.* 2:41-4, 1952.

34. Krain, L. W. Some epidemiologic variables in prostatic carcinoma in California. *Prev Med.* 3:154-9, 1974.

35. Steele, R., Lees, R.E.M., Kraus, A. S. et al. Sexual factors in the epidemiology of cancer of the prostate. *J Chronic Dis.* 24:29-37, 1971.

36. Schuman, L. M., Mandel, J., Blackard, C. et al. Epidemiologic study of prostatic cancer: preliminary report. *Cancer Treat Rep.* 61:181-6, 1977.

37. Rotkin, I. D. Epidemiologic studies in prostatic cancer. *Cancer Treat*

Rep. 61:173-80, 1977.

38. Berg, J. W. Can nutrition explain the pattern of international epidemiology of hormone-dependent cancers? *Cancer Res.* 35:3345-50, 1975.

39. Howell, M. A. Factor analysis of international cancer mortality data and per capita food consumption. *Br J Cancer.* 29:328-36, 1974.

40. Wynder, E. L., and Mabuchi, K. Etiological and preventive aspects of human cancer. *Prev Med.* 1:300-34.

41. Woolf, C. M. An investigation of the familial aspects of carcinoma of the prostate. *Cancer.* 13:739-44.

42. Morganti, G., Gianferrari, L., Cresseri, A. et al. Recherches clinico-statistiques et genetiques sur les neoplasies de la prostate. *Acta Genetica et Statistica.* 6:304-5, 1956.

43. Greenwald, P., Kirmss, V., Polan, A. K. et al. Cancer of the prostate among men with benign prostatic hyperplasia. *J Natl Cancer Inst.* 53:335-40, 1974b.

44. Armenian, H. K., Lilienfeld, A. M., Diamond, E. L. et al. Relation between benign prostatic hyperplasia and cancer of the prostate. *Lancet.* 2:7873-75, 1974.

45. Deaver, J. B. Etiology and predetermining factors of benign prostatic hypertrophy. In *Enlargement of the Prostate.* Philadelphia: Blakiston, 1922.

46. Glantz, G. M. Cirrhosis and carcinoma of the prostate gland. *J Urol.* 91:291-3, 1964.

47. Robson, M. C. Cirrhosis and prostatic neoplasms. *Geriatrics.* 21:150-4, 1966.

48. Marmorston, J., Lombardo, L. J. Jr., Myers S. M. et al. Urinary excretion of neutral 17-ketosteroids and pregnanediol by patients with prostatic cancer and benign prostatic hypertrophy. *J Urol.* 93:276-86, 1965.

49. Herbert, J. T., Birkhoff, J. D., Feorino, P. M. et al. Herpes simplex virus type 2 and cancer of the prostate. *J Urol.* 116:611-12, 1976.

50. Lang, D. J., and Kummer, J. F. Demonstration of cytomegalovirus in semen. *N Engl J Med.* 285:756-8, 1972.

51. Centifanto, Y. M., Zam, Z. S., Kaufman, H. E. et al. In vitro transformation of hamster cells by herpes simplex virus type 2 from human prostatic cancer cells. *Cancer Res.* 35:1880-6, 1975.

52. Gordon, T., Crittenden, M., and Haenszel, W. *Cancer Mortality Trends in the United States. End Results and Mortality Trends.* Washington: National Cancer Institute, Monograph No. 6, 1961, pp 133-298.

53. Nielsen, M. L., and Vestergaard, B. F. Virological investigations in chronic prostatitis. *J Urol.* 109:1023-5, 1973.

54. Centifanto, Y. M., Kaufman, H. E., Zam, Z. S. et al. Herpesvirus particles in prostatic carcinoma cells. *J Virol.* 12:1608-11, 1973.

55. Dmochowski, L., Maruyama, K., Obtsuki, Y. et al. Virologic and immunologic studies of human prostatic carcinoma. *Cancer Chemother Rep.* 59:17-31, 1975.

56. Farnsworth, W. E. Human prostatic reverse transcriptase and RNS-virus. *Urol Res.* 1:106-12, 1973.

57. Paulson, D. F., Rabson, A. S., and Fraley, E. E. Viral neoplastic transformation of hamster prostatic tissue in vitro. *Science.* 159:200-1, 1968.

58. Hesmat, M. Y., Herson, J., Kovi, J. et al. An epidemiologic study of gonorrhea and cancer of the prostate gland. *Med Ann District of Columbia.* 42:378-83, 1973.

59. Robbins, J., Kraemer, M. L., Festoff, B. W. et al. Xeroderma pigmentosum: an inherited disease with sun sensitivity, multiple cutaneous neoplasms, and abnormal DNA repair. *Ann Intern Med.* 80:221-48, 1974.

The Possible Viral Etiology of Human Prostatic Carcinoma

2

Robert F. Zeigel

Since the mid 1960s, when culmination of conceptually confluent thinking occurred regarding the need to examine the potential role of viruses and viral information in the induction of neoplasia in man, a broad spectrum of studies has been initiated and expedited and new techniques developed which undoubtedly will aid in the final resolution of this problem. A number of specific cancers have been targeted with this hypothesis in a relatively systematic fashion. Prominent among these are Burkitt lymphoma, the leukemias, osteosarcoma, melanoma, multiple myeloma, dermal squamous cell, and nasopharyngeal carcinoma. Cancers of specific internal organs have also been scrutinized for viral association. Spleen, pancreas, liver, lung, various regions of the alimentary tract, and endocrine organs have been probed by combined techniques in an attempt to detect any reproducible and persistent viral link. To date, all evidence indicates that although a few viral isolates have been made from human tumors, the "viral etiology of human cancer" hypothesis has been forced to retreat behind the concept that perhaps only viral "fragments" containing the "oncogene" are, in some direct or pseudogenetical fashion, linked with the cells' own heritable mechanism. The availability and accessibility of both diseased and control ("normal") cells and tissues, the success by which they can be maintained and cultivated in vitro, the level at which an understanding of their physiologic role and function exists, and the development of parallel model animal systems of the same tissue or organs from which to draw hopefully successful inferential leads has in part dictated which specific disease entities have come under the "investigative gun" sooner than others. Although human prostatic cancer has been widely recognized as a ubiquitous and dominant geriatric problem, it has only recently been included as a primary candidate for concerted investigation.[1-3] It has become abundantly apparent that a number of the problematic reasons listed above are germane to the fact that the human prostate has been deferred as a frequent experimental tissue of choice. A number of recent investigative and review articles have sufficiently defined the problems of research attendant to the human prostate.[4-7] It is, therefore, that with no

The author wishes to acknowledge the continued support and contributions of Dr Wm. F. McLimans, Dr S. Arya and Ms. L. Job of Roswell Park Memorial Institute.

small quanta of trepidation several laboratories have launched into virologic studies on the human prostate.

One of the overriding concerns not yet resolved is an attempt to determine the most suitable age of the prostatic tissue on which to concentrate virologic probes. Potential progress is currently limited by dependency on surgical specimens which are frequently traumatized by the biopsy process, often of unknown origin (with regard to its dorsal, ventral, lateral, or median nature), and usually of an advanced sarcomatoid state. Fresh, young, healthy prostatic tissue is exceedingly difficult to obtain. It is, therefore, a normal consequence that some investigators have turned to the acquisition of prostatic metastases to initiate their studies. Coupled with this difficulty has been the basic and difficult problem of definitive characterization of, for example, cellular outgrowths from organ culture obtained from primary cultures, or from clones or lines of cells derived from diseased prostatic tissue. Only very recently has there been some progress made in enzymologic and immunologic fields, from which specific techniques have been devised which can be utilized as marker or detection assays. Sophisticated virologic probes on these cells which have been definitively characterized as surviving functional prostatic epithelial cells will be significantly more interesting and important. For now, however, we remain content to review preliminary, frequently compromised and initial results with some fundamental conviction that viral association with oncogenesis is somewhat more than mere semantics. The following represents an attempt to present a summary of the development and evolution of thinking and research studies on the potential viral etiology of cancer of the prostate (CAP).

It has been customary in the past to search for intact, infectious, mature virus in diseased tissue by morphologic and other biologic methods. In recent years the conceptual separation of "virogene" from "oncogene" has led to the belief that only a portion of a virus may be required to produce neoplasia. There are indications that a fraction of a virus may remain in a transformed tissue long after the whole virus was introduced or following any possible replicative phase. Studies have also shown that "defective" oncogenic substrains of a virus may have been in contact with the tissue at some time.[8-12] Consideration of these complex possibilities necessitates careful deliberation as to what, when, and how to search for past, present, and even future expressions of the virus. The high priorities which have been given in recent years to allocation of research funds for study of the viral etiology of neoplasia is still another reason for minute examination of over-enthusiastic claims for virus "finds" which have been so common in the scientific arena. It is in this context that an attempt will be made to assess and draw inferences from recent reports and reviews of numerous lines of investigation of virologic research on carcinoma of the human prostate.

At this time it can safely be stated that although considerable efforts have been made to detect, identify, and isolate viruses in human prostatic tissue, with the exception of two instances of herpes-type virus identification, few strong leads have emerged. Data potentially focal to the possible viral etiology of the disease could conceivably come from several sources. No significant evidence has been derived from epidemiologic or demographic studies to suggest either a vertical (germ cell/viral/genetic) or lateral (viral/infectious) transmission parameter in the disease process. However, there are certain age, ethnic, and socioeconomic factors which appear to have exerted some influence on the statistics of the disease.[13-17] Whatever mechanisms are at work in the induction of this disease, they would appear to have a long latent period. As several recent reviews have noted, the incidence, distribution, and histopathologic character of prostatic cancer may be virtually inextricable from a large number of intercalated factors among which are the hormonal regulation of sexual maturity and activity, hygienic habits (ethnic or personal), contact with external stimuli, inadvertent exposure to environmental carcinogens, and spurious and incidental association with "household" viral infections.[4-6] Local tissue environment, particularly with regard to vascularity, hormonal and enzymic content, may play a definitive role in the triggering of the oncogenic process over long periods of time. Clinical studies have been oriented toward the problems of histopathologic staging, diagnosis, and treatment, and little if any inference regarding the possible affiliation of disease with virus has surfaced. A number of morphologic and pathologic studies of the prostate with both classical light and current electron microscopic procedures have not indicated substantive viral associations.[18-30]

Similarly, recent biochemical investigations directed at the hormonal and enzymologic characteristics of normal and neoplastic prostate have yielded no strong evidence for the association of viruses and prostatic cancer. Nor have studies designed to localize specific marker proteins (primarily enzymes) by immunologic means been productive.[31-43]

It should also be pointed out, if not emphasized, that prostatic carcinoma studies lack the conceptual input of the vast and extensive knowledge acquired from model animal studies. This is in contrast to the situation in the leukemias (avian, murine, guinea pig, feline), sarcomas (primate, avian, murine, rattus), lymphomas (primate, bovine), and mammary tumors (murine), etc. Well-defined and progressive technologic and philosophic concepts have been generated in these situations with regard to cell cultivation, viral isolation, viral proliferation, viral biology and purification, disease induction and pathology. The biology of such transmission parameters has been explored relatively exhaustively. The comparatively few examples of animal experiments involving prostatic tissue have been performed on dogs, hamsters, mice, and rats.[44-50]

A study implicating herpes virus in genital lesions in guinea pigs has been reported.[51] The human prostatic problem stands by comparison in a unique and somewhat isolated fashion, requiring that procedural and hypothetical approaches be extrapolated from other tissue studies. Some carryover concepts may be relevant while, frustratingly, some may not.

In lieu of extensive background from model systems, the recent approach to the problem of whether or not a virus or viruses are involved with human prostatic cancer has been a simplistic, unsubtle, frontal approach, wherein fresh surgical or autopsy prostatic tissue is examined directly by morphological and biochemical probes. Direct morphologic approaches, primarily employing electron microscopy, on both normal and neoplastic prostatic tissue, have supported and extended earlier and basic light microscopic histologic and cytologic studies. Differences between cell types, physiologic states, reflections of levels of hormonal stimulation and control, etc., have been documented. A significant study by Györkey[4] suggested that viral-like cytoplasmic inclusions were observed in several cases of CAP. Other than this, no other direct morphologic approach, has elicited evidence for the presence of virus, including our own.[6]

Concurrently, a number of attempts have been made to cultivate human prostate in vitro (see ref. 6 for bibliography). It is understood but frequently understated that it is imperative for the investigator to utilize a well defined and characterized system in order to perform significant experiments on prostatic tissue, whether to detect virus, identify enzymes, assay hormone levels, or eventually to elaborate hormones.[52] Any investigative study must have the morphologic and biochemical capability to assess the nature of the particular cells or tissues growing under artificial environmental conditions, and to conduct periodic karyologic analysis. More recently, it appears that several laboratories are on the brink of devising methods to maintain and sustain for longer periods of time, epithelioid cells derived from the prostate which possess several specific functional characteristics of prostatic epithelium. Primary among these characteristics are the isoenzymes, acid phosphatase and 5-α-reductase.

Significant contributions to this technology have been made by Seligman et al. and Chu et al., although confirmation and reproducibility of their immunospecific procedures must be awaited. The development and success of cell culture methodology become even more pertinent in the light of inherent difficulties encountered in experimental procedures on humans and the lack of an experimental model animal system. A broad review of recent and current endeavors of this nature has revealed limited but significant success and no small level of frustration precipitated by biologic or cellular contamination, the ubiquitous "fly in the ointment."[6,53,54] It should be noted that none of these studies on prostatic cells in vitro has revealed the occasional association with viruses.

Any serious attempt to induce the expression of, isolate, or characterize virus from prostatic cells is likely to depend upon the establishment of cell culture systems from the "proper" stage of the disease, the "right" patient at the "right" time, and under the most fortuitous circumstances. For example, a probable significant requirement could be that the donor has not been exposed to any immuno-chemotherapeutic or radiation regimen. Several new and novel tacks may provide the required impetus. These include development of long-term cell cultures under strict environmental conditions, utilization of pretreated microcarriers, suppression of fibroblastic growth, karyologic monitoring at frequent intervals, selective cell dissociation techniques, and conditioning of specific media or modification of serum.[52,55]

It is not within the scope of this chapter to present a comprehensive re-review of the current thinking or philosophy underlying the potential for viruses or viral information to act as "etiologic" agents for prostatic cancer or other human neoplasms. This has been accomplished in a number of readily available sources.[8-12,56-59] Suffice to state that a number of potential viral isolates, viral components (antigens, enzymes, fragments of genome, etc.), viral-specific by-products, viral-modified cell-antigens, etc., have been made or identified from representatives of diversified groups of vertebrates, including reptiles, subhuman primates, and man.[60] Perhaps just as important as these "viral finds" and inferences is the concomitant development of relatively sophisticated techniques and methodology for identification of low-titer viral antigens and short, but presumably characteristic, viral nucleic acid sequences. These include bioassay for high molecular weight RNA (60-70S), determination of viral genomic homology, detection of specific viral enzymes such as RNA-dependent-DNA-polymerase (RT'ase), and utilization of a putative high molecular weight RNA plus an RT'ase system activated in the presence of actinomycin D, which may produce an endogenous viral-specific high molecular weight RNA:DNA complex (known as the simultaneous detection test).[61-74] These molecular biologic procedures possess great potential for detecting particularly the endogenous RNA-containing "C"-type oncornaviruses which have been demonstrated to be involved with a variety of neoplasms in many model animal systems. Other similar assay techniques exist for isolation and identification of the potentially oncogenic DNA-containing viruses, such as herpes, adeno- and papovaviruses. It is fair to state that although these techniques have high sensitivity levels, and although "calibration test" results on cells or tissues with known or existing viral content are elegant, they have yet to culminate in detection of any new and as yet unclassified viral agents, as the morphologic and biologic techniques have done in the past two decades. Historically, morphologic and biologic techniques laid the groundwork for modern tumor virology, particularly through collaborative and original ultrastructural studies.

Considerable effort is being expended on the biology, genetics, and molecular biology of several representatives of DNA viruses with oncogenic potential. Primary among these are adeno-12 and -18, SV-40, and several herpes-type viral candidates.[75,76] The fact that their replicative cycle involves intimate association with the cell's genetic regulatory mechanism has fostered intensive investigations into their potential as prostatic tumor agents. As noted before, the herpes-type agents have more recently and frequently been demonstrated to be associated with human tumor cells and tissues. Because RNA tumor viral information may have "chosen" to remain largely "endogenous" within the genome of the human population, and apparently does not readily manufacture mature particles (virions), one may question the supportive role of morphologic approaches to human cancer studies. However, many experimental rationales involve the potential to "activate" endogenous agents, and ultrastructural analysis therefore would again be germane if not critical. However, if one chooses to consider these budding, intimately cell-associated anomalies, with their specific RT'ase enzymes (which also appear to be components, if perhaps at lower levels, of normal cells), as something other than "typical" viral agents, then one may predict that (futuristically) input may be technologically and conceptually asymptotic to that evolving in the field of somatic cell genetics. It is conceivable that many (all?) human cancers have a definitive genetic base and that parameters of the population genetics are as yet ill-defined and not well understood, possibly relating to the deregulation of specific genomic sites (viral?) through a sequential cascade of several coupled but statistically improbable events. Therefore in some instances at least, time, the fourth dimension (increasing age), would favor the expression of a relatively higher apparent incidence of disease. Prostatic cancer could fit this model.

The potential of viral association or expression in human prostate is extremely complex. Among the various complicating factors is the possibility of venereal transmission and vertical or the more typical lateral infective transmission. The concept that viral infection of certain tissues serving as reservoirs in the female could play some role in the initiation of infection in men, is always possible and a feasible consideration. This includes not only potential transmission through sexual experience but also through exposure to specific agents at birth or through other intimate physical contact such as nursing. Recent reviews have attempted to collate pertinent information from newer studies concerning any association of viruses with neoplasia or dysplasia in the female reproductive tract.[6,77-79] It is apparent that although some leads are thought-provoking, there are no data which suggest a strong etiologic correlation at present. The viral genomic information may well be ubiquitous, but its mere presence is cause for continuing consideration, particularly in the field of gene regulation.

There are two major approaches which are derived from direct virologic investigations on the human prostate. These relate to the two main groups of viral agents with reference to their nucleic acid content, either DNA or RNA. As noted previously, the DNA viruses which demonstrated in vivo and in vitro "transforming" potential include adeno-12 and -18, SV-40, other papovavirus representatives, and herpes-type viruses. As has been reported possibly the best case can be made for herpes-type viral agents.[6] Morriseau suggested an etiologic relationship might exist between herpes simplex and prostatitis in man.[80] Others have been more or less successful in demonstrating herpes-type viruses in prostatic fluids and in sera from cytomegalovirus-infected patients.[81-82] Immunofluorescence and electron microscopy studies by Centifanto suggested the presence of herpes virus in primary human prostatic adenocarcinoma cells.[83] Sanford has reviewed the potential role of DNA viruses in prostatic neoplasia and urged some caution in jumping from the level of detecting and identifying the "presence" of virus to suggesting an "etiologic role" for the virus.[84] Very recently Sanford and Rapp have reported new and extended evidence for the association of cytomegalovirus with human prostate-derived cells, thus reinforcing the potential role of a DNA-containing herpes-type viral agent.[85,57]

Other studies have attempted to utilize simian virus-40 (SV-40) to transform hamster prostatic cells in vitro.[86-88] Purportedly these cells produce tumors when reintroduced into young hamsters (homologous transplants). Other studies have reported the detection of SV-40 neutralizing antibody in humans with other urogenital disease.[89] Lecatsas indicated that papovaviruses may be present in human renal transplant patients who have received immunosuppressive therapy, however, other similar studies have not confirmed these observations.[90-92]

There have been a number of studies recording the possible association of RNA-containing viruses with CAP and other urogenital tumors in man.[93-95] A recent review has suggested caution in accepting these conclusions.[6] Many normal cellular constituents may "mimic" in several aspects, the RNA-A, B and C type viruses. Dmochowski reported observing C-type–like particles in 3 of 34 patients with CAP.[96] They did not record a concomitant positive assay for RT'ase nor for Rauscher Virus-specific homology of nucleic acid sequences. More recently Ohtsuki et al. published their observations on continued studies of human prostate.[97] They reported the presence of intracisternal (endoplasmic reticulum) particles in several biopsy specimens of human prostate and related the similarities to particles observed in a case of human breast cancer. Intracisternal A-type particles have heretofore been questioned as representing a stage in the successful replicative cycle of a virus. Only particles budding from peripheral plasma membranes of cells (or membranes destined to become peripheral membranes, as in the case of platelets forming from patches of the cytoplasm of megakaryocytes) have been demonstrated to be infectious or to contain *all* of the pertinent characteristics of C-type oncornaviruses. The current story of the intracytoplasmic A-type particles appears to suggest strongly that they are preinfectious precursors to the B-type murine mammary tumor virus. Our own observations resulting from electron microscopy studies on 19 prostatic specimens failed to reveal viral particles of any type, nor were there any indications of the presence of viral antigens, mycoplasma or other infectious agents.[6]

Definitive data have not been forthcoming from several biochemical and molecular biologic probes, but the following serious attempts to study the possibility of viral involvement are worthy of note. Farnsworth set out to detect RT'ase in crude extracts of 25 human prostate specimens and reported six positives.[98] No direct evidence was presented, however, to indicate that the RT'ase activity was specific for RNA tumor viruses. Some so-called "normal" cells which are presumably not viral-involved, or at least are not elaborating mature virus, have been demonstrated to possess systems which can mimic the viral RT'ase complex under certain specific conditions.[99] If an enzyme from a putatively viral-infected tumor cell is to be considered a viral RT'ase, it should be demonstrated that it can utilize $rC_n \cdot dG_0$ as well as $rA_n \cdot dT_0$, and should be able to copy natural or ecotropic viral RNA. However, because a convincing human viral RT'ase has not been characterized and its potential use of $rC_n \cdot dG_0$ has not been established, the utilization of a xenotropic viral RNA is, in the minds of some, not convincing evidence for the presence of a human viral enzyme and thus a new human oncornavirus. Arya et al. reported a series of studies utilizing template preferences and selective inhibitors of viral polymerase but did not convincingly confirm the presence of viral-specific RT'ase in solid tissues from human prostate.[100] Job et al. have more convincingly demonstrated a viral-like RT'ase activity in solid tissues from both human benign and malignant prostate.[101] Their results are based on evidence utilizing a new rapid, modified technique. Viral specificity of the enzyme was indicated by its inhibition with nucleotide inhibitors and more importantly its preference for poly(Cm). Other attempts by Arya et al. exploring other RNA tumor virus parameters, such as the potential banding density of "particles" at 1.15 to 1.18 g/cm^3 and the ability of potential product of an endogenous reaction of actinomycin D-resistant polymerase activity to form 70S RNA:DNA hybrids etc., have been equivocal.[102] Recent studies have suggested the potential isolation of "extracellular" particles from human prostate-derived fibroblastic cell cultures and epithelial explant cultures which resemble oncornavirus in several aspects including the presence of an RNA directed DNA polymerase.[103] Particles with a density of 1.15 to 1.18 g/cm^3, similar to known oncornaviruses, were recovered from cell culture supernatants after treatment with bromo-deoxy uridine (BUDR). These particles possess RNA and RT'ase with characteristics similar to those of RNA tumor viruses.[104] In addition, Arya tested several human prostatic tissue DNAs for possible content of simian sarcoma virus DNA.

No significant amount of a homologous sequence component was detected. Mickey and McCombs have employed immunologic assays in an attempt to detect the presence of the p30 core protein of known RNA tumor viruses in human benign and CAP tissues; their report is marginally supportive of its presence.[105,106] In parallel studies, Kind has attempted to localize p30 antigen in murine prostate with inconclusive results.[107]

As has been discussed, a number of modern techniques are beginning to be combined and employed with the idea of trying to show the association of virus with CAP.[6] These approaches include (1) ultrastructural examination of normal, benign prostatic hypertrophy (BPH) and CAP from different pathologic stages, from short- and long-term cell culture systems, and on cells from studies utilizing viral inducers and inhibitors of viral and/or cell nucleic acid synthetic processes; (2) biophysical analysis of particulates in cell-free media or supernatant fractions by density gradient procedures; (3) assessment of the presence of high molecular weight (60 to 70S) RNA which can be demonstrated to be homologous or complimentary to the RNA of known oncorna or oncogenic DNA viruses; (4) detection of the presence of RNA-directed DNA polymerase as evidence for the presence of RNA-containing tumor viruses; (5) utilization of potential functional endogenous high molecular weight RNA plus an RT'ase system capable of synthesizing a high molecular weight RNA:DNA hybrid; (6) immunologic tests for viral-specific antigens or viral-induced neoantigens or antibodies; (7) utilization of modern cell culture technology to combine with viral induction or potentiation procedures, such as the halogenated pyrimidines, dimethyl sulfoxide, or selective inhibitors such as actinomycin D or rifamycin derivatives, or streptovaricin; (8) cocultivation of prostate-derived cell cultures with other nonhomologous "permissive" cell systems to allow for the expression of viral genetic information; (9) investigation into the possibility that other bioactive agents such as mycoplasma may have some specific etiologic potential of their own, or through "immunosuppressive" parameters allow other, perhaps environmental factors, to trigger the transformational event.

To date a comprehensive review of results on studies employing these technologies indicates that there is no definitive evidence for the correlation of virus with prostatic disease. There is, however, the strong inference that herpes-type virus is the best candidate so far. There is a good possibility that herpes virus information is an integral part of many human cell systems. Additional evidence is required to deduce definitively the same likelihood for oncornaviral information in human CAP.[6,59]

In summary, it must be concluded that viral etiology of human cancer, although an attractive hypothesis, is as enigmatic now with several years of productive complexity and the development of knowledgeable "hindsight," as it was two decades ago. Although the attack on human prostatic cancer has been initiated only recently, utilizing the broader and relatively modern sophisticated collaborative technologies, only nonspecific ephemeral indications of viral association have emerged. It is indeed frustrating to realize that from a plethora of studies on the embryology, histocytology, and pathology of prostate and its related diseases, plus the relatively recent incantations of the tumor virologists, some definitive correlation has not yet emerged; but it hasn't. One must conclude that the level of viral involvement, if any, is at the same stage as gene expression and regulation within the individual cell, and resides, therefore, on a parallel with the question of what is the molecular modus which determines whether a cell will remain normal or lose its regulatory capacity and become neoplastic. We find ourselves coming full circle to the time when, four to five decades ago embryologists and cell biologists not so naively asked what are the mechanisms which control cell growth, differentiation, restriction of potency, cell-to-cell communication, and tissue organization. The level of impact of viral association is most likely to be very basic and not manipulable at a secondary or tertiary stage. In other words, if a viral etiology for human cancer is ultimately convincingly determined, a panacean vaccine targeted at ridding the cell of "replicative" virus may be totally ineffectual against the integrated or otherwise genetically linked "oncogene" matrix.

The search for "virus" in tumor tissues and basic study of various virus systems must continue, however, for knowledge gleaned with regard to regulation, control, and expression of virus in somewhat better defined and less complex systems than the intact cell may provide clues to follow with regard to the eventual understanding of the mechanisms of cellular neoplastic transformation.

REFERENCES

1. Franks, L. M. Etiology, epidemiology and pathology of prostatic cancer. *Cancer.* 32:1092-5, 1973.

2. The Veterans' Administration Cooperative Urological Research Group. Carcinoma of the prostate: a continuing cooperative study. *J Urol.* 91:590-4, 1964.

3. National Organ Site Programs; Div. of Cancer Research Resources and Centers: NCI: Natl. Prostatic Cancer Project. RPMI, G. P. Murphy, MD. Dir. NIH-DRG. *Newsletter* 9 (#9) September 1972.

4. Györkey, F. Some aspects of cancer of the prostate gland. Edited by H. Busch. In *Methods in Cancer Research.* New York: Academic Press, Inc., 10:279-368, 1973.

5. Blackard, C. E. The Veterans' Administration Cooperative Urological Research Group. Carcinoma of the prostate: a review. *Cancer Chemother Rep.* 59:225-7, 1975.

6. Zeigel, R. F., Arya, S. K., Horoszewicz, J. S. et al. A status report: hu-

man prostatic carcinoma, with emphasis on potential for viral etiology. *Oncology.* 34:29-44, 1977.

7. Cancer of the prostate (editorial). *N Eng J Med.* 278:848-9, 1968.

8. Todaro, G. J., and Huebner, R. J. The viral oncogene hypothesis: new evidence. *Proc Natl Acad Sci USA.* 69:1009-15, 1972.

9. Huebner, R. J., and Todaro, G. J. Oncogenesis of RNA tumor viruses as determinants of cancer. *Proc Natl Acad Sci USA.* 64:1087-94, 1969.

10. Temin, H. M. Nature of the provirus of Rous sarcoma. *Natl Cancer Inst Monogr.* 17:557-70, 1964.

11. Fischinger, P. J., and Haapala, D. K. Oncoduction. A unifying hypothesis of viral carcinogenesis. *Prog Exp Tumor Res.* 19:1-22, 1974.

12. Comings, D. E. A general theory of carcinogenesis. *Proc Natl Acad Sci.* 70:3324-8, 1973.

13. Huggins, C. D. Introduction, in Biology of the Prostate and Related Tissues. *Natl Cancer Inst Monogr.* 12:11-12, 1963.

14. Lilienfeld, A. M. Some limitations and problems for screening for cancer. *Cancer.* 33:1720-4, 1974.

15. King, H., Diamond, E., and Lilienfeld, A. M. Some epidemiological aspects of cancer of the prostate. *J Chronic Dis.* 16:117-53, 1963.

16. Wynder, E. L., Mabuchi, K., and Whitmore, W. F., Jr. Epidemiology of cancer of the prostate. *Cancer.* 28:344-60, 1971.

17. Hutchison, G. B. Etiology and prevention of prostatic cancer. *Cancer Chemother Rep.* 59:57-8, 1975.

18. Takayasu, H., and Yamaguchi, Y. An electron microscopic study of the prostatic cancer cell. *J Urol.* 87:935-40, 1962.

19. Fisher, E. R., and Sieracki, J. C. Ultrastructure of human normal and neoplastic prostate. Edited by E. P. Vollmer. In *Biology of the Prostate and Related Tissues.* Monograph 12. Washington: National Cancer Institute, 1963, pp 1-26.

20. Brandes, D., Kirchheim, D., and Scott, W. W. Ultrastructure of the human prostate: normal and neoplastic. *Lab Invest.* 13:1541-60, 1964.

21. Fisher, E. R., and Jeffrey, W. Ultrastructure of human normal and neoplastic prostate. *Am J Clin Path.* 44:119-34, 1965.

22. Kirchheim, D., and Bacon, R. L. Ultrastructural studies of carcinoma of the human prostatic gland. *Invest Urol.* 6:611-30, 1969.

23. Helminen, H. J., and Ericsson, J.L.E. Ultrastructural studies on prostatic involution in the rat. Mechanism of autophagy in epithelial cells with special reference to the rough surfaced endoplasmic reticulum. *J Ultrastruc Res.* 36:708-24, 1971.

24. Ishikawa, F. An electron microscopic study of the human prostatic cancer: With special references to lysosomal system in prostatic cancer and to high dose estrogen effect upon prostatic cancer. *Nippon Himyokika Gakki Zasshi.* 62:439-66, 1971.

25. Sinha, A. A., and Blackard, C. E. Ultrastructure of prostatic benign hyperplasia and carcinoma. *Urology.* 11:114-20, 1973.

26. Helminen, H. J., and Ericsson, J.L.E. Ultrastructural studies on prostatic involution in the rat. Changes in the secretory pathways. *J Ultrastruct Res.* 40:152-66, 1972.

27. Sinha, A. A., Blackard, C. E. et al. The in vitro localization of H_3 estradiol in human prostatic carcinoma. *Cancer.* 31:682-8, 1973.

28. Sarkar, K., Tolan, G., and McKay, D. E. Embryonal rhabdomyosarcoma of the prostate. An ultrastructural study. *Cancer.* 31:442-8, 1973.

29. Prout, G. R., Jr. Diagnosis and staging of prostatic carcinoma. *Cancer.* 32:1096-1103, 1973.

30. Byar, D. P., and Mostofi, F. K. Veterans' Adm. Coop. Urol. Res. Group: carcinoma of the prostate: prognostic evaluation of certain pathologic features in 208 radical prostatectomies examined by the step-section technique. *Cancer.* 30:5-13, 1972.

31. Li, M. C., Kanwal, G., and Kim, R. H. Prostatic tumor acid phosphatase production. *Urology.* 1:221-5, 1973.

32. Dow, D., and Whitaker, R. H. Prostatic contribution to normal serum acid phosphatase. *Br Med J.* 4:470-2, 1970.

33. Kent, J. R., Hill, M., and Bischoff, A. Acid phosphatase content of prostatic exprimate from patients with advanced prostatic carcinoma: a potential prognosis and therapeutic index. *Cancer.* 25:858-62, 1970.

34. Reynolds, R. D., Greenberg, B. R., Martin, N. D. et al. Usefulness of bone marrow serum acid phosphatase in staging carcinoma of the prostate. *Cancer.* 32:181-4, 1973.

35. Seligman, A. M., Sternberger, N. J., Paul, B. D. et al. Design of spindle poisons activated specifically by prostatic acid phosphatase (PAP) and new methods for PAP cytochemistry. *Cancer Chemother Rep.* 59:233-42, 1975.

36. Hein, R. C., Grayhack, J. T., and Goldberg, E. Prostatic fluid lactic dehydrogenase isoenzyme patterns of prostatic cancer and hyperplasia. *Trans Am Assoc Genitourin Surg.* 66:25-30, 1974.

37. Yam, L. T. Clinical significance of the human acid phosphatases: a review. *Am J Med.* 56:604-16, 1974.

38. Moncure, C. W., Johnson, C. L., Koontz, W. W. et al. Investigation of specific antigens in prostatic cancer. *Cancer Chemother Rep.* 59:105-10, 1975.

39. Reynoso, G., Chu, T. M., Guinan, P. et al. Carcino-embryonic antigen in patients with tumors of the urogenital tract. *Cancer.* 30:1-4, 1972.

40. Chu, T. M., Bhargava, A., Barnard, E. A. et al. Tumor antigen and acid phosphatase isoenzyme in prostatic cancer. *Cancer Chemother Rep.* 59:97-103, 1975.

41. Robinson, M.R.G., Nakhla, L. S., and Whitaker, R. H. A new concept in the management of carcinoma of the prostate. *J Urol.* 43:728-32, 1971.

42. Magarey, C. J., and Baum, M. Oestrogen as a reticulo-endothelial stimulant in patients with cancer. *Br Med J.* 2:367-70, 1971.

43. Merrin, C., Han, T., Klein, E. et al. Immunotherapy of prostatic carcinoma with *bacillus Calmett-Guerin. Cancer Chemother Rep.* 59:157-63, 1975.

44. Rudduck, H. B., and Willis, R. A. Malignant tumors in dogs. A description of 9 cases. *Am J Cancer.* 33:205-17, 1938.

45. Grant, C. A. Carcinoma of the canine prostate. *Acta Pathol Microbiol Scand.* 40:197-208, 1957.

46. Hill, H., and Maré, C. J. Genital disease in dogs caused by canine herpes virus. *Am J Vet Res.* 35:669-72, 1974.

47. Lear, I., Carazos, L. F., and Ofner, P. Fine structure and C_{19}-steroid metabolism of spontaneous adenocarcinoma of the canine prostate. *J Natl Cancer Inst.* 52:789-804, 1974.

48. Fortner, G., Faukhauser, J. W., and Cullen, M. R. A transplantable spontaneous adenocarcinoma of the prostate in the prostate in the Syrian (golden) hamster. *Natl Cancer Inst Monogr.* 12:371-9, 1963.

49. Paulson, D. F., Rabson, A. S., and Fraley, E. E. Viral neoplastic transformation of hamster prostate tissue in vitro. *Science.* 159:200-1, 1967.

50. Pollard, M., and Luckert, P. H. Transplantable metastasizing prostate adenocarcinomas in rats. *J Natl Cancer Inst.* 54:643-9, 1975.

51. Lukás, B., Wiesendanger, W., and Schmidt-Ruppin, K. H. Genital herpes in guinea pigs. An experimental model with herpes virus hominis–a brief re-

port. *Arch Gesamte Virusforsch.* 44:153-5, 1974.

52. McLimans, W. F., Kwasniewski, B., Robinson, F. et al. Culture of mammalian prostatic cells. *Cancer Treat Rep.* 61:161-5, 1977.

53. Nelson-Reese, W. A., Flandermeyer, R. R., and Hawthorne, P. K. Banded marker chromosomes as indicators of intraspecies cellular contamination. *Science.* 184:1093-6, 1974.

54. Culliton, B. J. Hela cells: Contaminating cultures around the world. *Science* 184:1058-9, 1974.

55. McLimans, W. F. Physiology of the cultured mammalian cell. Edited by G. L. Tritsch. In *Axenic Mammalian Cell Reactions.* New York: Marcel Dekker, 1969, pp 307-67.

56. Duff, R., and Rapp, F. The induction of oncogenic potential by herpes simplex virus. Edited by M. Pollard. In *Perspectives in Virology.* New York: Academic Press, 1973, pp 189-210.

57. Rapp, F., Geder, L., and Murasko, D. Long-term persistence of cytomegalovirus genome in cultured human cells of prostatic origin. *J Virol.* 16:982-90, 1975.

58. Rabson, A. S. Herpesviruses and cancer, Introduction. Pathology Society Symposium. *Fed Proc.* 31:1625-74, 1972.

59. Marx, J. L. RNA tumor viruses: getting a handle on transformation. *Science.* 199:161-4, 1978.

60. Gallo, R. C., and Levine, A. Meeting review, tumor viruses, Cold Spring Harbor. *Cell.* 2:295-304, 1974.

61. Schlom, J., and Spiegelman, S. Simultaneous detection of RT'ase and high molecular weight RNA unique to oncogenic RNA viruses. *Science.* 174:840-3, 1971.

62. Schlom, J., Spiegelman, S., and Moore, D. RNA-dependent-DNA-polymerase activity in virus-like particles isolated from human milk. *Nature.* 231:97-100, 1971.

63. Axel, R., Schlom, J., and Spiegelman, S. Presence in human breast cancer of RNA homologous to mouse mammary tumor virus RNA. *Nature.* 235:32-6, 1972.

64. Gulati, S. C., Axel, R., and Spiegelman, S. Detection of RNA-instructed-DNA-polymerase and high molecular weight RNA in malignant tissue. *Proc Natl Acad Sci USA.* 69:2020-4, 1972.

65. Schlom, J., and Spiegelman, S. Evidence for viral involvement in murine and human mammary adenocarcinoma. *Am J Clin Pathol.* 60:57-64, 1973.

66. Gallo, R. C., Yang, S. A., and Ting, R. C. RNA-dependent-DNA-polymerase of human acute leukemia cells. *Nature.* 228:927-9, 1970.

67. Moore, D. H., Charney, J., Kramarsky, B. et al. Search for a human breast cancer virus. *Nature.* 229:611-14, 1971.

68. Sarin, P. S., and Gallo, R. C. Biochemical approaches to detection of viral-related information in human acute leukemic cells. *Bibl Haematol.* 40:463-70, 1975.

69. Mondal, H., Gallagher, R. E., and Gallo, R. C. RNA-directed-DNA-polymerase from human leukemic blood cells and from primate type C virus-producing cells: high- and low-molecular weight forms with variant biochemical and immunological properties. *Proc Natl Acad Sci USA.* 72:1194-8, 1975.

70. Gallagher, R. E., and Gallo, R. C. Type C RNA tumor virus isolated from cultured human acute myelogenous leukemia cells. *Science.* 187:350-3, 1975.

71. Gilden, R. V., and Oroszlan, S. Group-specific antigens of RNA tumor viruses as markers for subinfectious expression of the RNA virus genome. *Proc*

Natl Acad Sci USA. 69:1021-5, 1972.

72. Howk, R. S., Rye, L. A., Killeen, L. A. et al. Characterization and separation of viral DNA-polymerase in mouse milk. *Proc Natl Acad Sci USA.* 70:2117-21, 1973.

73. Sarngadharan, M., Sarin, P., and Reitz, M. Reverse transcriptase activity of human acute leukemic cells: purification of the enzyme, response to AMV 70s RNA and characterization of the DNA product. *Nature New Biol.* 240:67-72, 1972.

74. Benveniste, R. E., and Todaro, G. J. Homology between type C viruses of various species as determined by molecular hybridization. *Proc Natl Acad Sci USA.* 70:3316-20, 1973.

75. Henle, W., and Henle, G. Evidence for a relation of the Epstein-Barr virus to Burkitt's lymphoma and nasopharyngeal carcinoma. Edited by Nakahara, Nishioka, Hirayama, and Ito. In *Recent Advances in Human Tumor Virology and Immunology.* Tokyo: University of Tokyo Press, 1971.

76. Sabin, A. B., and Tarro, G. Herpes simplex and herpes genitalis viruses in etiology of some human cancers. *Proc Natl Acad Sci USA.* 70:3225-9, 1973.

77. Nahmias, A. J., Naib, Z. M., and Josey, W. E. Epidemiological studies relating genital herpetic infections to cervical carcinoma. *Cancer Res.* 34:1111-17, 1974.

78. Aurelian, L. Persistence and expression of the herpes simplex virus type 2 genome in cervical tumor cells. *Cancer Res.* 34:1126-35, 1974.

79. Kessler, I. I., Kulcar, Z., Rawls, W. E. et al. Cervical cancer in Yugoslavia. 1. Antibodies to genital herpes virus in cases and controls. *J Natl Cancer Inst.* 52:369-76, 1974.

80. Morrisseau, P. M., Phillips, C. A., and Leadbetter, G. W. Viral prostatitis. *J Urol.* 103:767-9, 1970.

81. Nielsen, M. L., and Vestergaard, B. F. Virological investigations in chronic prostatitis. *J Urol.* 109:1023-5, 1973.

82. Lang, D. J., Kummer, J. F., and Hartley, D. P. Cytomegalovirus in semen: persistence and demonstration in extracellular fluids. *N Eng J Med.* 291:121-3, 1974.

83. Centifanto, Y. M., Kaufman, H. E., Zam, Z. S. et al. Herpes virus particles in prostatic carcinoma cells. *J Virol.* 12:1608-11, 1973.

84. Sanford, E. J., Rohner, T. J., and Rapp, F. Virology of prostatic cancer. *Cancer Chemother Rep.* 59:33-8, 1975.

85. Sanford, E. J., Geder, L., Laychock, A. et al. Evidence for the association of cytomegalovirus with carcinoma of the prostate. *J Urol.* 118:789-92, 1977.

86. Paulson, D. F., Fraley, E. E., Rabson, A. S. et al. SV-40 transformed hamster prostatic tissue. *Surgery.* 64:241-7, 1968.

87. Fraley, E. E., and Paulson, D. F. Morphological and biochemical studies of virus SV-40–transformed prostatic tissue. *J Urol.* 101:735-40, 1969.

88. Paulson, D. F., Bonar, R. A., Sharief, Y. et al. Properties of prostatic cultures transformed by SV-40. *Cancer Chemother Rep.* 59:51-5, 1975.

89. Shaw, K. V., Palma, L. D., and Murphy, G. P. The occurrence of SV-40 neutralizing antibodies in sera of patients with genitourinary carcinoma. *J Surg Oncol.* 3:443-50, 1971.

90. Lecatsas, G., Prozesky, O. W., Vanwyk, J. et al. Papovavirus in urine after renal transplantation. *Nature.* 241:343-4, 1973.

91. Gardner, S. D., Field, A. M., Coleman, D. V. et al. New human papovavirus (BK) isolated from urine after renal transplantation. *Lancet.* 1:1253-7, 1971.

92. Shaw, K. V., Daniel, R. W., Zeigel, R. F. et al. Search for BK and SV-40 virus reactivation in renal transplant recipients. *Transplantation.* 17:131-4, 1974.

93. Tannenbaum, M., Spiro, D., and Lattimer, J. K. Biology of the prostate gland: the electron microscopy of cytoplasmic filamentous bodies in human benign prostatic cells adjacent to cancerous cells. *Cancer Res.* 27:1415-17, 1967.

94. Tannenbaum, M., and Lattimer, J. K. Similar virus-like particles in cancers of the prostate and breast. *J Urol.* 103:471-5, 1970.

95. Elliott, A. Y., Fraley, E. E., Cleveland, P. et al. Isolation of RNA virus from papillary tumors of the human renal pelvis. *Science.* 179:393-5, 1973.

96. Dmochowski, L., Maruyama, K., Ohtsuki, Y. et al. Virologic and immunologic studies of human prostatic carcinoma. *Cancer Chemother Rep.* 59:17-31, 1975.

97. Ohtsuki, Y., Seman, G., Dmochowski, L. et al. Virus-like particles in a case of human prostate carcinoma. *J Natl Cancer Inst.* 58:1493-6, 1977.

98. Farnsworth, W. E. Human prostatic reverse transcriptase and RNA-virus. *Urol Res.* 1:106-12, 1973.

99. Weissbach, A. Eukaryotic DNA polymerases. *Annu Rev Biochem.* 46:25-47, 1977.

100. Arya, S., Zeigel, R. F., Carter, W. A. et al. RNA tumor virus-like activities in human solid tissues; endogenous RNA; DNA polymerase activities in the prostate. *J Surg Oncol.* (In press)

101. Job, L., Carter, W. A. and Arya, S. K. Reverse transcriptase activity in extracts of human prostate. (In preparation)

102. Arya, S. K., Carter, W. A., Zeigel, R. F. et al. The search for "Virogene" in human prostatic tissues: Prostatic DNA polymerases. *Cancer Chemother Rep.* 59:39-46, 1975.

103. Job, L., Arya, S. K., Carter, W. A. et al. Oncornavirus-like particles released by human prostatic explants cultures. (In preparation)

104. Arya, S. K., Job, L., Horoszewicz, J. S. et al. RNA tumor virus-like activities in human prostate: possible novel pharmacologic approaches. *Cancer Treat Rep.* 61:113-17, 1977.

105. Mickey, D. D., Stone, K. R., Stone, M. P. et al. Morphologic and immunologic studies of human prostatic carcinoma. *Cancer Treat Rep.* 61:133-8, 1977.

106. McCombs, R. M. Role of oncornaviruses in carcinoma of the prostate. *Cancer Treat Rep.* 61:131-2, 1977.

107. Kind, P. P-30 antigen in mouse prostate. *Cancer Treat Rep.* 61:129-30, 1977.

Immunologic Factors in Prostate Cancer

3

Ruben F. Gittes and Pierluigi E. Bigazzi

There has been extensive speculation but little convincing progress on the role of immunologic reactions in prostatic diseases. This chapter will attempt to review in a critical fashion the recent immunologic research on the prostate, with emphasis on its relation to prostatic cancer.

CANCER OF THE PROSTATE

The observed high incidence of clinically inapparent foci of carcinoma found at autopsy in old men and the capricious behavior of clinical prostate cancer nodules has raised speculation that the immune system might play a peculiar role in both incidence and dormancy of early prostatic cancer.[1,2] The hypothesis that the prostatic parenchyma is an immunologically privileged site has been forwarded (see below), but any firm evidence relative to human carcinoma is lacking.

At the other end of the clinical spectrum, the rare observation of spontaneous regression of metastases associated with cryotherapy of the primary prostatic lesion has raised speculation that somehow the immune system can be stimulated to destroy advanced tumors by the in situ denaturation of tumor cells.[3] Again, the experimental approach to this hypothesis has failed to get a start in the absence of demonstrable tumor-specific antigens in human prostate tumors or in the available animal tumor models (see below).

TISSUE-SPECIFIC ANTIGENS OF THE PROSTATE

Immunologic studies with prostate tissue were first performed by Flocks et al. who immunized rabbits with human prostatic tissue and obtained antibodies against prostate-specific antigens.[4] These studies were

---

Supported in part by Grant #CA 19213-03, the Thornburg Medical Research Foundation, and the Brigham Surgical Group Foundation, Inc.

pursued by several investigators who had identified tissue-specific antigens of the prostate.[5-7] One of the most interesting of these is acid phosphatase (PAP), one of the first tumor markers to be used for diagnostic purposes. The recent introduction of sensitive and specific procedures for detection of PAP in the serum has greatly increased its diagnostic value. Using a solid-state radioimmunoassay, Foti et al. have detected elevations of PAP in 33%, 79%, 71%, and 92% of patients with stage I, II, III and IV prostatic cancer, respectively.[8] In contrast, the enzyme assay which is commonly used detected increases of the enzyme in only 12%, 15%, 29%, and 60% of the same patients. Other studies in progress utilize both radioimmunoassay and counter-immunoelectrophoresis with promising results. Thus, investigations of tissue-specific antigens of the prostate may have provided an effective way for mass screening and detection of patients with prostatic tumors in early stages, increasing their chances of survival.

HUMORAL IMMUNITY TO AUTOLOGOUS PROSTATIC ANTIGENS IN HUMANS

Serum antibodies to prostatic antigens have been detected by indirect immunofluorescence and mixed hemadsorption.[7,9] In one study these antibodies were detected in 54% of patients with prostatic tumors and in 10% of controls.[7] Sera from these patients reacted with membranes or intercellular areas of benign autologous prostate and normal monkey prostate. It has been reported that they were bound in vivo to the prostate, as demonstrated by acid elution experiments. They were obviously not directed against tumor-associated antigens, but against normal components of prostate.

CELL-MEDIATED IMMUNITY TO PROSTATIC TUMOR ANTIGENS

Delayed hypersensitivity reactions to prostatic tumor antigens have been observed both in vivo and in vitro. Positive skin tests were noted in 4 of 10 patients injected with extracts of their own prostatic tumor.[10] Production of MIF (or LIF) was obtained when lymphocytes from patients with malignant tumors of the prostate were stimulated with extracts of prostate cancer.[7] Significant migration inhibition was observed in 35% of patients vs 8% of controls. Similarly, reduction of leukocyte adherence was noted when leukocytes from tumor patients were incubated with autologous tumor. When the sera of the same patients were added to their leukocytes, leukocyte adherence was found to be normal, which was interpreted as evidence of the presence of "blocking" factors in the serum of patients with tumors.[11] Inhibition of leukocyte migration and leukocyte adherence were also observed by Evans and Bowen when lymphocytes from patients with carcinoma of the prostate were stimulated with an extract of prostatic carcinoma.[12] There was no correlation with the stage of the tumor.

THE PROSTATE AS AN IMMUNOLOGICALLY PRIVILEGED SITE

Laboratory studies in the rat and the rabbit have supported in part the concept that bacterial or tumor antigens within the substance of the prostate enjoy a relative shelter from the immune system. This is similar to, but less marked than, the immunologically privileged sites of the anterior chamber of the eye or the testis. The humoral immunity was unimpaired but the measured cellular immunity was significantly decreased, compared to that elicited in other sites when BCG mycobacterial walls were injected into the rabbit prostate and the systemic immune response was measured at 21 days.[13] Using tumor cell allografts in rats, nodules grew after injection of cells into the prostate and the anterior chamber but not into muscle.[14] More recent work with allografts of skin or parathyroids transplanted across strong histocompatability barriers have failed to show significant shelter from rejection within the substance of the prostate.[15,16]

An explanation for the diminished cellular immunity elicited by some antigens placed in the prostate may be a relative lack of lymphatic uptake from the prostatic parenchyma. Such an afferent block in the cellular immune response is suggested by (a) the extremely delayed clearance of lymphangiographic emulsion or patent blue dye injected in the rat's ventral prostate, compared to the rapid uptake from subcutaneous or intratesticular injections; and, (b) uncertainty as to the presence of lymphatic channels within the prostate, although the pericapsular area is rich in them.[17,18] Using radioactive colloidal gold injection into the prostates of dogs, however, Catalona and coworkers have shown excellent uptake into a retroperitoneal lymph node, thus failing to support the hypothesis of an afferent arc defect.[19] Further work by W. F. Whitmore and W. Kaplan (unpublished observations, 1978) is in progress with lymph node scanning agents injected into the prostate.

Speculation that the human prostate may also shelter antigens from a cellular response has suggested the hypothesis that the common incidentally found cancers of the prostate may represent oversights of the immune surveillance system.[1,14] Further speculation is that the nodules may be "dormant" for years due to the humoral response that is elicited by presumptive tumor-associated antigens. It is known that in some immunologic responses humoral antibodies can hinder but not kill target cells. Sudden growth of a nodule to a clinical lesion and the successful seeding of metastases to lymph nodes and bones could be related not to a sudden fall in immune responsiveness, but to the development of blocking antibody activity by the titer and affinity of the long-stimulated humoral antibodies.[20]

Unfortunately, quantitative measurements of cellular or blocking antibody activity against prostate cancer are not yet feasible. Tumor antigens are not defined even in tumor models, and tissue culture of prostatic cancers is so difficult and unpredictable that tests for cellular cytotoxicity, colony inhibition, etc., needed to quantitate specific immunity are not applicable.

NONSPECIFIC IMMUNE RESPONSIVENESS IN PATIENTS WITH CANCER OF THE PROSTATE

A number of investigations, aimed at the determination of immune responsiveness in patients with prostatic tumors, have yielded rather inconclusive results. From a humoral point of view decreases of IgG and IgM and increases in IgA and C3 have been reported; however, such findings were obtained by comparing tumor-bearing patients with a small sample of normal subjects, and the differences noted may have little meaning.[7] As far as delayed hypersensitivity is concerned, there have been somewhat contrasting findings. Catalona et al.[21] using DNCB skin sensitization, found a greater reduction of immunocompetence in patients with localized tumors than in those with metastatic tumors. On the other hand, other investigators observed a correlation between reduction of DNCB reactivity and increase of stage and grade of prostatic malignancy.[22-25] Robinson et al. observed a reduced lymphocyte stimulation by PHA in advanced cases of prostatic cancer and an increased response in patients with more limited disease, while other investigators have reported a reduced PHA stimulation irrespective of stage of disease.[7,26,27]

When attempts to correlate generic immune responsiveness and clinical stage have been made, it has been found that patients with a higher clinical stage have poor immune responses.[7]

SUMMARY

Speculation and hypotheses have abounded in the immunologic considerations of cancer of the prostate. The investigation of prostate-specific normal antigens has led to the development of a very sensitive radioimmunoassay for acid phosphatase that holds promise of improving the case finding of early carcinoma of the prostate. Tumor-specific antigens are being sought and the techniques for specific immunologic manipulation or evaluation of patients with cancer of the prostate await more convincing findings of such antigens and the development of tissue culture techniques to carry out tests of cytotoxicity. There is some evidence to support the concept that the widespread incidence of incidental carcinoma of the prostate in old men and the variable natural history of prostatic cancer are related to the peculiar response of the immune system to antigens in prostatic substance. Work is in progress with animal models of prostatic cancer and with tissue culture of human prostatic cancer that may make possible rapid advances in the immunologic study of this common disease.

REFERENCES

1. Scott, R., Jr., Mutchnik, D., Laskowski, T., and Schmalhorst, W. R. Carcinoma of the prostate in elderly men: incidence, growth characteristics and clinical significance. *J Urol.* 101:602-7, 1969.
2. Whitmore, W. F., Jr. The natural history of prostatic cancer. *Cancer.* 32:1104-12, 1973.
3. Soanes, W. A., Albin, R. J., and Gonder, M. J. Remission of metastatic lesions following cryosurgery in prostatic cancer: immunologic considerations. *J Urol.* 104:154-59, 1970.
4. Flocks, R. H., Urich, V. C., Patel, C. A. et al. Studies on the antigenic properties of prostatic tissue. *J Urol.* 84:134-43, 1960.
5. Shulman, Sidney. *Reproduction and Antibody Response.* Cleveland: C.R.C. Press, 1975.
6. Prout, G. R., Jr. and Ornellas, E. P. Immunology of the prostate. *Urol Clin North Am.* 2:93-104, 1975.
7. Ablin, R. J. Immunobiology of the prostate. Edited by M. Tannenbaum. In *Urologic Pathology: The Prostate.* Philadelphia: Lea & Febiger, 1977.
8. Foti, A. G., Cooper, J. F., Herschman, H. et al. Detection of acid phosphatase by solid phase radioimmunoassay of serum prostatic acid phosphatase. *N Engl J Med.* 297:1357-61, 1977.
9. Dmochowski, L., Maruyama, K., Ohtsuki, Y. et al. Virologic and immunologic studies of human prostatic carcinoma. *Cancer Chemother Rep.* 59:17-31, 1975.
10. Brannen, G. E., and Coffey, D. S. Tumor-specific immunity in patients with prostatic adenocarcinoma of benign prostatic hyperplasia. *Cancer Treat Rep.* 61:211-16, 1977.
11. Bhatti, R. A., and Ablin, R. J. Leukocyte adherence inhibition: the detection of cellular responsiveness and serum "blocking" factors in malignancy. *Allergol et Immunopath.* 3:357-66, 1976.
12. Evans, C. M., and Bowen, J. G. Immunological tests in carcinoma of the prostate. *Proc R Soc Med.* 70:417-20, 1977.
13. Whitmore, W. F. III, and Gittes, R. F. Afferent lymphatics: their importance to immunologically privileged sites. *Surg Forum.* 26:338-40, 1975.

14. Gittes, R. F., and McCullough, D. L. Occult carcinoma of the prostate: an oversight of immune surveillance–working hypothesis. *J Urol.* 112:241-4, 1974.

15. Whitmore, W. F. III, and Gittes, R. F. The fate of skin allografts within the prostate. *J Urol.* 117:4-51, 1977.

16. Whitmore, W. F. III, and Gittes, R. F. Studies on the prostate and testis as immunologically privileged sites. *Cancer Treat Rep.* 61:217-22, 1977.

17. McCullough, D. L. Experimental lymphangiography–experience with direct medium injection into the parenchyma of the rat testis and prostate. *Invest Urol.* 13:211-19, 1975.

18. Rodin, A. E., Larson, D. L., and Roberts, D. K. Nature of the perineural space invaded by prostatic carcinoma. *Cancer.* 20:1772-9, 1967.

19. Menon, M., Menon, S., Strauss, H. W. et al. Demonstration of existence of canine prostatic lymphatics by radioisotope techniques. *J Urol.* 118:274-7, 1977.

20. Hellstrom, I., and Hellstrom, K. E. Cell-mediated immune reactions to tumor antigens with particular emphasis on immunity to human neoplasms. *Cancer.* 34:1461-8, 1974.

21. Catalona, W. J., Chretien, P. B., and Trahan, E. E. Abnormalities of cell-mediated immunocompetence in genitourinary cancer. *J Urol.* 11:229-32, 1974.

22. Brosman, S., Hausman, M., and Shacks, S. Immunologic alterations in patients with prostatic carcinoma. *J Urol.* 113:841-5, 1975.

23. Huus, J. C., Kursh, E. D., Poor, P. et al. Delayed cutaneous hypersensitivity in patients with prostatic adenocarcinoma. *J Urol.* 114:86-7, 1975.

24. Adolphs, H. D., and Steffens, L. Correlations between tumor stage, tumor grade, and immunocompetence in patients with carcinoma of the bladder and prostate. *Eur Urol.* 3:23-25, 1977.

25. Robinson, M.R.G., Nakhla, L. S., Whitaker, R. H. Lymphocytic transformation in carcinoma of the prostate. *Br J Urol.* 43:480-6, 1971.

26. Catalona, W. J., Tarpley, J. L., Chretien, P. B. et al. Lymphocyte stimulation in urologic cancer patients. *J Urol.* 112:373-7, 1974.

27. McLaughlin, A. P. III, Kessler, W. O., Triman, K. et al. Immunologic competence in patients with urologic cancer. *J Urol.* 11:233-7, 1974.

Histologic Grading of Prostatic Cancer: Background and Possibilities

4

John F. Gaeta and William A. Gardner, Jr.

Despite the high frequency of human prostatic cancer, statistics indicate a certain disparity between its clinical incidence and its frequency as a direct cause of death, ranking only third after pulmonary and bowel cancers. An important factor which accounts for such disparity is the wide biological potential of the disease as demonstrated by frequent cases in which the original diagnosis is followed by rapid dissemination and death, in contrast to others who die of unrelated causes many years after the original diagnosis following a successful "arrest" of their disease by a wide range of therapeutic approaches.

Investigators associated with the National Prostatic Cancer Project, addressing themselves to an evaluation of prevalent hormonal and surgical treatment modalities, soon became aware of the difficulty of comparing groups of patients who in the same stage of their clinical disease showed a significant lack of uniformity in their response to an essentially identical therapeutic approach. It was natural to assume that the histologic features of prostatic cancer should be a significant factor to explain differences of clinical behavior and therapeutic response when all other parameters are equal. When attention was focused on the morphology of prostatic cancer, it could easily be corroborated that there is no universal method of assessing the degree of malignancy of this type of adenocarcinoma. On the other hand, the question as to whether differentiation of the tumor affects prognosis has been repeatedly raised. Criteria for histologic classification of prostatic cancer have been advanced as a response to this question, and while some authors claim that the histology of prostatic disease correlates more or less closely with prognosis, there are others who found a poor correlation, or who maintain that no such correlation exists.[1-8]

Most criteria have been based on methods for assessment of the structure and arrangement of the malignant glands, or on the degree of anaplasia of the tumor cells.[4-9] Unfortunately, however, none of these criteria have been applied on a universal basis either because they have been deemed subjective, or because it is the common tendency of many prostatic cancers to show varying degrees of differentiation and structure within a single section, and frequently within a single microscopic field.

Finally, the question has been raised as to whether the differentiation of this tumor can be realistically assessed by examination of the limited amount of material provided by a needle biopsy or transurethral resection (TUR).

Recognizing these factors, several attempts have been made recently to propose a method of grading that hopefully, will be universally accepted. The most significant of them, because of departure from conventional methods of grading in tumors of other organs, is that of Gleason which is based on recognition of at least two predominant patterns within the tumor.[2] These he called primary and secondary patterns, the latter generally representing the less differentiated portion of the neoplasm. He recognizes five basic patterns, roughly corresponding to (1) very well differentiated, (2) well differentiated, (3) moderately differentiated, (4) poorly differentiated, and (5) very poorly differentiated types. Distinction of each of these types is generally based on size, configuration and presence of glands, and on their relationship to the stroma. Although his correlation between patterns and survivals in the Veterans Administration Study was fairly accurate, he improved the accuracy of his system by the addition of stage numbers to grade numbers, resulting in a sum that he called "categories." His results indicate five-year survivals of approximately 75% for low sum categories 3 to 7, 60% for categories 8 to 9, 25% for categories 10 to 12, and no survivals for high-grade and patients in categories 13 to 14. Furthermore the recognition of two different patterns in each tumor identified a group with no cancer deaths—the pure pattern one case—and at the same time his system demonstrated that, at least for cancer of the prostate, the biologic malignancy of the lesion correlated better with "average" histologic pattern rather than with its "best" or "worst" patterns.

Limitations to the above system include (a) the need of histologic expertise in the field of prostate pathology for an accurate application, and some familiarity with the system, especially for proper classification of patterns 3, 4 and 5; (b) resistance to its application by clinicians because of lack of familiarity with the terms; (c) objections to mixing grading and staging within the same system, thus obscuring the separate influence of each on prognosis; and (d) small needle biopsies which may easily miss at least one pattern, thus placing the lesion in a false, low category.

Mostofi, emphasizing conceptual differences between anaplasia and differentiation, has proposed a system of classification of prostatic cancer in which he includes a composite evaluation of glands, individual tumor cells, and stroma.[10] The degree of anaplasia is evaluated by a scaled assessment of nuclear characteristics of the tumor cells such as nuclear size, hyperchromatism, pleomorphism, presence and characteristics of nucleoli, and mitotic activity. His concept of differentiation refers to recording of the tendency of the tumor to form glands and to their characteristics as compared to normal prostatic glands. This system seems to solve the problem of classifying minimally anaplastic tumors that grow in solid sheets with no gland formation, and more cytologically anaplastic lesions forming well developed glands.

In a preliminary report Harada et al. compared Gleason's classification of the same cases to which they applied his classification criteria.[11] They learned, not surprisingly, that there was significant reproducibility among themselves on repeat readings using Gleason's system, although there was lesser correlation between their readings and Gleason's readings of the same slides. They also applied two of the criteria from the Mostofi system, ie, nuclear anaplasia and glandular differentiation, and their data suggested prognostic usefulness of this simplified approach.

There is a conspicuous absence of similar comparative analytical approaches between various grading schemata. Such data would seem to be desirable.

Although Mostofi and Price outlined their system in 1973, their final data and correlation to survivals have not been published to this date.[12] In their recent study of the characteristics of prostatic carcinoma in pelvic lymph nodes, Saltzstein and McLaughlin used the above system for their assessment of prostatic disease and reported the presence of differentiated tumor in 20% of pelvic lymph node metastases, whereas the incidence of undifferentiated disease was 56%.[13] Following the same system and using anaplasia as the only parameter, in the same group of cases they reported 22% Grade I, 36% Grade II, and 60% Grade III in the primary tumor, thus demonstrating a satisfactory correlation between grade and metastatic spread in a prospective study.

Kempson and Levine, while considering the Mostofi and Price system as "the most comprehensive and objective yet suggested," found it very complex on account of its combination of several factors including a separate evaluation of three elements: cells, glands, and stroma.[14] Devising their own system, they set up four grades, each of them combining the degree of gland formation with the degree of cellular anaplasia on a scale of increasing malignancy. Their attempt to simplify Mostofi's method seems to fail when they introduce a quantitation in approximate percentages of differentiating or anaplastic features for the definition of each grade, thereby jeopardizing its reproducibility.

Analyzing a series of 266 patients, they found no patient deaths in their category I, but among 35 patients in their worst category (Grade IV), they found 7 (20%) who were alive and free of tumor with follow-up up to five years.

McNeal used a new approach for the study of the anatomy of the prostate gland, and in an effort to correlate prostatic carcinoma with the structural site of origin, concluded that most adenocarcinomas fall into one of three types: medullary-alveolar, tubular-scirrhous, and mixed.[15,16]

In an attempt to use McNeal's method of classification, Epstein and

Fatti studied 146 cases of prostatic cancer, correlating them with five-year survivals.[17] Their study, however, demonstrated significant survival differences correlating with the presence or absence of well defined cytoplasmic borders among tumor cells. This feature also correlated to some extent with the degree of differentiation, since most of the medulloalveolar types of lesions showed distinct cytoplasmic borders, whereas the tubular-scirrhous only showed the same feature sparingly. Tumors with distinct cytoplasmic borders demonstrated a five-year survival of 44% compared to 21% for the second group. A third group of lesions which demonstrated a mixed pattern of distinct and indistinct combinations of cytoplasmic features showed an intermediate survival of 46%.

This system has the advantage of high reproducibility, but with a limited stratification into only three categories, it fails to identify prospectively the extreme categories one and four, clearly identified by the systems of Gleason and Mostofi as lesions with excellent and poor prognosis respectively.

An additional factor noted in the above paper was the correlation between prognosis and the presence or absence of lymphocytic infiltration. Although interesting, the significance of these almost ubiquitous cells is unclear.

The question has been raised whether the degree of differentiation of a tumor is one of its intrinsic characteristics or whether it worsens as part of continued growth. In keeping with the latter postulate, McNeal demonstrated that the greater the size of the microscopic lesion, the greater the tendency to be poorly differentiated.[16] Scott et al. also showed that the proportion of poorly differentiated lesions increases with the tumor size.[18] Conversely, the common finding of good differentiation among small lesions can represent either the early appearance of a progressively deteriorating neoplasm or simply a process of natural selection as postulated by others.[19]

Gaeta, in his analysis (unpublished) of 377 cases of Stage D prostatic cancer from the files of the National Prostatic Cancer Project, found approximately 60% incidence of poorly differentiated lesions. Using the same grading criteria he found an incidence of 36% for the poorly differentiated group in a series of 233 unselected cases of prostatic cancer of all stages. The presence of such a significant number of high-grade lesions in the first group seems to indicate that at least a substantial number of poorly differentiated or anaplastic lesions demonstrate a high-grade histology from the onset. The fact that incidental carcinomas (Stage A) can give evidence of progressive disease when observed in long follow-up also corroborates the same principle.[7]

Despite the presence of these varied schemata for histologic grading of carcinoma of the prostate, it is our distinct impression that in standard practice the diagnosis of "adenocarcinoma of the prostate" is frequently made without any reference to a histologic grade; the only evidence of an attempted grade is often only an adjective of "well," "moderately," or "poorly" differentiated. The multiplicity of approaches to histologic grading and the lack of general acceptance is probably symptomatic of our lack of understanding of basic tumor biology of prostatic cancer, including its origins and its precursors.

There is strong evidence to indicate that prostatic adenocarcinoma is frequently multicentric in origin, although it is not always easy to determine whether a tumor is in a single focus or in multiple foci even in radical prostatectomy specimens.[6] The presence of multifocal neoplastic disease can also be explained on the basis of intraprostate extension or metastases. Recent scanning-microscopy studies of prostatic cancer indicate that intraglandular extension is a pathway for neoplastic spread within the glands, at least in some of the better differentiated types.[20] Multicentricity, however, could possibly explain the presence of several patterns within the same prostatic lesion, following simultaneous neoplastic transformation of multiple clones of cells which have not necessarily reached the same level of differentiation.

Most epithelial tumors in other organs seem to go through an in situ stage for a significant period of time before the tumor cells invade into underlying tissues or into the surrounding stroma. Although not clinically detectable, we should assume that prostatic cancer also exhibits a similar sequence of events. Mostofi refuses to accept "carcinoma in situ" as a morphologic entity, but alerts our attention to the finding of "atypical hyperplasia" because it can be easily mistaken for carcinoma.[12] Whether atypical hyperplasia represents a transition from pure hyperplasia into carcinoma in situ and how it differs from noninvasive cancer remains obscure. Tannenbaum has suggested criteria for their histological differentiation.[9,21] He apparently diagnoses carcinoma in situ by identifying the presence of one or multiple foci of prostatic glands with a back-to-back arrangement and with small residual stroma interposed between the abnormal glands. Despite the lack of stromal invasion, the epithelial cells show faintly acidophilic cytoplasm and abnormal nuclei, the latter remaining as the best single criterion for their neoplastic identification. The exact incidence of this lesion is largely unknown because when overlooked, the possibility of complete removal in a TUR is quite high. On the other hand, when the lesion is recognized by the pathologist it is frequently diagnosed as "carcinoma" without further specification. The lack of generally accepted criteria for such terms as "carcinoma in situ" and "atypical hyperplasia" probably contributes to the wide divergence in frequency of incidental prostatic cancer in TUR specimens.[5]

Finally, an ideal grading system should make a further attempt to find morphologic parameters that may identify prostatic cancers which are sensitive to hormonal therapy. It would be tempting to concoct a grading system which would bring to bear the full armamentarium of modern technology, including histochemical and immunochemical studies, precise morphometric determinations, scanning and transmission electron microscopy, cell and organ cultures, etc. The search for the ideal system, however, should be tempered by the realization that in order to have wide acceptance, any grading system must be based on a readily available data base, ie, derived from routinely stained sections by light microscopy. A contribution of Gleason's system, ie, recognizing the presence of at least two patterns in a significant number of prostatic lesions, has not yet been followed by a corresponding characterization of differing functional profiles. The character and extent of acid phosphatase secretion and its exact correlation with the different patterns of prostate cancer as well as to their variations of clinical response, have not been defined.

In summary, there is a need for a concerted effort to formulate a system of prostatic cancer grading before we can make a final evaluation of prevalent therapeutic attitudes by comparison of different treatment groups. Some of the previously outlined systems have proven to be effective, but their validity has been somewhat limited by lack of reproducibility when used in general practice. Further efforts are needed to arrive at a method with sufficient flexibility to separate significant groups of prostatic cancer patients with different prognoses and therapeutic responses, regardless of the stages of their disease. The possibility of including objective histochemical features that could enhance its predictive value should be also considered.

REFERENCES

1. Bailar, J. C., Mellinger, G. T. and Gleason, D. F. Survival rates of patients with prostatic cancer, tumor stage and differentiation. Preliminary report. *Cancer Chemother Rep.* 50:129-36, 1966.

2. Gleason, D. F. Histologic grading and clinical staging of prostatic carcinoma. Edited by M. Tannenbaum, in *Urologic Pathology: The Prostate.* Lea and Febiger, 1977, pp 171-98.

3. Hanash, K. A., Utz, D. C., Cook, E. N. et al. Carcinoma of the prostate, a 15 year follow-up. *J Urol.* 107:450-3, 1972.

4. Mobley, T. L. and Frank, I. N. Influence of tumor grade on survival and on serum acid phosphatase levels in metastatic carcinoma of the prostate. *J Urol.* 99:321-3, 1968.

5. V. A. Cooperative Urological Research Group. Factors in the prognosis of carcinoma of the prostate—a cooperative study. *J Urol.* 100:59-65, 1968.

6. Byar, D. P., Mostofi, F. K. and the V. A. Cooperative Urological Research Group. Carcinoma of the prostate—prognostic evaluation of certain pathogenic features in 208 radical prostatectomies. *Cancer.* 30:5-13, 1972.

7. Schoones, R., Palma, L. D., Gaeta, J. F. et al. Prostatic carcinoma treated at categorical center. *NY State J Med.* 72:1021-7, 1972.

8. Franks, L. M., Fergusson, J. D. and Murraghan, G. F. An assessment of factors influencing survival in prostatic cancer. The absence of reliable prognostic features. *Br J Cancer.* 12:321-6, 1958.

9. Tannenbaum, M. Diagnostic criteria for histopathologic evaluation of prostatic tissue sections. *Urology.* 5:407-8, 1975.

10. Mostofi, F. K. Carcinoma of the Prostate. Edited by Eric Riches. In *Modern Trends in Urology.* London, Butterworths, 1970, pp 231-63.

11. Harada, M., Mostofi, F. K., Corle, D. K., et al. Preliminary studies of histologic prognosis in cancer of the prostate. *Cancer Treat Rep.* 61:223-5, 1977.

12. Mostofi, F. K. and Price, E. B. Malignant tumors of the prostate. In *Tumors of the Male Genital System, Atlas of Tumor Pathology,* Second Series, Fascicle 8, Washington, D.C.: Armed Forces Institute of Pathology, 1973, pp 218.

13. Saltzstein, S. L. and McLaughlin, A. P. Clinicopathological features of unsuspected regional lymph node metastasis in prostatic adenocarcinoma. *Cancer.* 40:1212-21, 1977.

14. Kempson, R. L. and Levine, G. The relationship of grade to prognosis in carcinoma of the prostate. *Front Rad Therap Oncol.* 9:267-73, 1974.

15. McNeal, J. E. Regional morphology and pathology of the prostate. *Am J Clin Path.* 49:347-57, 1968.

16. McNeal, J. E. Origin and development of carcinoma in the prostate. *Cancer.* 23:24-34, 1969.

17. Epstein, N. A. and Fatti, L. P. Prostatic carcinoma. Some morphological features affecting prognosis. *Cancer.* 37:2455-65, 1976.

18. Scott, R., Jr., Mutchnik, D. L., Laskowski, T. Z. et al. Carcinoma of the prostate in elderly men. Incidence, growth characteristics and clinical significance. *J Urol.* 101:602-7, 1969.

19. Whitmore, W. F. The natural history of prostatic cancer. *Cancer.* 32:1104-12, 1973.

20. Gaeta, J. F., Berger, J. E. and Gamarra, M. C. Scanning microscopy of prostatic cancer. *Cancer Treat Rep.* 61:227-53, 1977.

21. Tannenbaum, M. Atypical epithelial hyperplasia or carcinoma of the prostate gland. The surgical pathologist at an impasse? *Urology.* 4:758, 1974.

Steroid Receptors and Prostatic Cancer

5

James P. Karr and Avery A. Sandberg

An extensive literature exists on high-affinity, specific hormone binding to intracellular protein molecules called receptors. The interactions of these macromolecules with steroid hormones have been characterized to varying degrees in many target and nontarget tissues. The human prostate has not been an exception in this regard and in this chapter the role and possible significance of such receptors in both the normal and diseased (cancerous) gland will be examined. Since the biochemical nature and mechanism of action of receptors in the human prostate have not been documented, a number of gaps will be bridged with data from other species, particularly the rat. It is not our intent to review the very extensive literature on steroid receptors, but only to discuss and evaluate (1) those parameters related to intracellular steroid receptors that are of significance and cogency to the possible role they may play in cancer of the prostate and, (2) the utilization of receptor measurements in the therapy of this condition in a manner, for example, similar to the approaches being utilized in cancer of the breast. For those readers who wish to consider in detail the biochemistry of hormone receptors and their function in cell biology, major reviews are listed as general references at the end of this chapter.

STEROID HORMONE RECEPTORS

The use of estrogenic therapy,[1] particularly of diethylstilbestrol (DES), in the treatment of prostatic cancer was recognized with the awarding of a Nobel Prize to Professor Huggins in 1966.[2] As significant contributions to the understanding of the endocrine and molecular mechanisms which regulate the prostate, Huggins' accomplishments in retrospect represent early milestones linking up with current interest in steroid receptors as potential aids in diagnosis and therapeutic management of prostatic disease. Synthesis of radioactive hexestrol and estradiol of sufficient specific activity and the demonstration of selective retention

The work emanating from our laboratory alluded to in this chapter has been supported in part by grants CA-20459 and CA-15436 from the National Cancer Institute (National Prostatic Cancer Project).

of estrogens by target tissues gave investigators the technological breakthrough needed to probe hormonal mechanisms on a molecular basis within the cellular cytoplasmic and nuclear compartments.[3-6] The research which followed saw widespread application of isotopically labeled hormones and general acceptance of a common mechanism involving specific receptor proteins by which steroid hormones interact with target cells to elicit a biologic response. However, before discussing this mechanism and some of its vagaries, a description of receptor terminology and parameters may be of value. As the term will be used in this chapter, a receptor is a steroid-binding protein which, in addition to being localized in target cells, must satisfy several criteria.

Specificity

Even though steroids circulating in the plasma can be isolated from nearly all the tissues in the body (Figure 1), specific biologic responses to each steroid are initiated only in target tissues and organs. The process of entry into target cells is believed to be primarily one of simple diffusion of free steroids although the possibility that the process is facilitated by a cell surface carrier mechanism involving a specific membrane protein has yet to be resolved.[7-15] Once inside the cell, only those steroids with a stereochemical configuration which complements the binding sites of the receptor particular to the target cell will be bound to form a steroid-receptor complex. Studies on androgen analogs and the structural requirements for steroid-receptor binding suggest that the steroid is almost totally enveloped by the receptor and it is this association that accounts for the specificity of a receptor.[16-17] The specificity of androgen receptors in prostatic tissue is demonstrated by the fact that only androgenic compounds displace 5α-dihydrotestosterone (DHT) from binding sites; other steroid classes, such as aldosterone and corticosterone, are not competitive for these sites.[18] It should be noted, however, that in addition to binding specifically to receptor proteins, steroids also bind to various nonspecific binding sites in target cell preparations. Since the number of specific binding sites is low in comparison to the very large nonspecific steroid binding capacity encountered in most systems, it is essential that these two types of binding be distinguished to ensure accurate assessment of receptor concentrations and steroid-receptor interactions. This can be accomplished by measurement of binding affinities.

High Affinity

The physiologic concentrations of steroid hormones in plasma and tissues are generally low (10^{-10} to 10^{-8} molar) and therefore the affinity or strength with which a receptor specifically binds a steroid must be high. High- and low-affinity binding sites can be distinguished by the fact that the latter do not become saturated even in the presence of high steroid concentrations (10^{-5} to 10^{-4} molar). Thus the binding of a radioactive steroid in the presence and absence of a 100-fold excess of unlabeled competitor will result in a measurable displacement of labeled steroid from the high-affinity (low-capacity) sites, but not from the low-affinity (high-capacity) binders. Steroid-binding data obtained in this fashion are usually evaluated by Scatchard plot analysis in which specifically bound-steroid/free-steroid is plotted against specifically-bound steroid; such data can also be analyzed with a modification of the method of Lineweaver and Burk known as the double reciprocal plot in which the reciprocal of the number of occupied receptor sites (bound) is plotted against the reciprocal of the concentration of unbound (free) steroid.[19,20] Plotting of binding data by either method will yield the physical constants which express the affinity of a receptor for its specific ligand, ie, K_a, the association constant, or its reciprocal, K_d, the dissociation constant. Examples of these calculations based on the binding of estradiol-17β (E_2) in the baboon prostate will be given in a later section dealing with estrogen receptors. A perusal of the literature will show that the

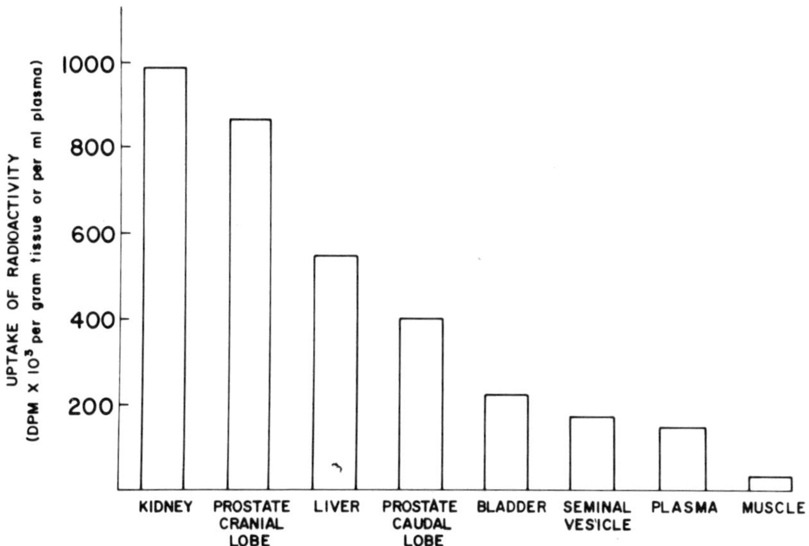

Figure 1. Distribution of radioactivity in various tissues and organs following in vivo infusion of [^{3}H]-E_2 into hypogastric arteries of a male baboon. Except for organs that metabolize and/or excrete E_2, highest levels of radioactivity were present in caudal and cranial lobes of the prostate.

terms "high affinity" and "low affinity" are frequently used synonymously with specific and nonspecific binding since the relationship has been proven to be valid for most steroid-receptor interactions.

Saturability

An extension of the concept that responses of target tissues to steroids are limited is the finding that steroid hormone receptors in target cells are finite in number. This does not mean that the number of specific binding sites in a cell cannot vary, but it does indicate that this number is limited. Therefore, receptor evidence frequently includes the demonstration that the binding sites can be saturated with low concentrations (10^{-9}M) of a specific ligand.

Translocation

Once a steroid binds to its receptor in the cytoplasm, the resulting complex undergoes a temperature dependent modification of its physicochemical properties which, in the case of the cytosol DHT-receptor complex, is noted by a pronounced shift in sedimentation coefficient from 8S to 4.2S.[21] This process is called activation and is associated with the transfer of the steroid receptor complex at physiologic temperatures to the nucleus, where it binds to a restricted number of specific acceptor sites associated with the basic, nonhistone protein components of chromatin.[22]

Translocation can be monitored by the temporal dissociation in labeling of cytosol and nuclear receptors. Using the rat ventral prostate, Rennie and Bruchovsky demonstrated a reciprocal relationship of cytoplasmic and nuclear receptor concentrations, ie, when rats were injected with radioactive DHT, the label appeared in the cytosol before it was detected in the nuclei, but as the nuclear receptor concentration increased there was a concomitant decrease in receptor-bound steroid in the cytoplasm.[23,24] Autoradiographic localization of labeled steroids has also provided evidence for the temperature-dependent translocation of cytoplasmic receptors to prostatic nuclei.[25] Binding of the steroid-receptor complex in the nucleus initiates transcriptional and subsequently cytoplasmic translational activities as measured by increased RNA synthesis in selected parts of the genome and increased protein synthesis, but the understanding of these events as well as of the fate of the nuclear receptor in terms of retention, dissociation, or possible return to the cytoplasm is far from complete.[26]

Other Criteria

The proteinaceous nature of receptors is evidenced by destruction of binding activity with proteolytic enzymes (pronase) and the inability of ribonuclease and deoxyribonuclease to produce any degradative effects. Receptors are also heat labile and at temperatures of 40° C and above their binding capacities are destroyed.

In addition to characterizing a specific steroid receptor satisfactorily according to the above criteria, care must be exercised to ensure that receptor preparations have not been contaminated with plasma containing transcortin or testosterone-estradiol binding globulin (TeBG). These plasma proteins are specific high-affinity steroid binders, and failure to account for their presence in tissues can result in grossly exaggerated assessment of receptor concentrations. Transcortin can be distinguished, however, from glucocorticoid receptors by the fact that it does not bind dexamethasone and from progesterone receptors by virtue of its insignificant binding with the synthetic progestin R5020.[27-29] Similarly, TeBG, which has a high affinity ($K_d = 10^{-10}$ to 10^{-8}M) for DHT, testosterone (T) and E_2, can be distinguished from estrogen and androgen receptors by its inability to bind the synthetic estrogen DES.[29-31]

PROSTATIC ANDROGEN RECEPTORS

Rat Prostate

The study of androgen receptors in the rat ventral prostate (VP) has been extensive and exceeds the amount of research devoted to any other prostatic receptor. A comprehensive review of these studies has been published and therefore only those features essential to an appreciation of the human prostate will be presented here.[32]

The direct control by testicular hormones over prostatic growth and function is well documented, as is evidenced by rapid regression of the normal rat prostate following castration.[33-35] Androgen withdrawal results in the elimination of a large number of prostatic cells, a few of which persist and regenerate if androgen is restored.[36] These cells of the atrophied prostate require, in the same manner as do cells in the normal prostate, an initial interaction of androgen with a specific cytoplasmic receptor before the hormonal-biologic effects (restoration) are registered. Before this occurs, however, T is rapidly reduced upon entering the prostate by the enzyme Δ^4-3-ketosteroid-5α-reductase (5α-reductase) to 5α-androstan-17β-ol-3-one (DHT).[37] In fact, the biologic effects of androgens on the prostate are not only closely related to their conversion to

DHT, but it is this metabolite which binds to the cytoplasmic receptor and is the major steroid found in prostatic nuclei following administration of T to intact rats.[38-40] DHT has also been shown to play an important role in the retention of the androgen receptor by prostatic nuclei in vivo. This retention process in cell-free systems is inhibited by the potent antiandrogen, cyproterone acetate (CA).[41] This, of course, is why CA could be of significant clinical importance, since it is the binding of the DHT-receptor complex to chromatin which triggers the nuclear activities that orchestrate the biologic responses of prostatic cells to androgen. Since there is some evidence that castration may cause a discharge of nuclear receptor into the cytoplasm, it has been further suggested that prolonged retention of receptor-steroid complex in the nucleus may prevent prostatic regression.[42]

Estimates of the number of receptor sites for DHT in the rat VP vary considerably and range from 57 fmoles/mg cytosol protein to 171 fmoles.[43,44] Expressed in different units, receptor concentrations have been reported as 8,000 nuclear receptor molecules per resting cell and 11,500 binding sites per cell, over 80% of which were in the nucleus.[42,45] The varying conditions under which receptor measurements have been made may account for some of the differences reported in the literature. For example, aging is associated with a progressive reduction in detectable androgen receptor content in the VP.[46] Castration also produces variable effects, as noted by the apparent decrease in receptor concentration three to four days following orchiectomy.[47-50] However, within 8 to 10 days after castration, the receptor concentration in the VP exceeds that of intact animals and 24-hour castrates.[49,50] These castration effects on androgen receptor concentrations are not always observed; Bruchovsky and Craven reported that VP androgen receptors were virtually undetectable in the seven-day castrate.[51]

The cytosol DHT-receptor complex of the VP sediments as a 7-12S unit and is transformed to a 3-5S unit by heating at 20° to 30°C; the smaller form is similar to that retained by the cell nuclei.[52] The high-affinity nuclear acceptor sites reside in the basic DNA-associated nonhistone fraction of chromatin and are highly specific for complexes of DHT and its receptor.[53,54] Measurements of the DHT-receptor complex affinity constants fall within the expected range, ie, $K_d = 1\text{–}2 \times 10^{-9}$M and $K_a = 1 \times 10^9$ liters/mole.[43,45] It will become apparent when we consider the human prostate that the ease with which these data were obtained was greatly facilitated by the fact that TeBG is not a component of rat serum.

Human Prostate

In many respects the mechanism of androgen action in the rat and human prostate are similar, ie, T, the principle testicular androgen, is first converted by the enzyme 5α-reductase to DHT, the androgen primarily responsible for stimulating the prostate. Transfer of cytosol DHT-receptor complexes to chromatin binding sites in hypertrophied human prostates (benign prostatic hypertrophy BPH) has been shown to be associated with a shift in the sedimentation coefficient (Figure 2) and an increase in RNA polymerase activity and transcription.[55] DHT is found in high concentrations in the prostate, particularly in BPH where it accumulates mainly in the periurethral tissue rather than in the peripheral stroma.[56] In spite of the fact that the human prostate concentrates and retains large amounts of DHT and that binding of this hormone to macromolecules is readily demonstrated, consistent identification of androgen receptors in human prostatic tissue has been difficult.[57] The main sources of aggravation have been (1) the similarity with which androgens specifically bind to intracellular receptors and TeBG, and (2) the high endogenous (20nM) DHT in the human prostate which results in its occupation of most receptor sites.[58-61]

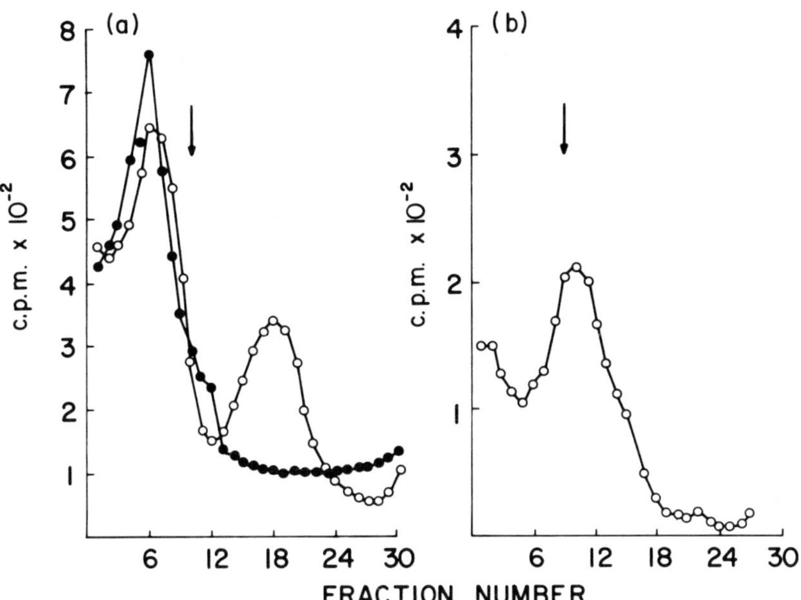

Figure 2 a. Analysis of cytoplasmic binding of [^{3}H]-DHT by sucrose density gradient centrifugation. Direction of centrifugation was from left to right. Sedimentation marker (arrows) was bovine serum albumin ($S_{20,w}$4.6S). Cytosol was labeled with [^{3}H]-DHT (4nM) in absence (●) and presence (○) of 400nM-unlabeled DHT. The higher molecular weight binding protein (7.5 to 8.5S) was specific for DHT and of low capacity, as indicated by displacement of radioactivity in this zone by 100-fold excess of unlabeled DHT. The 3-4S component was nonspecific and of high capacity, as shown by inability of 100-fold excess DHT to decrease the radioactivity in this region.

Figure 2 b. Sucrose density gradient analysis of retention of [^{3}H]-DHT by extracts of BPH nuclei previously incubated with [^{3}H]-labeled cytosol from BPH yielded a definite peak of protein-bound radioactivity with sedimentation coefficient of 4-5S.[81]

The first problem is readily identified by virtue of the fact that the two steroid-binding components have distinct profiles as shown by sucrose density gradient centrifugation of prostatic cytosol incubated with [^{3}H]-DHT (Figure 2); the sedimentation coefficient of TeBG is approximately 4S whereas that of the DHT-receptor complex ranges from 8-10S.[62-66] The plasma origin of significant concentrations of bound DHT in cytosol from BPH is revealed by the data of Jung-Testas et al. who calculated that there are 5,000 DHT-receptor sites/cell vs 8,000 DHT-TeBG sites/cell.[65] Steins et al., who found no physicochemical differences in androgen-binding properties of plasma and prostate cytosols of 13 patients with BPH, reported that cytosols had a higher DHT-binding than could be related to plasma contamination and raised the question of whether the augmented prostatic DHT binding they measured was related to a cellular increase of TeBG.[67] The complex nature of the human prostatic androgen receptor may be part of the reason why numerous procedures have been used to characterize it.[61,68] As a result, the variability of data is a reflection both of different methodologies and actual differences in the prostatic specimens analyzed.

Nijs et al. using agar gel electrophoresis, detected androgen receptors in two samples of prostatic cancer (one primary and one metastatic) and in none of 23 specimens of BPH analyzed following retropubic prostatectomy.[69] In a later study Hawkins et al. using both agar gel electrophoresis and sucrose density gradient centrifugation, described a high affinity (charcoal stable) 8S form of [^{3}H]-DHT binding in a cervical lymph node containing metastatic prostatic tissue; in contrast to cancer containing tissue ($N=3$), no saturable [^{3}H]-DHT binding was detected in any of the BPH samples ($N=25$) analyzed.[64] On the other hand, Geller et al. identified androgen receptors in 80% (14 of 17 patients) of BPH samples analyzed by gel filtration.[70] However, prior treatment of patients can affect receptor measurements, as shown by later work of Geller et al. who detected no [^{3}H]-DHT-receptor complexes in four out of six patients treated with megestrol acetate.[71] Other factors including possible destruction of receptors by electroresection of prostatic specimens[72] and prostate samples from noncastrated men in which available receptor sites are limited,[66] may also preclude demonstration of androgen receptors. Recently Mobbs et al. reported that TeBG contamination of prostatic cytosol can be partly resolved with the use of CA as a means of distinguishing between DHT binding to the androgen receptor and serum components.[73] Moreover these investigators demonstrated that the total high-affinity, CA-inhibitable prostate receptor binding of DHT was correlated with the endocrine status of the patient.

Definition of the androgen receptor in terms of its high-affinity binding characteristics and its concentrations in the human prostate is given in Table 1. Since a number of factors can contribute to variations in reported receptor concentrations it is important to distinguish whether available or total number of receptor sites have been measured. The number of available sites will be affected by the endocrine status of the patient. For example, Mobbs et al. found that in untreated patients the number of free androgen-receptor sites was on the average 0.5 fmole/mg tissue.[77] This value represented only 5.8% of the total [^{3}H]-DHT high-affinity sites and reflected the occupation of available sites by endogenous androgens. On the other hand, orchiectomized and/or estrogen-treated cancer patients have lower levels of circulating testosterone and thus the free receptor sites measured in these patients ranged from 0.5 to 2.5 fmole/mg tissue, a value representing a higher proportion of the total number of receptors.

Table 1
Concentrations and Dissociation Constants of Androgen Receptors in Human Prostate Cytosols

Receptor Concentration[1]		Dissociation Constant
45.8 ± 4.7	fmol/mg protein[2]	$0.9 \pm 0.2 \times 10^{-9}$M
9 – 26	fmol/mg protein[3]	$0.3 - 1.8 \times 10^{-9}$M
50	fmol/mg protein[4]	
27	fmol/mg protein[5]	
120	fmol/mg protein[6,10]	
25 – 50	fmol/gm tissue[4,11]	
100 – 700	fmol/gm tissue[8,12]	$1 - 5 \times 10^{-9}$M
2.6	pmol/gm tissue[9,10]	

1. Number of high-affinity binding sites
2. Menon et al. 1978
3. Snochowski et al. 1977
4. Jung-Testas et al. 1976
5. Wagner et al. 1975
6. Bonne & Raynaud 1976[75]
7. Menon et al. 1977a
8. Menon et al. 1977b
9. Rosen et al. 1975
10. Total binding sites
11. Measured by sucrose density gradient centrifugation. Nuclear extract receptor concentrations were 100-150 fmol/gm tissue
12. Measured by protamine sulfate precipitation. Nuclear extract receptor concentrations were 10-60 fmol/gm tissue

Specificity of the androgen receptor has been demonstrated by competitive steroid binding studies, the results of which are not in total accord. Shimazaki et al. found that the androgen receptor in normal and BPH tissues had similar affinities (K_a) and that T, CA, and E_2 competed with [^{3}H]-DHT for receptor sites.[78] Fang and Hsu also reported that the 9.5S cytosol receptor had a high affinity for DHT, but that this receptor did not bind T, E_2, progesterone, or cortisol at concentrations up to 10^{-7}M.[63] Other studies have shown that estrogens inhibit in vitro binding of [^{3}H]-DHT to the cytosol receptor, and that E_2 or CA, but not cortisol, inhibited nuclear binding.[79-80] The contrasting report of Mainwaring and Milroy that nuclear binding of [^{3}H]-DHT (5nM) in vitro was not diminished significantly by E_2 (0.5μM) (a 17% decrease was determined) may therefore be a matter more of degree rather than absolute difference.[58] The important point that emerges is that any degree of E_2 inhibition of androgen binding may be clinically significant with regard to estrogen treatment of human prostatic cancer.

The suggestion that androgen receptors in all organs and species are similar has been offered by several groups. Davies and Griffiths demonstrated that cytosol preparations from androgen-dependent tissues (human prostate) were able (1) to transfer protein-bound [^{3}H]-DHT to nuclei of other androgen-dependent tissues (rat prostate) and, (2) to stimulate RNA polymerase activity of the rat prostatic nuclei.[81] However, this transfer of [^{3}H]-DHT could not be made to androgen-independent tissue. It was concluded therefore that the DHT-receptor complex and its activities are not species-specific. Recently Attramadal et al. reported no difference in physicochemical properties of androgen receptors measured in non-neoplastic and neoplastic tissue, but showed a drastic reduction of DHT formation in tissue from prostatic cancer as compared to normal and hyperplastic prostatic tissue.[82] They concluded that differences in steroid binding by androgen receptors in different organs are not due to differences in steroid specificity of receptors but rather to specific differences in tissue metabolism (levels of 5α-reductase activity, for example). The role of androgen receptors in hormone-dependent and -independent prostatic tissues certainly needs further clarification, and the task should be facilitated by the apparent similarity of these receptor molecules in different organs and species.

PROSTATIC ESTROGEN RECEPTORS

Human Prostate

Even though treatment of prostatic cancer with estrogens has been practiced for over three decades, our understanding of the mechanism(s) through which estrogens effectively lead to regression of certain prostatic tumors is still not complete. It has generally been assumed that the effects of estrogens are mediated indirectly via the hypothalamic-hypophyseal-gonadal axis, though some direct effects have been reported.[83] In 1973 Sinha et al., using autoradiographic techniques, demonstrated both cytoplasmic and nuclear binding of [^{3}H]-E_2 in five patients with prostatic cancer.[84] Their discovery that the tritium was preferentially incorporated into basal and invasive cells and that little isotope was localized in the differentiated cells of carcinomatous acini, could be related to the varying degrees with which hormonal therapy affects prostatic cancer. In the same year, E_2 receptors were identified in 3 of 15 prostatic adenomas; 13 of these specimens also had specific DHT binding sites.[85] The simultaneous presence of both androgen and estrogen receptors in the human prostate has since been confirmed by several other groups.[74,86,87] Unfortunately, no consistent pattern has emerged to date regarding the occurrence of estrogen receptors in the normal and diseased gland. Thus, in a preliminary report, the estrogen receptor concentration (M/mg tissue protein) in BPH was found to be twice as high (0.29×10^{-13}) as that in normal tissue (0.8×10^{-13}).[74] In contrast, however, Hawkins et al. found the receptor in only 4 of 23 BPH specimens taken at autopsy.[86] In another specimen from a patient with both chronic prostatitis and BPH (no cancer cells were detected), no estrogen receptors were identified, whereas the presence of DHT receptors was demonstrated.[87]

Evidence that prostatic androgen and estrogen receptors are indeed separate identities is seen in sucrose density gradient analyses of labeled cytosols. In both BPH and cancer the sedimentation coefficient of the estrogen receptor is approximately 4S vs the 8-10S profile registered by the androgen receptor complex.[86,87] Furthermore, the estrogen receptor in BPH binds natural estrogens with high affinity ($K_d = 1.73 \times 10^{-9}$M), and its low number of specific binding sites (12×10^{-15}M/mg cytosol protein) are saturable.[86,88,89] Whether or not the receptor has similar properties in cancerous tissue is not known and, therefore, it would be quite significant to establish this in future studies.

Baboon Prostate

The effects of estrogens are different in the anterior and posterior regions of the human prostate and may be related to the propensity for BPH to originate in the periurethral region in contrast to the peripheral origin of cancer of the prostate.[90] Thus, characterization of estrogen receptors in the inner and outer zones of the gland would be of great interest. Since normal human tissues are not always ideal or available for experimentation, this question was examined by us in a series of studies on adult baboons, an animal thought to serve as a surrogate for the human.[91] In these studies prostatectomies were performed 40 hours after the animals had been bilaterally orchiectomized so as to increase the numbers of demonstrable receptor sites in the caudal and cranial lobes.

Determination of total, nonspecific and specific estradiol binding sites was accomplished by incubation of cytosol samples with decreasing concentrations (20×10^{-9}M to 0.2×10^{-9}M) of [^{3}H]-E_2 in the presence or absence of a 100-fold molar excess of the competitor, DES. Bound and free steroid were then separated by gel filtration on Sephadex G-25 columns. Sephadex G-25 filtration was selected over other commonly used methods for the assay of cytoplasmic receptors since it is known to give the highest measure of E_2 receptor concentrations.[92] The fractionated void volume containing the bound steroid was counted for radioactivity, and the bound steroid concentrations were normalized to a mg of cytosol protein basis.[93] The unlabeled DES, under the conditions described above, occupied the specific, high-affinity, low-capacity receptor sites, but did not compete appreciably with the high-capacity, low-affinity nonspecific binding sites. Thus, as shown in Figure 3, the quantity of specifically bound steroid in the caudal lobe is equal to the difference between the nonspecific (the amount of labeled E_2 measured in the presence of DES) and the total (nonspecific and specific binding sites combined) binding. This figure clearly shows a nonsaturable binding component as depicted by the linearity of the nonspecific binding and the saturability of the estrogen receptor. Linearization of these data with double reciprocal plots of bound and free steroid or Scatchard analysis (Figure 4) yields the specific binding constants (calculated from the

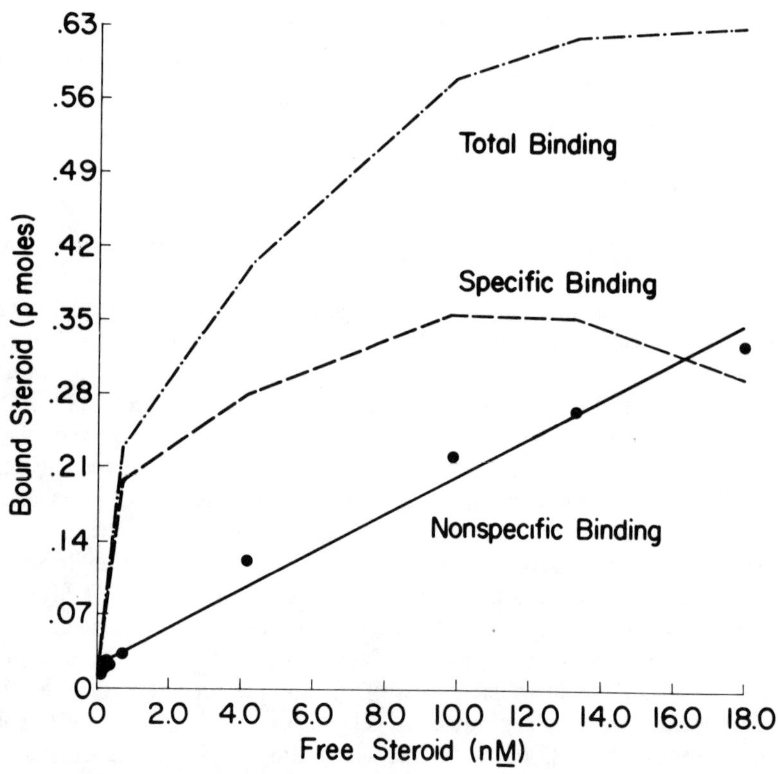

Figure 3. Titration of specific estrogen-binding sites in cytosol from caudal lobe of baboon prostate.

slopes) and the number of specific binding sites (calculated from the intercepts). In the case of the Scatchard plot, the dissociation constant (slope $= {}^{-1}/K_d$) for the caudal lobe was calculated to be 8.3×10^{-10}M, and the number of high affinity E_2 binding sites (N), as determined by the intercept with the abscissa, was 265 femtomoles per mg of cytosol protein. The K_a value calculated from the double reciprocal plot (slope$= {}^{1}/nK_a$) was 1.2×10^9M. Corresponding values for the cranial lobe were markedly different, ie, $K_d = 1.3 \times 10^{-10}$; $K_a = 7.7 \times 10^9$; N=168 femtomoles per mg of cytosol protein.

Hormone specificity of the estrogen cytosol receptor was demonstrated by measuring the binding of [^{3}H]-E_2 in the presence of various unlabeled steroids which were added in 1-, 10- and 100-fold molar excess to the labeled E_2-cytosol mixture (1×10^{-9}M in 0.5 ml cytosol). The results of the 2-hour incubations carried out at 30°C are given in Table 2

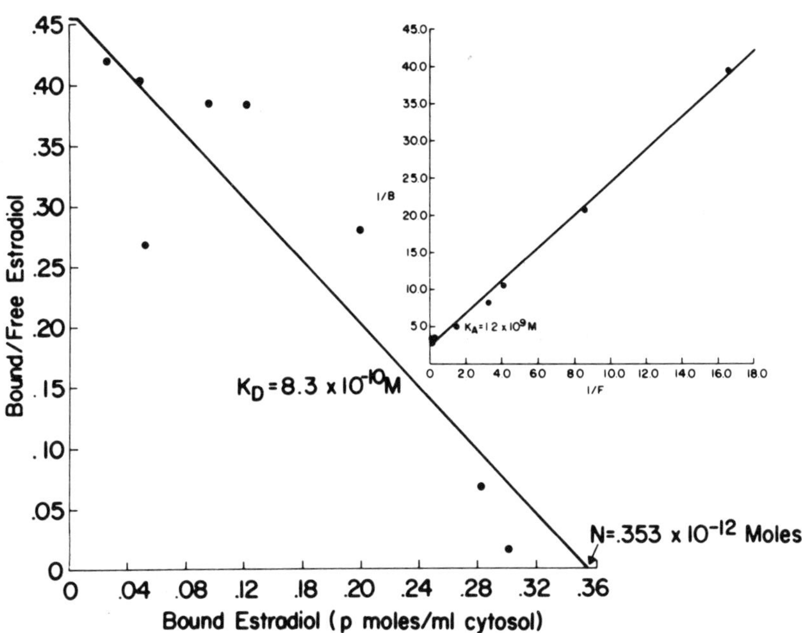

Figure 4. Scatchard plot of E_2-binding data from baboon caudal prostate cytosol showing ratio of bound/free-labeled E_2 as a function of amount of bound-labeled E_2. The straight line (r=0.90) indicates single class of binding sites (n=265 fmol per mg protein) and apparent K_d value of 8.3×10^{-10}M.
Inset: Double reciprocal plot (r=0.99) of binding data showing ratio of 1/bound-labeled E_2 as function of 1/free-labeled E_2 and association constant of $1.2 \times$ 10M. Best fit of line through points was determined by linear regressional analysis.

Table 2
In Vitro Competition of Various Unlabeled Steroids With [^{3}H]-estradiol for Cytosol Estrogen Receptors in the Caudal Lobe of the Baboon Prostate

Steroid added	Molar ratio to estradiol	Caudal ^{3}H-estradiol bound DPM/mg protein	% of control
^{3}H-estradiol–control	—	3036	100
17β-estradiol (E_2)	100	1705	56
	10	2295	76
	1	2465	81
Diethylstilbestrol (DES)	100	1678	55
	10	2443	80
	1	2624	86
Testosterone (T)	100	3168	100
	10	2934	97
	1	2957	97
Dihydrotestosterone (DHT)	100	3081	100
	10	3168	100
	1	3063	100

and clearly illustrate the specificity of the E_2 receptor in the baboon caudal prostate. Addition of unlabeled E_2 or DES reduced the amount of labeled complexes to 56% and 55%, whereas no competitive binding was demonstrated by the addition of T or DHT. Data similar to these were also obtained in parallel studies on cytosols from the cranial lobe.

Translocation of the estrogen receptor complex to the nucleus was demonstrated following 1) in vivo perfusion of the hypogastric arteries with radioactive estrogen, 2) in vitro incubation of prostatic tissue slices with labeled E_2, and 3) in vitro incubation of prostatic cytosol with labeled E_2 followed by recombination of the cytosol-E_2 mixture with pure nuclei prepared from the same prostate. The radioactivity associated with the labeled E_2 was transferred to the nucleus in two bound forms. One complex was readily extracted with 0.4M KC1 buffer and the other, whose binding to the nucleus was enhanced with elevated temperature (0°C vs 37°C), was nonextractable and probably represented the more tightly bound estrogen receptor complex which regulates gene activity.

Rat Prostate

The rat prostate is comprised of anatomically distinct lobes in which the estrogen receptor concentrations may differ. To date, however, only the VP has been examined for estrogen receptors. Specific E_2 binding has been demonstrated in the VP and investigators have carefully shown that this does not occur on the androgen receptor sites.[94-96] The receptor has a high affinity for E_2, ie, $K_a = 1-4 \times 10^9M$ and sediments at 3.5S as does the human cytoplasmic estrogen-receptor complex.[97,98] Unlike the 10-11S DHT-receptor complex in VP cytosol which disappears when the animals become one to two years of age, the 3.5S E_2 receptor is readily detected in retired (10- to 12-month old) breeders.[98,99] Whether or not significant changes occur in estrogen receptor concentrations of 2-year-old rats is not known. The simultaneous occurrence of distinct prostatic androgen and estrogen receptors has also been demonstrated in calves and pigs but it is doubtful that these species can serve as useful experimental models for receptor research in prostatic cancer.[100] This is not the case, however, for the guinea pig. In a recent study on these animals saturable DHT and E_2 binding in prostate cytosols was demonstrated.[101] From the authors' data the impression is gained that the androgenic receptors are primarily localized in the epithelial cells and the estrogenic receptors in the fibromuscular compartment; thus it is possible that these anatomic compartments may be under androgenic and estrogenic controls respectively.

OTHER HORMONES

Even though the bulk of receptor research on the human prostate has been focused primarily on androgens and estrogens, there have been several reports which suggest that other hormone receptors may also be found in the gland. The exact nature of this binding is not clear, but we mention these studies here in anticipation that future work will determine their possible significance in the normal and diseased prostate. In a preliminary report a corticosterone-binding protein has been found in prostatic tissues removed from patients with BPH, but not in human skin, skeletal muscle, breast, thyroid, uterus and liver.[102] This protein had a very high specificity for corticosterone but behaved differently from transcortin both electrophoretically and on sucrose gradients. The puzzling aspect of this hormone binder was that corticosterone, cortisol, and deoxycorticosterone were only weak competitors for [^{3}H]-corticosterone binding sites, whereas other steroids, notably cortisone, dexamethasone, and dihydrocortisone, did not displace any of the radiolabel. In another study a cortisol binding protein (transcortin-like) had the unique feature of being localized only in the stromal but not in the epithelial tissue of BPH, suggesting that this protein is preferentially localized in the interstitial fluid of the stromal compartment only.[103]

These studies are intriguing, but the presence of glucocorticoid receptors in the human prostate is an unsettled question. A slightly stronger case for glucocorticoid receptors in laboratory animals is developing. For example, Roth identified glucocorticoid receptors in the prostates of Sprague-Dawley rats.[104] In this study the number of specific high-affinity binding sites increased progressively between sexual maturity (2 to 3 months) and 13 months of age, after which they decreased through 25 months of age. In contrast, Ballard et al. were unable to demonstrate the presence of specific cytoplasmic receptors for glucocorticoids in the prostates of Buffalo rats (42 to 45 days old) and New Zealand White rabbits (10 to 11 weeks old).[105] Baxter and Forsham reported without mention of species, that prostatic glucocorticoid binding was very weak or undetectable, in various animals.[106]

Another puzzling receptor has been described by Asselin et al. who found that the potent synthetic-androgen methyltrienolone (R1881) was displaced from BPH-cytosol–binding sites more effectively by progesterone and R5020, a potent progestin, than by 19-nortestosterone.[107] Their data, which are similar to those of Menon et al. suggest the presence of a progesterone receptor or an atypical androgen receptor in human BPH.[76]

HORMONE RECEPTORS AND CANCER

The observation that specific steroid receptors, and particularly those which bind androgens, have intrinsic properties which are remarkably similar among various target organs and different species has been widely reported.[108-110] There may be a simple genetic explanation for this, as deduced from studies of the congenital defect in rats, mice, and men, known as the testicular feminization syndrome.[111-113] This condition is due to a single gene mutation which does not affect normal conversion of T to DHT, but does cause a deficiency of T and DHT receptors.[114,115] Thus it can be inferred that if the androgenic receptors are under the control of one gene, then all receptors for androgens are identical.[116]

The preceding descriptions of steroid interactions with target cells encompasses a general mechanistic scheme which is not unique to the prostate. In fact the intracellular role played by cytoplasmic and nuclear receptors in hormonally responsive tissues seems to have a basically universal nature which even extends to certain tumors. The ongoing search for a correlation of prostatic cancer with steroid receptors is an outgrowth of the presence of estrogen receptors in certain breast tumors and the response of the patients to hormone therapy.[117] Today steroid receptor assays are used clinically for screening estrogen-dependent tumors of the breast and glucocorticoid-sensitive acute human leukemia cells.[118,119] Unfortunately these receptor tests do not predict unequivocally whether a cancer condition will respond to exogenous or ablative endocrine therapy. Thus a beneficial response to endocrine therapy is achieved in only about 65% of the breast cancer patients who tested positively for estrogen receptors.[120] Conversely, about 5% of the E_2 receptor-negative breast carcinomas also respond to hormonal treatment. It follows, therefore, that the presence of cytoplasmic receptors alone is not necessarily an exclusive indicator of in vivo hormonal dependency.[121] This suggestion is supported not only by clinical evidence but by experimental evaluation of the Shionogi mouse mammary carcinoma as well.[122] In studies of nine variant lines of this tumor, two were androgen-dependent and seven autonomous. However, two of the autonomous lines contained androgen receptors, as did the two dependent lines.

Experimental tumors of the prostate have also been developed and have shed some insight on the variable nature of hormonal dependency in prostatic cancer. One such tumor is a spontaneous, transplantable prostatic adenocarcinoma in aged rats.[123,124] Administration of DES for eight weeks to rats with implanted tumors led to more than a 50% decrease of the tumor weight and a reduced incidence of metastases. Receptors in the Pollard tumor have yet to be characterized. Another spontaneous tumor of probably greater interest is the R-3327 rat papillary adenocarcinoma, probably of the dorsolateral gland, initially reported in 1973 by Dunning and later shown to be androgen-sensitive and transplantable.[125,126] The first report which correlated the presence or absence of androgen receptors in this tumor of the prostate with androgen sensitivity appeared in 1975.[127] This study followed the development of a line (R-3327-A) of androgen-insensitive squamous cell carcinomas established from the R-3327 androgen-responsive tumors, and clearly demonstrated the presence of DHT-receptors in the latter (androgen-sensitive) but not in the former tumor. Moreover, receptor concentrations were higher in tumors borne by male than female rats, and castration of the males decreased tumor binding of DHT. The recent finding that the R-3327 tumor also contains a specific receptor for E_2 further explains its hormone sensitivity; no progesterone- or glucocorticoid-binding sites were observed in this study.[128] Two additional spontaneous and transplantable adenocarcinomas have been produced in the dorsal lobe of the prostate in Nb rats with prolonged T and/or T-estrone treatment.[129] Both tumor lines metastasize readily, but are uniquely distinguished by the fact that one line is autonomous and the other is estrogen-dependent. It is hoped that these tumor lines, along with the others already mentioned, will prove to be useful in future research of receptor roles in prostatic carcinoma.

Since DHT is directly responsible for androgenic stimulation of the prostate and has also been implicated as the key androgen in some pathologic states of the prostate in the human and animals, knowledge of steroid-receptor mechanisms was used advantageously for the development and testing of antiandrogens.[37,56,67,130,131] The latter were designed to block the target organ effects of androgens by inhibiting the binding of DHT to the cytosol receptor.[132-134] Compounds of this nature have been reviewed by Sandberg and Gaunt, and some have been administered clinically.[83] Other steroid agents to which antimetabolites have been attached have been developed and theoretically serve a dual purpose: 1) they interfere with hormone-receptor binding, and 2) they may carry the antimetabolite "piggyback" into prostatic cell compartments. One such agent is estramustine phosphate (Estracyt), an E_2-conjugate with an alkylating agent. This compound has been shown to compete for E_2 receptors in BPH (N=8) and human cancer (N=4). It also binds to DHT receptors, thereby explaining its effectiveness in treatment of prostatic cancer after estrogenic compounds lose their effectiveness.[135]

The application of steroid receptor technology to the diagnosis, therapeutic management, and prognosis of prostatic cancer is still in its infancy; some investigators feel that it is unlikely that the measurement of androgen receptors will prove to be a useful tool in this regard.[136] Even measurements of the proportion of glandular constituents and binding characteristics in the hyperplastic prostate show no correlation.[78] The fact that neoplastic cells may be surrounded by or adjacent to normal cells, and that both benign and malignant tissues within a given prostate may have significant receptor concentrations, is undoubtedly one of the major hindrances to obtaining a consistent correlation between prostatic cancer and its receptor concentration. This does not negate the two important factors which up to this point have established the plausibility of receptor measurements as potentially valuable tools to the clinician, that is, 1) responsiveness of normal prostatic cells requires the presence of receptors which bind and retain hormones in physiologic levels in cytoplasmic and nuclear compartments, and 2) normal prostatic processes can be blocked by agents which occupy receptor sites but do not exert a hormonal effect; they may also be cytotoxic.

The value of future receptor analyses of prostatic specimens and their correlation to cancer will be improved by inclusion of histologic classification and 1) assessment of the entire receptor profile for androgens, estrogens, and possibly other hormones. These measurements ideally would include assessment of total as well as unoccupied receptor sites. Currently most receptor measurements are of available sites and do not assess the sites occupied by endogenous hormone in situ in the cytoplasm and nuclei. 2) Measurement of a prostatic receptor profile would be of limited value without a thorough analysis of the patient's endocrine status. This is of particular importance for those hormones which are known to induce the synthesis of their own cytoplasmic receptor or which control the concentration of another receptor.[137,138]

Continuing advances in receptor methodology, such as the 400- to 600-fold purification of the prostatic DHT-receptor complex and the development of antibodies for the characterization of steroid receptors certainly brighten the prospects of a needle biopsy providing sufficient material for a total receptor profile.[139-141] Thus it is hoped that the clinical usefulness of receptor determinations in guiding the management of leukemia, breast, and endometrial cancers will find its counterpart in the near future in prostatic cancer.

REFERENCES

1. Huggins, C., and Hodges, C. V. Studies on prostatic cancer. I. The effect of castration, of estrogen, and of androgen infection on serum phosphatases in metastatic carcinoma of the prostate. *Cancer Res.* 1:293-7, 1941.
2. Huggins, C. Endocrine-induced regression of cancers. Stockholm: Les Prix Nobel in 1966, p 172.
3. Glascock, R. F., and Hoekstra, W. G. Selective accumulation of tritium-labelled hexoestrol by the reproductive organs of immature female goats and sheep. *Biochem J.* 72:673-82, 1959.
4. Jensen, E. V. Studies of growth phenomena using tritium-labelled steroids. *Proceedings 4th International Congress of Biochemistry. Vienna:* 1958, 15:119, 1960.
5. Jensen, E. V., and Jacobsen, H. I. Fate of steroid estrogens in target tissues. Edited by G. Pincus and E. P. Vollmer. In *Biological Activities of Steroids in Relation to Cancer.* New York: Academic Press, 1960, pp 161-78.
6. Jensen, E. V., and Jacobsen, H. I. Basic guides to the mechanism of estrogen action. *Recent Prog Horm Res.* 18:387, 1962.
7. Vermeulen, A., Stoica, T., and Verdonck, L. The apparent free testosterone concentration, an index of androgenicity. *J Clin Endrocrinol Metab.* 33:759-67, 1971.
8. Lasnitzki, I., and Franklin, H. R. The influence of serum on uptake, conversion, and action of testosterone in rat prostate glands in organ culture. *J Endocrinol.* 54:333-42, 1972.
9. Giorgi, E. P., Grant, S. K., Stewart, J. C. et al. Androgen dynamics in vitro in the canine prostate gland. *J Endocrinol.* 55:421-39, 1972.
10. McMahon, M. J., Butler, A.V.J., and Thomas, G. H. Testosterone metabolism in cultured hyperplasia of the human prostate. *Acta Endocrinol* (Copenhagen). 77:784-93, 1974.
11. Giorgi, E. P., Stewart, J. C., Grant, J. K. et al. Androgen dynamics in vitro in the human prostate gland. Effect of oestradiol 17-*β*. *Biochem J.* 126:107-21, 1972.
12. Giorgi, E. P., Shirley, I. M., Grant, J. K. et al. Androgen dynamics in vitro in the human prostate gland. Effect of cyproterone and cyproterone acetate. *Biochem J.* 132:465-74, 1973.
13. Giorgi, E. P., Moses, T. F., Grant, J. K. et al. In vitro studies on the regulation of androgen-tissue relationship in canine normal and human hyperplastic prostate. *Mol Cell Endocrinol.* 1:271-84, 1974.
14. Milgrom, E., Atger, M., and Baulieu, E. E. L'entrée des oestrogènes dans les cellules utérines dépendelle d'une protéine? *C R Acad Sci.* 274:2771-4, 1972.
15. Milgrom, E., Atger, M., and Baulieu, E. E. Studies on estrogen entry into uterine cells and on estradiol-receptor attachment to the nucleus. Is the entry of estrogen into uterine cells a protein mediated process? *Biochim Biophys Acta* 320:267-83, 1973.
16. Liao, S., Liang, T., Fang, S. et al. Steroid structure and androgenic activity. Specificities involved in the receptor binding and nuclear retention of various androgens. *J Biol Chem.* 248:6154-62, 1973.

17. Smith, H. E., Smith, R. G., Toft, D. O. et al. Binding of steroids to progesterone receptor proteins in chick oviduct and human uterus. *J Biol Chem.* 249:5924-32, 1974.

18. Mangan, F. R., and Mainwaring, W.I.P. An explanation of the antiandrogenic properties of 6α-Bromo-17β-hydroxy-17α-methyl-4-oxa-5α-androstane-3-one. *Steroids.* 20:331-43, 1972.

19. Scatchard, G. The attraction of proteins for small molecules and ions. *Ann NY Acad Sci.* 51:660-72, 1949.

20. Lineweaver, H., and Burk, D. The determination of enzyme dissociation constants. *J Am Chem Soc.* 56:658-66, 1934.

21. Mainwaring, W.I.P., and Peterken, B. M. A reconstituted cell-free system for the specific transfer of steroid-receptor complexes into nuclear chromatin isolated from rat ventral prostate gland. *Biochem J.* 125:285-95, 1971.

22. Nozu, K., and Tamaoki, B. Incorporation of ^{131}I-labeled androgen-receptor into nuclei of rat prostates. *Biochem Biophys Res Commun.* 58:145-50, 1974.

23. Rennie, P., and Bruchovsky, N. In vitro and in vivo studies on the functional significance of androgen receptors in rat prostate. *J Biol Chem.* 247:1546-54, 1972.

24. Rennie, P., and Bruchovsky, N. Studies on the relationship between androgen receptors and the transport of androgens in rat prostate. *J Biol Chem.* 248:3288-97, 1973.

25. Sar, M., Liao, S., and Stumpf, W. E. Nuclear concentration of androgens in rat seminal vesicles and prostate demonstrated by dry-mount autoradiography. *Endocrinology.* 86:1008-10, 1970.

26. Mohla, S., DeSombre, E. R., and Jensen, E. V. Tissue-specific stimulation of RNA synthesis by transformed estradiol-receptor complex. *Biochem Biophys Res Commun.* 46:661-7, 1972.

27. Munck, A., and Brinck-Johnsen, T. Specific and nonspecific physiochemical interactions of glucocorticoids and related steroids with rat thymus cells in vitro. *J Biol Chem.* 243:5556-65, 1968.

28. Chan, D. W., and Slaunwhite, W. R. Jr. The binding of a synthetic progestin, R5020, to transcortin and serum albumin. *J Clin Endocrinol Metab.* 44:983-5, 1977.

29. Karr, J. P., Kirdani, R. Y., Murphy, G. P. et al. Sex hormone globulin and transcortin in human and baboon males. *Arch Androl.* (In press) 1978.

30. Rosner, W. The binding of steroid hormones in human serum. Edited by G. A. Jamieson and T. J. Greenwalt. In *Trace Components of Plasma: Isolation and Clinical Significance.* New York: Alan R. Liss, Inc., 1976, p 377.

31. Gardner, D. G., and Wittliff, J. L. Specific estrogen receptors in the lactating mammary gland of the rat. *Biochemistry.* 12:3090-6, 1973.

32. Liao, S. Receptors and the mechanism of action of androgens, Edited by Jorge R. Pasqualini. In *Receptors and Mechanism of Action of Steroid Hormones. Part 1.* New York: Marcel Dekker, Inc., 1976, pp 159-214.

33. Greene, R. R., and Thompson, D. M. Effects of estrogen on androgen stimulation of the prostate and seminal vesicle of the rat. *Endocrinology.* 30:85-8, 1942.

34. Grayhack, J. T. Effect of testosterone-estradiol administration on citric acid and fructose content of the rat prostate. *Endocrinology.* 77:1068-74, 1965.

35. Karr, J. P., Kirdani, R. Y., Murphy, G. P. et al. Effects of testosterone and estradiol on ventral prostate and body weights of castrated rats. *Life Sci.* 15:501-13, 1974.

36. Bruchovsky, N., Lesser, B., Van Doorn, E. et al. Hormonal effects on cell proliferation in rat prostate. *Vitam Horm.* 33:61-102, 1975.

37. Bruchovsky, N., and Wilson, J. D. The conversion of testosterone to 5α-androstan-17β-ol-3-one by rat prostate in vivo and in vitro. *J Biol Chem.* 242:2012-21, 1968a.

38. Bruchovsky, N., Wilson, J. D. The intranuclear binding of testosterone and 5α-androstan-17β-ol-3-one by rat prostate. *J Biol Chem.* 243:5953-60, 1968b.

39. Bruchovsky, N. Comparison of the metabolites formed in rat prostate following the in vivo administration of seven natural androgens. *Endocrinology.* 89:1212-22, 1971.

40. Nozu, K., Yitoh, H., and Tamaoki, B.-I. Direct evidence on incorporation of the receptor into the nuclei of rat ventral prostate in the form of the complex with dihydrotestosterone. *Endocrinol Jpn.* 22:537-48, 1975.

41. Fang, S., and Liao, S. Androgen receptors. Steroid- and tissue-specific retention of a 17β-hydroxy-5α-androstan-3-one-protein complex by the cell nuclei of ventral prostate. *J Biol Chem.* 246:16-24, 1971.

42. Van Doorn, E., Craven, S., and Bruchovsky, N. The relationship between androgen receptors and the hormonally controlled responses of the ventral prostate. *Biochem J.* 160:11-21, 1976.

43. Verhoeven, G., Heyns, W., and DeMoor, P. Ammonium sulfate precipitation as a tool for the study of androgen receptor proteins in rat prostate and mouse kidney. *Steroids.* 26:149-67, 1975.

44. Krieg, M., Dennis, M., and Voight, K. D. Comparison between the binding of 19-nortestosterone, 5 alpha-dihydrotestosterone and testosterone in rat prostate and bulbocavernosus/levator ani muscle. *J Endocrinol.* 70:379-87, 1976.

45. Blondeau, J. P., Corpéchot, C., and Robel, P. Androgen binding proteins in the rat prostate: methodological problems and regulation. *Ann Endocrinol.* (Paris) 37:95-6, 1976.

46. Shain, S. A., Boessel, R. W., and Axelrod, L. R. Aging in the rat prostate. Reduction in detectable ventral prostate androgen receptor content. *Arch Biochem Biophys.* 167:247-63, 1975.

47. Baulieu, E.-E., and Jung, I. A prostatic cytosol receptor. *Biochem Biophys Res Commun.* 38:599-606, 1970.

48. Mainwaring, W.I.P., and Mangan, R. F. A study of the androgen receptors in a variety of androgen-sensitive tissues. *J Endocrinol.* 59:121-39, 1973.

49. Sullivan, J. N., and Strott, C. A. Evidence for an androgen-independent mechanism regulating the levels of receptor in target tissue. *J Biol Chem.* 248:3202-8, 1973.

50. Blondeau, J. P., Corpéchot, C., LeGoascogne, C. et al. Androgen receptors in the rat ventral prostate and their hormonal control. *Vitam Horm.* 33:319-45, 1975.

51. Bruchovsky, N., and Craven, S. Prostatic involution: effect on androgen receptors and intracellular androgen transport. *Biochem Biophys Res Commun.* 62:837-43, 1975.

52. Liao, S., Tymoczko, J. L., Castañeda, E. et al. Androgen receptors and androgen-dependent initiation of protein synthesis in the prostate. *Vitam Horm.* 33:297-317, 1975.

53. Mainwaring, W.I.P., Symes, E. K., and Higgins, S. J. Nuclear components responsible for the retention of steroid-receptor complexes, especially from the standpoint of the specificity of hormonal responses. *Biochem J.* 156:129-41, 1976.

54. Klyzsejko-Stefanowicz, L., Chiu, J. F., Tsai, Y. H. et al. Acceptor proteins in rat androgenic tissue chromatin. *Proc Natl Acad Sci USA.* 73:1954-8, 1976.

55. Davies, P., and Griffiths, K. Influence of steroid-receptor complexes on transcription by human hypertrophied prostatic RNA polymerases. *Mol Cell Endocrinol.* 5:269-88, 1976.

56. Siiteri, P. K., and Wilson, J. D. Dihydrotestosterone in prostatic hypertrophy. 1. The formation and content of dihydrotestosterone in the hypertrophic prostate of man. *J Clin Invest.* 49:1737-45, 1970.

57. Hansson, V., Tveter, K. J., Attramadal, A. et al. Androgenic receptors in human benign nodular prostatic hyperplasia. *Acta Endocrinol.* (Copenhagen) 68:79-88, 1971.

58. Mainwaring, W.I.P., and Milroy, E.J.G. Characterization of the specific androgen receptors in the human prostate gland. *J Endocrinol.* 57:371-84, 1973.

59. Cowan, R. A., Cowan, S. K., and Grant, J. K. The specificity of 5α-dihydrotestosterone binding in human prostate cytosol preparations. *Biochem Soc Trans.* 3:537-40, 1975.

60. Mobbs, B. G., Johnson, I. E., and Connolly, J. G. In vitro assay of androgen binding by human prostate. *J Steroid Biochem.* 6:453-8, 1975.

61. Menon, M., Tananis, C. E., McLoughlin, M. G. et al. Androgen receptors in human prostatic tissue: a review. *Cancer Treat Rep.* 61:265-71, 1977a.

62. Rosen, V., Jung, I., Baulieu, E. E. et al. Androgen-binding proteins in human benign prostatic hypertrophy. *J Clin Endocrinol Metab.* 41:761-70, 1975.

63. Fang, S., and Hsu, R. S. Characterization of androgen binding components in human prostate cytosol. *Fed Proc.* 34:348, 1975.

64. Hawkins, E. F., Nijs, M., and Brassinne, C. Steroid receptors in the human prostate. Detection of tissue-specific androgen binding in prostate cancer. *Clin Chim Acta* 75:303-12, 1977.

65. Jung-Testas, I., Mercier-Bodard, C. H., and Robel, P. Androgen binding proteins in human prostate. *Ann Endocrinol.* (Paris) 37:97-8, 1976.

66. Menon, M., Tananis, C. E., McLoughlin, M. G. et al. The measurement of androgen receptors in human prostatic tissue utilizing sucrose density gradient centrifugation and a protamine precipitation assay. *J Urol.* 117:309-12, 1977b.

67. Steins, P., Krieg, M., Hollmann, H. J. et al. In vitro studies of testosterone and 5α-dihydrotestosterone binding in benign prostatic hypertrophy. *Acta Endocrinol.* (Copenhagen) 75:773-84, 1974.

68. Walsh, P. C., McLoughlin, M. G., Menon, M. et al. Measurement of androgen receptors in human prostatic tissue: methodological considerations. *Prog Clin Biol Res.* 6:159-68, 1976.

69. Nijs, M., Hawkins, E. F., and Coune, A. Binding of 5α-dihydrotestosterone in human prostatic cancer: examination by agar gel electrophoresis. *J Endocrinol.* 69:18-19, 1976.

70. Geller, J., Cantor, T., and Albert, J. Evidence for a specific dihydrotestosterone-binding cytosol receptor in the human prostate. *J Clin Endocrinol Metab.* 41:854-62, 1975.

71. Geller, J., Albert, J., Geller, S. et al. Effect of megestrol acetate (Megace) on steroid metabolism and steroid-protein binding in the human prostate. *J Clin Endocrinol Metab.* 43:1000-8, 1976.

72. Snochowski, M., Pousette, A., Ekman, P. et al. Characterization and measurement of the androgen receptor in human benign prostatic hyperplasia and prostatic carcinoma. *J Clin Endocrinol Metab.* 45:920-30, 1977.

73. Mobbs, B. G., Johnson, I. E., Connolly, J. G. et al. Evaluation of the use of cyproterone acetate competition to distinguish between high-affinity binding of [^{3}H]-dihydrotestosterone to human prostate cytosol receptors and to sex hormone-binding globulin. *J Steroid Biochem.* 8:943-9, 1977.

74. Wagner, R. K., Schulze, K. H., and Jungblut, P. W. Estrogen and androgen receptor in human prostate and prostate tumor tissue. *Acta Endocrinol.* (Copenhagen) 193 (suppl):52, 1975.

75. Bonne, C., and Raynaud, J.-P. Assay of androgen binding sites by exchange with methyltrienolone (R-1881). *Steroids.* 27:497-507, 1976.

76. Menon, M., Tananis, C. E., Hicks, L. L. et al. Characterization of the binding of a potent synthetic androgen, Methyltrienolone (R-1881) to human tissues. *J Clin Invest.* 61:150-62, 1978.

77. Mobbs, B. G., Johnson, I. E., and Connolly, J. G. High-affinity binding of androgen by human prostate. *Proc Am Assoc Cancer Res.* 17:9, 1976.

78. Shimazaki, J., Kadoma, T., Wakisaka, M., et al. Dihydrotestosterone-binding protein in cytosols of normal and hypertrophic human prostates, and influence of estrogens and anti-androgens on binding. *Endocrinol Jpn.* 24:9-14, 1977.

79. Geller, J., and Worthman, C. Characterization of a human prostate cytosol receptor protein. *Acta Endocrinol.* (Copenhagen) 177 (suppl):4, 1973.

80. Fraser, H. M., Mitchell, A.J.H., Anderson, C. K. et al. The interaction of dihydrotestosterone and oestradiol-17β with macromolecules in human hyperplastic prostate tissue. *Acta Endocrinol.* 76:773-82, 1974.

81. Davies, P., and Griffiths, K. Similarities between 5α-dihydrotestosterone-receptor complexes from human and rat prostatic tissue: effects on RNA polymerase activity. *Mol Cell Endocrinol.* 3:143-64, 1975.

82. Attramadal, A., Weddington, S. C., Naess, O. et al. Androgen receptors in male sex tissues of rats and humans. *Prog Clin Biol Res.* 6:189-203, 1976.

83. Sandberg, A. A., and Gaunt, R. Model systems for studies of prostatic cancer. *Semin Oncol.* 3:177-87, 1976.

84. Sinha, A. A., Blackhard, C. E., Doe, R. P. et al. The in vitro localization of ^{3}H estradiol in human prostatic carcinoma. An electron microscopic autoradiographic study. *Cancer.* 31:682-8, 1973.

85. Wirtz, A., Wiedman, M., Raith, L. et al. Studies on the estradiol and 5α-dihydrotestosterone receptors in mammary and prostatic tissues. *Acta Endocrinol.* (Copenhagen) 177 (suppl):8, 1973.

86. Hawkins, E. F., Nijs, M., Brassinne, C. et al. Steroid receptors in the human prostate. I. Estradiol-17β binding in benign prostatic hypertrophy. *Steroids.* 26:458-69, 1975.

87. Bashirelahi, N., and Young, J. D. Specific binding protein for 17 β estradiol in prostate with adenocarcinoma. *Urology.* 8:553-8, 1976.

88. Bashirelahi, N., O'Toole, J. H., and Young, J. D. A specific 17 β-estradiol receptor in human benign hypertrophic prostate. *Biochem Med.* 15:254-61, 1976.

89. Hawkins, E. F., Nijs, M., and Brassinne, C. Steroid receptors in the human prostate. 2. Some properties of the estrophilic molecule of benign prostatic hypertrophy. *Biochem Biophys Res Commun.* 70:854-61, 1976.

90. Huggins, C., and Webster, W. O. Duality of human prostate in response to estrogen. *J Urol.* 59:258-66, 1948.

91. Karr, J. P., Sufrin, G., Kirdani, R. Y. et al. Prostatic binding of estradiol-17β in the baboon. *J Steroid Biochem.* 9:87-94, 1978.

92. Jungblut, P. W., Hughes, S., Hughes, A. et al. Evaluation of various methods for the assay of cytoplasmic oestrogen receptors in extracts of calf uteri and human breast cancers. *Acta Endocrinol.* 70:185-95, 1970.

93. Lowry, O. H., Rosebrough, N. J., Farr, A. L. et al. Protein measurement with folin phenol reagent. *J Biol Chem.* 193:265-75, 1951.

94. Unjhem, O. Metabolism and binding of oestradiol-17β by rat ventral

prostate in vitro. Edited by M. Finkelstein, A. Klopper, C. Conti, and C. Cassano. In *Research on Steroids.* Oxford, Pergamon Press, 1970, pp. 139-43.

95. O'Toole, J. H., Young, J. D., and Bashirelahi, N. The use of an anti-androgenic agent to distinguish between estrogen and androgen-binding proteins in rat ventral prostate. *Biochem Med.* 14:297-304, 1975.

96. Robinette, C. C., Thomas, J. A., Mawhinney, M. G. Dihydrotestosterone and estradiol-17β receptors in the rat ventral prostate and seminal vesicle. *Pharmacologist.* 18:249, 1976.

97. Smírnova, O. V., Smirnov, A. N., Khodakova, T. K. et al. Estradiol receptors in the sex organs and some other organs of male rats. *Probl Endokrinol.* (Moscow) 21:71-6, 1975.

98. Armstrong, E. G., Bashirelahi, N. A specific protein for 17β-estradiol in retired breeder rat ventral prostate. *Biochem Biophys Res Commun.* 61:628-34, 1974.

99. Shain, S. A., and Axelrod, L. R. Reduced high affinity 5α-dihydrotestosterone receptor capacity in the ventral prostate of the aging rat. *Steroids.* 21:801-12, 1973.

100. Jungblut, P. W., Hughes, S. F., Görlich, C. et al. Simultaneous occurrence of individual estrogen and androgen receptors in female and male target organs. *Hoppe-Seylers Z Physiol Chem.* 352:1603-10, 1971.

101. Belis, J. A., Blume, C. D., and Mawhinney, M. G. Androgen and estrogen binding in male guinea pig accessory sex organs. *Endocrinology.* 101:727-40, 1977.

102. Hawkins, E. F., Nijs, M., Brassinne, C. et al. Enigmatic binding of corticosterone to protein in cytosols of human benign prostatic hypertrophy tissue. *J Endocrinol.* 69:17P, 1976.

103. Cowan, R. A., Cowan, S. K., Giles, C. A. et al. Prostatic distribution of sex hormone binding globulin and cortisol-binding globulin in benign hyperplasia. *J Endocrinol.* 71:121-31, 1976.

104. Roth, G. Age-related changes in specific glucocorticoid binding by steroid-responsive tissues of rats. *Endocrinology.* 94:82-90, 1974.

105. Ballard, P. L., Baxter, J. D., Higgins, S. J. et al. General presence of glucocorticoid receptors in mammalian tissues. *Endocrinology.* 94:998-1002, 1974.

106. Baxter, J. D., and Forsham, P. H. Tissue effects of glucocorticoids. *Am J Med.* 53:573-89, 1972.

107. Asselin, J., Labrie, F., Gourdeau, Y. et al. Binding of [^{3}H] methyltrienolene (R-1881) in rat prostate and human benign prostatic hypertrophy (BPH). *Steroids.* 28:449-59, 1976.

108. Mainwaring, W.I.P., and Mangan, F. R. A study of the androgen receptors in a variety of androgen-sensitive tissues. *J Endocrinol.* 59:121-39, 1973.

109. Hansson, V., Tveter, K. J., Unhjem, O. et al. Androgen binding in male sex organs, with special reference to the human prostate. Edited by M. Goland. In *Normal and Abnormal Growth of the Prostate.* Springfield, Ill.: Charles C Thomas, 1974, pp 676-711.

110. Heyns, W., Verhoeven, G., and DeMoor, P. A comparative study of androgen binding in rat uterus and prostate. *J Steroid Biochem.* 7:987-91, 1976.

111. Gehring, U., Tomkins, G. M., and Ohno, S. Effect of the androgen-insensitivity mutation on a cytoplasmic receptor for dihydrotestosterone. *Nature New Biol.* 232:106-7, 1971.

112. Bullock, L. P., and Bardin, W. C. Androgen receptors in testicular feminization. *J Clin Endocrinol Metab.* 35:935-7, 1972.

113. Attardi, B., and Ohno, S. Cytosol androgen receptor from kidney of normal and testicular feminized (Tfm) mice. *Cell.* 2:205-12, 1974.

114. Bardin, C. W., Bullock, L. P., Sherins, R. J. et al. Androgen metabolism and mechanism of action in male pseudohermaphroditism: a study of testicular feminization. *Recent Prog Horm Res.* 29:65-109, 1973.

115. Bullock, L. P., and Bardin, C. W. In vivo and in vitro testosterone metabolism by the androgen insensitive rat. *J Steroid Biochem.* 4:139-51, 1973.

116. Bullock, L. P., and Bardin, C. W. Androgen receptors in mouse kidney: a study of male, female, and androgen-insensitive (Tfm/y) mice. *Endocrinology.* 94:746-56, 1974.

117. Jensen, E. V., Block, G. E., Smith, S. et al. Estrogen receptors and breast cancer response to adrenalectomy. *Nat Cancer Inst Monograph.* 34:55-70, 1971.

118. McGuire, W. C., Vollmer, E. P., and Carbone, P. P. (eds). *Estrogen Receptors in Human Breast Cancer.* New York: Raven Press, 1975.

119. Lippman, M. E. Glucocorticoid Receptor. Edited by G. S. Levey. In *Hormone-Receptor Interaction: Molecular Aspects.* New York: Marcel Dekker, Inc., 1976, pp 221-42.

120. Jensen, E. V., Polley, T. Z., Smith, S. et al. Prediction of hormone dependency in human breast cancer. Edited by W. C. McGuire, P. P. Carbone and E. P. Volmer. In *Estrogen Receptors in Human Breast Cancer.* New York: Raven Press, 1975, pp 37-55.

121. Bruchovsky, N., and Lesser, B. Control of proliferative growth in androgen responsive organs and neoplasms. *Adv Sex Horm Res.* 2:1-55, 1976.

122. Bruchovsky, N., Sutherland, D.J.A., Meakin, J. W. et al. Androgen receptors: relationship to growth response and to intracellular androgen transport in nine variant lines of the Shionogi mammary carcinoma. *Biochim Biophys Acta.* 381:61-71, 1975.

123. Pollard, M. Spontaneous prostate adenocarcinomas in aged germ-free Wistar Rats. *J Natl Cancer Inst.* 51:1235-41, 1973.

124. Pollard, M., and Luckert, P. H. Transplantable metastasizing prostate adenocarcinomas in rats. *J Natl Cancer Inst.* 54:643-9, 1975.

125. Dunning, W. F. Prostate cancer in the rat. *Natl Cancer Inst Monogr.* 12:351-69, 1973.

126. Voight, W., and Dunning, W. F. In vivo metabolism of testosterone-^{3}H in R-3327, an androgen-sensitive rat prostatic adenocarcinoma. *Cancer Res.* 34:1447-50, 1974.

127. Voight, W., Feldman, M., and Dunning, W. F. 5α-dihydrotestosterone-binding proteins and androgen sensitivity in prostatic cancers of Copenhagen rats. *Cancer Res.* 35:1840-6, 1975.

128. Markland, F. S., and Lee, L. Steroid hormone receptor characterization of the Dunning R-3327 prostatic adenocarcinoma. *Proc Am Assoc Cancer Res.* 18:151, 1977.

129. Noble, R. L. The development of prostatic adenocarcinoma in Nb rats following prolonged sex hormone administration. *Cancer Res.* 37:1929-33, 1977.

130. Anderson, K. M., and Liao, S. Selective retention of dihydrotestosterone by prostatic nuclei. *Nature.* 219:277-97, 1968.

131. Mainwaring, W.I.P. A review of the formation and binding of 5 alpha-dihydrotestosterone in the mechanism of action of androgens in the prostate of the rat and other species. *J Reprod Fert.* 44:377-93, 1975.

132. Fang, S., and Liao, S. Antagonistic action of anti-androgens on the formation of a specific dihydrotestosterone-receptor protein complex in rat ventral prostate. *Mol Pharmacol.* 5:420-431, 1969.

133. Skinner, R.W.S., Pozderac, R. V., Counsell, R. E. et al. The inhibitive effects of steroid analogues in the binding of tritiated 5α-dihydrotestosterone to

receptor proteins from rat prostate tissue. *Steroids.* 25:189-202, 1975.

134. Pita, J. C. Jr., Lippman, M. E., Thompson, E. B. et al. Interaction of spironolactone and digitalis with the 5 alpha-dihydrotestosterone (DHT) receptor of rat ventral prostate. *Endocrinology.* 97:1521-7, 1975.

135. Nilsson, I., Liskowski, L., and Nilsson, T. Inhibition by estramustine phosphate on estradiol and androgen binding in benign and malignant prostate in humans. *Urology.* 8:118-21, 1976.

136. Mainwaring, W.I.P. The relevance of studies on androgen action to prostatic cancer. Edited by K. M. Menor and J. R. Reel. In *Steroid Hormone Action and Cancer.* New York: Plenum Press, 1976, pp 152-71.

137. Sarff, M., and Gorski, J. Control of estrogen binding protein concentrations under basal conditions and after estrogen administration. *Biochemistry.* 10:2557-63, 1971.

138. Milgrom, E., Atger, M., Perrot, M. et al. Progesterone in uterus and plasma: VI. Uterine progesterone receptors during the estrous cycle and implantation in the guinea pig. *Endocrinology.* 90:1071-8, 1972.

139. Ichii, S. 5 alpha-dihydrotestosterone binding protein in rat ventral prostate: purification nuclear incorporation and subnuclear localization. *Endocrinol Jpn.* 22:433-7, 1975.

140. Castañeda, E., and Liao, S. A new method for characterization of the androgen receptors by use of a steroid antibody. *Endoc Res Commun.* 1:271-81, 1974.

141. Castañeda, E., and Liao, S. The use of anti-steroid antibodies in the characterization of steroid receptors. *J Biol Chem.* 250:883-9, 1975.

GENERAL REFERENCES

1. Goland, M. (ed). *Normal and Abnormal Growth of the Prostate.* Springfield, Ill: Charles C Thomas, 1974.

2. King, R.J.B. and Mainwaring, W.I.P. (eds). *Steroid-Cell Interactions.* Baltimore: University Park Press, 1974.

3. Levey, G. S. (ed). *Hormone-Receptor Interaction: Molecular Aspects.* New York: Marcel Dekker, Inc., 1976.

4. O'Malley, B. W. and Means, A. R. (eds). *Receptors for Reproductive Hormones.* New York: Plenum Press, 1973.

5. Pasqualini, J. R. (ed). *Receptors and Mechanism of Action of Steroid Hormones.* New York: Marcel Dekker, Inc., 1976.

6. Wittliff, J. L. Steroid-binding proteins in normal and neoplastic mammary cells. Edited by H. Busch. In *Methods in Cancer Research XI.* New York: Academic Press, 1975.

Cell and Organ Culture in Prostatic Cancer

6

Donald J. Merchant

Most of our knowledge and understanding of neoplastic disease of the prostate is based on its natural history and has been derived from astute clinical observations and from anecdotal and retrospective studies of the disease. Significant observations have been made relating to carcinogenesis, androgen dependence, hormone response, and action of chemotherapeutic agents using animal models or animal prostatic tissue in vitro. Nevertheless, interpretation and extrapolation of results from such systems must be guarded due to recognized variation in the comparative embryology, histology, and biochemistry of the prostate among animal species.[1,2]

Despite the early report by Burrows, Burns, and Suzuki that they had successfully grown cells from a tissue specimen obtained from benign prostatic hypertrophy, the development of in vitro systems utilizing human prostatic tissue has progressed at a very slow pace.[3] Röhl published the first study involving culture of large numbers of prostate specimens.[4] In this report he was able to cite as references only two limited studies in addition to the original paper by Burrows, et al. and it is only since 1970 that frequent reports on the culture of human prostatic tissue have appeared.[3,5,6] It may be of significance in this regard that the National Prostatic Cancer Project was organized in 1973.

POTENTIAL USES OF CELL AND ORGAN CULTURE SYSTEMS

Although cultures of animal prostate tissue will continue to provide useful information, elucidation of specific problems related to prostatic cancer is more likely to result from use of human tissue. The following discussion will be limited to systems using human tissue except for reference to potential interplay between human and animal systems.

There are a number of questions regarding prostatic cancer as well as prostate biology which might be investigated using cell or organ culture alone or in conjunction with animal models.[7] Several of these will be explored briefly to point up both the potential and the limitations of in vitro systems.

An aspect of prostatic cancer which appears to be particularly susceptible to investigation with in vitro methods is etiology. Some of the targets of current research in this area are 1) alterations in the host's immune surveillance mechanisms, 2) viral agents, 3) chemical carcinogens, and 4) changes in hormone sensitivity.

To understand the role of host immunity in the initiation and progression of neoplastic change it will be necessary to have culture systems of host cells to serve as targets for assay of both humoral and cellular immune components. In addition the identification and isolation of tumor-specific antigens will be enhanced significantly by production of expanded populations of tumor cells freed of stromal elements. While pilot studies or experimental models might be achieved with animal material, definitive answers must come from human systems.

Investigations of the role of viruses in the initiation of prostatic cancer is almost completely dependent on cell and organ culture.[8] Requirements include the ability to develop cultures of a single cell type which will permit detection of viral effects such as CPE, cell transformation, etc. Proliferation of host cells can also significantly increase the probability of activation of a latent or cryptic viral agent or of the expression of viral genome. Culture can provide sufficient quantities of cells for analysis by electron microscopic, biochemical, and immunologic techniques. If a candidate virus should be identified, demonstration of its role as an etiologic agent would depend to a significant degree upon its ability to transform normal prostatic cells in culture.

Kinetic studies of prostatic tumor cell populations could yield valuable information related to tumor immunity, chemotherapy, radiotherapy, and endocrine responsiveness. Although a number of workers have attempted to establish models by injection of human tissue into "nude" mice, the results to date have not been sufficiently reproducible to permit kinetic studies.[9] Establishment of cells in culture and the use of cloning techniques would make possible a wide range of investigations providing a sufficient number of genetic markers can be defined.

SPECIMENS FOR CULTURE

A number of factors related to selection of prostate tissue specimens for culture have been discussed in an earlier publication.[10] It was pointed out that benign or nodular hyperplasia and prostatic adenocarcinoma arise in quite distinctly different tissues.[11] Nodular hyperplasia has its origin in periuretheral gland tissue which is sometimes referred to as the cranial lobe and is located between the ejaculatory ducts and the urethra.[12,13] Prostatic carcinoma, on the other hand, arises from the long branching glands of the prostate proper in areas referred to as the peripheral zone or the posterior lobes.[11,14]

It is obvious, therefore, that in vitro culture systems addressed to investigation of nodular hyperplasia or carcinoma must be derived from appropriate tissue samples, and that satisfactory controls must be derived from the same areas as the respective tumors. With regard to nodular hyperplasia, this is not too difficult in most instances since surgical intervention is a relatively common procedure. Close cooperation between surgeon, pathologist, and those doing the culture should make it possible to establish procedures which will assure proper tissue samples. Adequate specimens for routine histologic study are necessary for confirmation.

Adequate tissue specimens are much less accessible from prostatic carcinoma. Prostatectomy is considerably less common as a therapeutic procedure in carcinoma of the prostate than it formerly was, and is performed much less frequently than in nodular hyperplasia. The normal procedures for obtaining specimens for pathologic diagnosis of carcinoma are transurethral resection or perineal needle biopsy. Both methods provide limited amounts of material for culture, and the accuracy of sampling, though satisfactory for diagnosis in more advanced stages of the disease, leaves a great deal to be desired in terms of tissue identification for culture, and obtaining proper normal control tissue is very uncertain. In stage 4, stage 3, and probably in many instances of stage 2 disease, palpation of the lesion is relatively accurate and adequate pathologic specimens should be obtained.[15] Use of a hot wire for cauterization to obtain specimens by transurethral resection, however, renders the tissue almost useless for culture.

The microscopic architecture of the prostate is such that great variability can exist between samples depending on the size of the specimen, the orientation of the specimen, and the location from which the tissue is obtained. This is due in part to the variable distribution of glands and fibromuscular stromal tissue which differs from prostate to prostate, from one location to another within the organ, and changes significantly in the presence of hyperplasia or carcinoma.

Prostatic fluid has a high content of enzymes, especially proteases with high specific activity. Thus the length of time which elapses between procurement of tissue and establishment of culture, as well as the conditions of collection, transport, and processing, may be of critical importance.

A major potential source of variation in viability, growth capacity, and possibly in the qualitative cell composition of donor tissue, is the prior therapeutic history of the patient. Röhl presents very suggestive evidence of significant differences in growth potential and patterns of growth of prostatic carcinoma depending upon whether or not the patient had received prior estrogen therapy.[4] We have found no study which has examined the effect of chemotherapy or radiotherapy on subsequent behavior of tissue in vitro, nor have we found any expression of concern in this regard in the current literature, although our own studies suggest that prior therapy may play a significant role (Merchant, unpublished data).

NUTRITIONAL AND PHYSIOLOGIC REQUIREMENTS FOR CULTURE

No definitive studies have been made of the specific nutritional or physiologic requirements for growth or maintenance of the human prostate in vitro. Early tissue culture studies employed natural products such as serum, plasma, ascitic fluid, and tissue extracts. With development of the science of cell and tissue culture it has become common practice to utilize a chemically defined mixture containing various combinations of amino acids, vitamins, hormones, and other known growth or regulatory factors. With few exceptions these are supplemented with serum, varying considerably as to species of origin and concentration in the final medium. For a recent review of the general aspects of nutrition of mammalian cells in culture the reader is referred to the text by Paul.[16]

If one reviews the literature relative to the culture of prostatic tissue it is obvious that each investigator has been influenced either by prior experience in the culture of other types of cells or tissues, or has been influenced by colleagues working in the field. There is no uniformity in the media formulations employed and no rationale is presented for the choice of components with few exceptions. Various studies have utilized Eagle BME or MEM, Ham's F-10 or F-12, CMRL 1066, or RPMI 1640.[17-22] These have been supplemented with fetal calf, calf, bull, human, or horse serum which has been either heat-inactivated or noninactivated. The sera have been used alone or in combination, and in concentrations varying from 10% to 40%. Supplements have been primarily testosterone or insulin.

The only efforts to date to define specific aspects of the nutritional or physiologic requirements involve studies comparing horse serum and human serum, the role of testosterone in cell growth, and an effort to establish steady-state-conditions of growth.

Webber used horse serum and fetal calf serum as supplements for CMRL 1066 and reported that horse serum favored epithelial growth, with only a few cultures initially showing fibroblastic outgrowth.[23] On the other hand, initial growth was reported to be fibroblastic in more than half of cultures grown in fetal calf serum. This latter observation is at variance with the majority of published reports which indicate predominately epithelial outgrowth in fetal calf serum medium. This difference may be due to the fact that Webber's cultures were derived entirely from the prostate of one six-year-old donor, and extrapolation to diseased prostates of aged adults seems unwarranted and questionable. The findings of Webber are also entirely descriptive. Quantitative, well-controlled experiments will be required to assess the differential effects of sera.

Schröeder and Mackensen wished to assess the role of testosterone in prostatic growth in vitro, but were confronted with the presence of unknown quantities of hormones in the serum supplement.[24] They used extraction procedures to produce "androgen-free" fetal calf serum and judged the retention of its general growth-supporting properties by assay with HeLa cells. Growth of prostate was inhibited in the presence of "androgen-free" fetal calf serum, but was only partially restored by supplementation with testosterone. McLimans et al. are attempting development of a "steady-state" system for maintenance of populations of prostate cells which can be used to produce replicate cultures.[25] The approach is appealing on a theoretical basis, but its practicality and reliability remain to be demonstrated.

Perhaps the most significant point which can be made at present concerning nutritional and physiologic requirements is that in spite of an extreme range of variables, the results obtained to date by the majority of workers are surprisingly consistent. The length of time required to attain outgrowth, the extent of outgrowth, the type of cells and patterns of growth noted, and the length of time or number of passages which cultures can be maintained, generally are quite comparable not only among current studies but also between current and earlier studies which used much less refined nutrients such as plasma and embryonic extract.

There would appear to be two major reasons for failure to note greater differences in response to variation in nutritional and physiologic parameters. Perhaps the most important is that the questions being asked and the indicators being applied are much too unrefined; we are not yet at the point of asking sophisticated questions. A second reason is that studies to date have been highly descriptive, and in a number of cases have been inadequately planned and reported. As a result, other parameters are very difficult to evaluate despite relatively consistent patterns of cell growth. In too many instances the materials-and-methods section of the protocol lists a series of variables which are not subsequently related to the observations made, either in the experimental section of the paper or in the discussion.[26] If useful data are to be derived from future studies, the work must be more scientifically done.

Finally, it should be emphasized that nutritional and physiologic conditions which are optimal for cellular proliferation probably are not optimal for expression of differentiated cell functions. Thus the design of systems must be related to the aims of investigation.

PRIMARY CELL CULTURE

Primary cell cultures are those which consist of the initial outgrowth prior to subculture or transfer. Cultures may consist of outgrowth from a fragment of tissue (explant), or may be the progeny of cells separated from the tissue by chemical or mechanical means.

The chief advantage of primary cultures is that there is limited multiplication and therefore the cells should be more representative of the in situ cell population. Although the population may be either mixed or represent the cell type(s) most adaptable to the particular culture conditions, it will not have been subjected to the strong selective pressures exerted by continuous proliferation.

Although the explant technique probably has been used most extensively to study the prostate it currently lacks the desired refinement and precision. The earliest studies used the classical plasma clot procedure which immobilizes explants against the surface of the culture vessel and thus permits viable cells to establish contact, adhere, and migrate. However, prostate is characterized by high protease activity so that clots usually are lysed within a short time. This, coupled with slow rate of emergence of cells from the explants, minimizes the effectiveness of the plasma clot.

Current practice utilizes the principle of protein denaturation which classically has been applied to fixation of histologic sections to a microscopic slide with albumin. As applied in cell culture, explants are suspended in medium containing a relatively high content of serum, and are transferred to the culture vessel and planted with a minimal volume of medium bathing each explant. The vessel is allowed to sit for an hour or more allowing droplets of medium around the explants partially to evaporate. Thus serum proteins are denatured and attach the explants to the vessel wall prior to addition of the final medium volume. The method is very imprecise! The degree of attachment depends upon concentration and type of serum proteins, volume of fluid left on the explants, conditions and time of drying, etc. Moreover, the effects of drying, particularly with regard to osmotic changes and concentration of medium components, are unknown and may vary from one tissue specimen to another.

Several practical considerations influence efforts to establish reproducible and replicate primary explant cultures. Particular care should be given to the cutting of explants to insure minimal tearing and cell damage. If fragments are quite uneven in contour, points of contact with the growth surface will be minimal and the percentage of successes will be reduced. Another significant variable is the microscopic architecture of differing fragments. The relative proportions of muscle, connective tissue stroma, and glandular structure is quite varied even in the normal prostate. This is best envisioned by microscopic examination of tissue sections with comparison of adjacent $1mm^2$ areas (the usual explant is $1mm^3$). Similar examination of sections from benign hyperplasia or carcinoma will show even greater sources of variation. Moreover, in cutting a series of explants it is almost impossible to keep exact note of which explants were adjacent to each other in situ.

An interesting effort to take advantage of observed behavior of tissue to improve the reproducible growth of prostatic epithelium has been reported by Stonington and Hemmingsen.[27] Noting the tendency of acinar epithelial cells to emerge from the ducts and spread over the unattached surfaces of explants, they fostered this by preliminary incubation in a high serum concentration during which frequent agitation prevented attachment to the surface. They reported complete coating of most of the explants within 7 to 14 days. When these "epithelialized" explants were then planted in conventional culture, they adhered readily to the culture surface and gave rise to extensive outgrowth. These experiments were restricted to benign prostatic hyperplasia and it is not known whether similar results would be obtained with either normal prostate or prostatic carcinoma.

A second method for preparation of primary cultures involves the dispersal of tissue fragments into cell suspensions with enzymes or chemicals. Such procedures make possible the preparation of cell suspensions which can be plated to provide replicate cultures. Enzymes which have been used for prostate culture include trypsin, collagenase, and pronase, alone or in combination. While enzymes generally act to disaggregate tissues yielding cell suspensions, Stone, Stone and Paulson have reported the separation of acinar ducts from stromal elements by the use of collagenase.[28] The acinar structures remained intact with this procedure and, when planted in conventional culture, gave rise to epithelial outgrowth. The studies utilized tissue from benign prostatic hyperplasia.

Despite the apparent success of separation of acinar tissue with collagenase and the preparation of cell suspensions for culture by treatment with trypsin or collagenase by several groups, the majority of investigators continue to report complete or variable refractoriness of prostate to enzymatic digestion.[29-32] Obviously much work remains to be done to define optimal conditions and to standardize procedures.

There are a number of important variables which must be taken into account when preparing primary monolayer cultures from dispersed tissue samples. Enzymes and chelating agents vary in effectiveness depending upon cell type and their extracellular products. Thus there are likely to be marked differences in the ease of dispersal between normal, hyperplastic, and neoplastic tissue, between tissue from different patients, and between portions of a given specimen. More important, however, is the fact that composition of the resulting cell suspension with regard to cell type is likely to be highly variable. The reader is referred to the excellent review of this topic by Waymouth.[33]

Most enzyme preparations used are crude mixtures which may vary in composition from batch to batch and which certainly vary from one manufacturer to another.[34] These are used under markedly different physiologic conditions (ionic, pH, temperature, etc.) by different investigators. Finally, when cell suspensions are plated the ability of particular cells to attach to the surface and grow depends upon cell type, nature and condition of the culture surface, and physiologic status of the cells.

Recital of the variables involved is not intended to discourage the use of primary monolayer cultures, but to emphasize the need for caution in interpreting results and particularly in comparing results between laboratories, unless the techniques employed are carefully coordinated. Replicate primary cultures, either explant or monolayer, prepared from transurethral resection (TUR) or biopsy specimen might provide a system for analyzing sensitivity of a particular tumor to hormones, radiation, or chemotherapeutic agents as a guide to therapy, or might serve as prognostic indicators. Combined with sensitive immunologic, biochemical, cytochemical, and cytologic techniques, primary cultures offer one of the most promising means of study of the basic biology of the prostate and for assessing the status of specific tumors.

SERIALLY PASSAGED CELLS

There are a number of questions concerning prostatic cancer which can best be answered with in vitro systems but which will require large quantities of reproducible cell populations. These include the search for viral components, either as etiologic or contributing factors, purification of tumor specific antigens, and isolation and study of hormone receptors. Such investigations require extensive expansion of cell populations. In some instances the production of confluent monolayers in the original flasks is adequate, but generally it is necessary to propagate continuously by transplanting and subdividing the population. For many purposes an established line of cells which can be stored in the frozen state for reference and which can be expanded and replicated at will is highly desirable.

All of those concerns about specimen selection, preparation, and population selection, both for explants and primary monolayers apply and are magnified here. With each subculture differential selection of a mixed population can occur and, with continued proliferation, differing nutritional and physiologic requirements, as well as differences in inherent growth capacity, can serve to select for specific variants in the population. The question becomes: what portion of the cell population of the original tissue has grown and survived and what relation, if any, does it have to the in situ tissue?

For the purpose of understanding BPH and carcinoma it is presumed that the cell of primary interest is the acinar epithelial cell of the periurethral gland or of the posterior lobes, respectively. There is very suggestive evidence that replenishment of acinar cells in normal prostatic function is by division of basal, less differentiated cells, which then undergo maturation to become the secreting acinar cells. Thus it is possible that only a very small fraction of the cells of the normal prostate, which are representative of the cell type desired for study, actually are capable of division. It is thought that these cells expand to varying degrees in BPH and carcinoma, presumably following transformation. Whether this is a general transformation or consists of single or multiple events followed by clonal development is unknown.

If longterm culture of prostatic cells is to play an important role as a model system in research on BPH and carcinoma, it will be imperative to define markers of the normal and transformed acinar cells. These will be required to determine whether desired cell types have been isolated from the tissue and maintained in culture. In addition, it will be necessary to select the specific cell desired from among cells which grow in culture, and to monitor continually for its identity and continued function in vitro.

Three experimental methods have been applied to prostate tissue in an effort to derive pure cultures of acinar epithelial cells. Stone et al. attempted to separate the glandular portions of prostate tissue from the stromal elements, and then to culture the acini.[28] While the limited data which they presented indicated a degree of success, it is not certain that this method could be relied upon to free the acinar tissue of fibroblasts completely, and there is no evidence of the effectiveness of the procedure either with normal prostate or with carcinoma. Kaighn and Babcock have approached the purification by use of cloning techniques which provide a great deal of confidence as to the purity of the derived cell lines.[32] Again, their studies have been limited to a few specimens of BPH, and the reproducibility as well as the applicability to normal prostate and/or prostatic carcinoma remains to be demonstrated. Finally, Pretlow et al. have utilized the Ficoll procedure of velocity sedimentation in isokinetic gradients to separate acinar epithelial cells from other prostate cellular components.[34] It is uncertain as yet whether this method alone can yield an adequate separation to assure purity in longterm culture. Similarly, the degree of damage to the cells and the extent to which they will demonstrate continuous proliferation have not been clearly defined. This procedure warrants careful consideration, particularly if it can be combined with cloning methods.

With one or more of these methods or others still to be developed, it seems likely that success will be attained in establishing cell lines from normal prostate, BPH, and prostatic carcinoma. The primary deterrent to use of such cell lines at the present time is lack of suitable markers for identifying the cells as being those desired. The only specific marker yet available is prostatic acid phosphatase.[35] If several reliable markers can be identified, it will be possible to identify the specific cell desired, and clone for that cell type. Genetic drift in the population then can be controlled by the application of pure culture technology. The ability to store cells for indefinite periods in the frozen state will extend the usefulness of such systems significantly.

Although it should be possible theoretically to derive pure cultures of desired cell phenotypes and maintain them for experimental purposes, it is necessary to point out the limitations of such systems. The most important of these is that the very process of selection and purification lessens the possibility that the derived cell line can be considered as broadly representative of the tissue of origin. Perhaps of equal importance is the fact that prostatic tumors, like other tumors, vary greatly in their biologic properties from one host to another. Thus a cell line derived from one tumor might respond quite differently in a particular test from a cell line derived from another tumor. It is even possible that significant differences might exist in lines derived from the same host if multiple transformations occurred initially.

For these reasons it will be necessary to use extreme caution in interpreting results of studies based on a single cell line. It may even be necessary to utilize multiple cell lines derived from tumors in different hosts to yield significant results.

To date two widely used continuously propagated cell lines have been established which are purported to be prostatic epithelium. These are the MA-160 cell line derived from a case of benign prostatic hypertrophy by Fraley, Ecker and Vincent and the EB33 cell line derived from a case of prostatic carcinoma by Okada and Schröeder.[36,37] According to the authors, MA-160 underwent spontaneous neoplastic transformation in vitro. Based on karyologic and enzyme profile analysis both lines have been reported to be contaminated with or replaced by HeLa cells. Although the MA-160 line recently was shown by Ofner et al. to have a C_{19}-steroid metabolic pattern different from HeLa cells and more comparable to that of normal prostate, Nelson-Rees has countered with the observation that the line lacks the Y chromosome and contains a complex of HeLa cell chromosome markers.[38,39] It is clear from these observations that the matter is not yet settled to everyone's satisfaction, but it also emphasizes the fact that possible cross-contamination of continuous cell lines is a danger and that careful and continuous monitoring is required. The history of the MA-160 line has been reviewed recently.[40]

ORGAN CULTURE

Unlike cell or "tissue" culture methods which depend in varying degree upon cell proliferation, "organ" culture methods are designed to foster or maintain differentiation and functional activity of tissue fragments. Only in the case of early embryonic organ rudiments is a whole organ maintained. Except for studies with scanning electron microscopy, morphologic changes in explanted tissue fragments must be evaluated by sectioning and staining procedures. Biochemical assay can be carried out provided sufficiently sensitive techniques are available.

Since tissue relationships are maintained, artifacts introduced by population selection do not pertain to the organ culture system. Nevertheless, the same difficulties apply in selection of tissue fragments for study as have been reported for primary explant cultures, the most important being the variation in histologic architecture within the prostate and marked differences between the normal prostate, BPH, and prostatic carcinoma.

Since evaluation of results is based in large measure on morphologic changes which can be assessed only by sacrificing the culture fragment, the need for large numbers of replicate fragments is apparent. The difficulties encountered in attempting to obtain truly replicate fragments even under the most ideal conditions have been detailed above. In the case of carcinoma this becomes very difficult due to the relatively small amounts of tissue available.

On the other hand, it is possible to maintain tissue in a state of differentiation and function by using completely defined culture media. This makes possible sensitive biochemical assay and facilitates assays which cannot be made in the presence of serum. Particularly, studies of hormones, which commonly are present in serum are made easier. A drawback to organ culture classically has been the short duration of experiments. In most instances tissue fragments begin to show degenerative changes within a very few days. Recently Edwards, Bates and Yuspa, working with rodent prostates, have been able to maintain normal histology and viability up to 14 days as contrasted to the two to four days usually reported.[41] Success appeared to be due to use of a combination of spermine and testosterone in the culture medium.

In organ culture the aim is to discourage outgrowth and thereby maintain the cells in their normal functional relationships. The classical technique was placing tissue fragments on the surface of a plasma clot rather than imbedding them as is done in the explant method of primary culture. The presumed critical difference is that, with explants on the clot surface, cells were not encouraged to migrate out and attach. In fact early clot techniques involved rolling the explants about on the surface at frequent intervals. While this was intended in part to prevent lysis of the clot, the chief aim was to prevent attachment.

Current procedures utilize a support structure for the tissue fragments which is so designed and positioned as to keep the tissue at the interface between the fluid medium and the gaseous atmosphere of the culture vessel. Much higher oxygen tensions are generally employed than is the case with cell cultures. The effectiveness of higher oxygen tensions may be related to penetration of the gas to the interior of the tissue.

Organ culture studies are particularly suited to the study of endocrine relationships, studies of chemotherapeutic agents, analysis of carcinogenesis, and similar problems. The development of sensitive radioimmunoassay methods in particular offer opportunities to combine biochemical and cytologic parameters in imaginative ways. Much work has been done with this technique using rodent tissues. Although the method has not been fully exploited a number of studies also have been published over the past few years using human prostate tissue in organ culture.[42-47]

Addendum: Since this manuscript was prepared, cell lines of human prostatic origin have been reported by three laboratories[48-50] and by T. I. Malinin of the University of Miami School of Medicine (personal communication).

REFERENCES

1. Brandes, D. Fine structure and cytochemistry of male sex accessory organs. Edited by D. Brandes. In *Male Accessory Sex Organs.* New York: Academic Press, 1974, pp 17-44.
2. Price, D. Comparative aspects of development and structure in the prostate. *Natl Cancer Inst Monogr.* 12:1-27, 1963.
3. Burrows, M. T., Burns, J. E. and Suzuki, Y. Studies on the growth of cells. The cultivation of bladder and prostatic tumors outside the body. *J Urol.* 1:3-15, 1917.
4. Röhl, L. Prostatic hyperplasia and carcinoma studied with tissue culture technique. *Acta Chir Scand.* 240(suppl):1-88, 1959.
5. Allgöwer, M. The cultivation of human prostate adenomata in vitro. *Exper Cell Res.* 1(suppl):456-9, 1949.
6. Cone, R. E., Hooks, C. A., Pomerat, C. M. et al. Correlation studies on prostatic fluid, prostatic tissue, and the testis with histopathological, Papanicolaou smear and tissue culture technique. *Tex Rep Biol Med.* 7:462-7, 1949.
7. Merchant, D. J. Model systems for the study of prostatic cancer. *Oncology.* 34:100-1, 1977.
8. Zeigel, R. F., Arya, S. K., Horoszewicz, J. S. et al. A status report: human prostatic carcinoma, with emphasis on potential for viral etiology. *Oncology.* 34:29-44, 1977.
9. Sato, G., Desmond, W. and Kelly, F. Human prostatic tumors in conditioned animals and culture. *Cancer Chemother Rep.* 59:47-59, 1975.
10. Merchant, D. J. Prostatic tissue cell growth and assessment. *Semin Oncol.* 3:131-40, 1976.
11. Scott, W. W. Growth and development of the human prostate. *Natl Cancer Inst Monogr.* 12:111-19; 1963.
12. McNeal, J. E. Age-related changes in prostatic epithelium associated with carcinoma. Edited by K. Griffiths and C. G. Purripoint. In *Third Tenovus Workshop: Some Aspects of the Aetiology and Biochemistry of Prostatic Cancer.* Cardiff, Wales: Tenovus Workshop Publications, 1970, pp 23-32.
13. Narbaitz, R. Embryology, anatomy and histology of the male sex accessory glands. Edited by D. Brandes. In *Male Accessory Sex Organs.* New York: Academic Press, 1974, pp 3-15.
14. McNeal, J. E. The prostate and prostatic urethra: a morphologic synthesis. *J Urol.* 107:1008-16, 1972.
15. Kirchheim, D., Brandes, D. and Bacon, R. L. Fine structure and cytochemistry of human prostatic carcinoma. Edited by D. Brandes. In *Male Accessory Sex Organs.* New York: Academic Press, 1974, pp 397-405.
16. Paul, J. *Cell and Tissue Culture.* 5th Ed. Edinburgh: Churchill Living-

ston, 1975.

17. Eagle, H. Nutritional needs of mammalian cells in tissue culture. *Science.* 122:501-4, 1955.

18. Eagle, H. Amino acid metabolism in mammalian cell cultures. *Science.* 130:432-7, 1959.

19. Ham, R. G. An improved nutrient solution for diploid Chinese hamster and human cell lines. *Exper Cell Res.* 29:515-26, 1963.

20. Ham, R. G. Clonal growth of mammalian cells in a chemically defined synthetic medium. *Proc Natl Acad Sci USA.* 53:288-93, 1965.

21. Parker, R. C. *Methods of Tissue Culture.* 3rd Ed. New York: Paul B. Hoeber, Inc., 1961, pp 62-77.

22. Moore, G. E., Garner, R. E., and Franklin, H. A. Culture of normal human leukocytes. *JAMA.* 199:519-24, 1967.

23. Webber, M. M. Effects of serum on the growth of prostatic cells in vitro. *J Urol.* 112:798-801, 1974.

24. Schröeder, F. H., and Mackensen, S. J. Human prostatic adenoma and carcinoma in cell culture. The effects of androgen-free culture medium. *Invest Urol.* 12:176-81, 1974.

25. McLimans, W. F., Kwasniewski, B., Robinson, F. O. et al. Culture of mammalian prostatic cells. *Cancer Treat Rep.* 61:161-5, 1977.

26. Webber, M. M., and Stonington, O. G. Stromal hypocellularity and encapsulation in organ cultures of human prostate: application in epithelial cell isolation. *J Urol.* 114:246-8, 1975.

27. Stonington, O. G., and Hemmingsen, H. Culture of cells as a monolayer derived from the epithelium of the human prostate: a new cell growth technique. *J Urol.* 106:393-400, 1971.

28. Stone, K. R., Stone, M. P., and Paulson, D. F. In vitro cultivation of prostatic epithelium. *Invest Urol.* 14:79-82, 1976.

29. Bregman, R. U., and Bregman, E. T. Tissue culture of benign and malignant human genitourinary tumors. *J Urol.* 86:642-9, 1961.

30. Brehmer, B., Marquardt, A., and Madsen, P. O. Growth and hormonal response of cells derived from carcinoma and hyperplasia of the prostate in monolayer cell culture. A possible in vitro model for clinical chemotherapy. *J Urol.* 108:890-6, 1972.

31. Rose, N., Choe, B.-K., and Pontes, J. E. Cultivation of epithelial cells from the prostate. *Cancer Chemother Rep.* 59:147-9, 1975.

32. Kaighn, M. E., and Babcock, M. S. Monolayer cultures of human prostatic cells. *Cancer Chemother Rep.* 59:59-63, 1975.

33. Waymouth, C. To disaggregate or not to disaggregate. Injury and cell disaggregation, transient or permanent? *In Vitro.* 10:97-111, 1974.

34. Pretlow, T. G., II, Brattain, M. G., and Kreisberg, J. I. Separation and characterization of epithelial cells from prostates and prostatic carcinomas: a review. *Cancer Treat Rep.* 61:157-60, 1977.

35. Choe, B. K., Pontes, E. J., McDonald, I. et al. Immunochemical studies of prostatic acid phosphatase. *Cancer Treat Rep.* 61:201-10, 1977.

36. Fraley, E. E., Ecker, S., and Vincent, M. M. Spontaneous in vitro neoplastic transformation of adult human prostatic epithelium. *Science.* 170:540-2, 1970.

37. Okada, K., and Schröeder, F. H. Human prostatic carcinoma in cell culture: preliminary report on the development and characterization of an epithelial cell line (EB33) *Urol Res.* 2:111-21, 1974.

38. Ofner, P., Vena, R. L., Barowsky, N. J. et al. Comparative C_{19}-radiosteroid metabolism by MA-160 and HeLa cell lines. *In Vitro.* 13:378-88, 1977.

39. Nelson-Rees, W. A. Letter to the editor. *In Vitro.* 13:525, 1977.

40. Webber, M. M., Horan, P. K. and Bouldin, T. R. Present status of MA-160 cell line. Prostatic epithelium or HeLa cells. *Invest Urol.* 14:335-43, 1977.

41. Edwards, W. D., Bates, R. R. and Yuspa, S. H. Organ culture of rodent prostates; effects of polyamines and testosterone. *Invest Urol.* 14:1-5, 1976.

42. Dilley, W. G. and Birkhoff, J. D. Hormone response of benign hyperplastic prostate tissue in organ culture. *Invest Urol.* 15:83-6, 1977.

43. Vakarakis, M. J., Gaeta, J. F., Mirand, E. A. et al. Morphological responses of benign prostatic hypertrophic tissue to chemotherapeutic agents in an in vitro culture system. *J Med.* 15:65-71, 1975.

44. Lasnitzki, I., Whitaker, R. H. and Withycombe, J.F.R. The effect of steroid hormones on growth pattern and synthesis in human benign prostatic hyperplasia in organ culture. *Br J Cancer.* 32:168-78, 1975.

45. McMahon, M. J., and Thomas, G. H. Morphological changes in benign prostatic hyperplasia in culture. *Br J Cancer.* 27:323-35, 1973.

46. Harbitz, T. B. Organ culture of benign nodular hyperplasia of human prostate in chemically defined medium. *Scand J Urol Nephrol.* 7:6-13, 1973.

47. McMahon, M. J., Butler, A.V.J., and Thomas, G. H. Morphological responses of prostatic carcinoma to testosterone in organ culture. *Br J Cancer.* 26:388-94, 1972.

48. Stone, K. R., Mickey, D. D., Wunderli, H. et al. Isolation of a human prostate carcinoma cell line (DU 145). *Int J Cancer.* 21:274-81, 1978.

49. Kaighn, M. E., Lechner, J. R., Narayan, K. S. et al. Prostatic carcinoma: tissue culture cell lines. *Natl Cancer Inst Monograph.* (In Press) 1978.

50. Lechner, J. F., Narayan, K. S., Chnuki, Y. et al. Replicative epithelial cell cultures from normal human prostate. *J Natl Cancer Inst.* 60:797-801, 1978.

7

Animal Models for the Study of Prostatic Cancer

Donald S. Coffey, John T. Isaacs,
and Robert M. Weisman

THE IMPORTANCE OF ANIMAL MODELS

Many important therapeutic concepts have been derived from studies utilizing animal models of cancer. Among these accomplishments are the development and utilization of principles of tumor growth and cell kinetics, the testing of new concepts in combination and adjuvant therapy, and the preliminary screening of new cancer chemotherapeutic agents. In addition, these animal tumor models have been of value in elucidating basic principles of radiation and immunotherapy. Others have questioned the advantages of animal models and have stressed the limitations and difficulties in extrapolating useful information from animal studies to man.[1] Indeed, comparing similar human clinical studies has often yielded conflicting results because of the biologic variations of the tumor and host. The ultimate evaluation of any therapeutic modality will require careful randomized and controlled clinical studies; however, to define all therapeutic parameters and principles only in human studies would be prohibitively expensive, time consuming, and would in many cases involve ethical limitations. Waiting for clinical studies to resolve basic therapeutic questions has often been frustrating. For example, the simple question of the benefits of hormonal manipulation for the management of human benign prostatic hyperplasia started over 75 years ago with what appeared at that time to be a most successful study of 200 patients.[2,3] However, a recent review of numerous ensuing clinical studies still leaves the basic question of hormonal sensitivity of benign prostatic hyperplasia unresolved at the present time.[4] The inability of many different investigators using hundreds of patients on study to resolve this basic question within the last 75 years only emphasizes some of the difficulties encountered in the study of the human prostate. In contrast, recent canine studies of the condition have yielded important concepts that have shed new insight into the most common diseases even though the canine model has many obvious dissimilarities in comparison to the human.[5]

Even with extensive clinical experience utilizing estrogen therapy for human prostatic cancer for over 30 years, it has only recently become evident that no real estrogen dose-response data for benefit and risk were available to guide the clinician. In addition, the timing and beneficial effects of castration in the different disease states of prostatic cancer have not been resolved in a very compelling manner. In spite of these uncertainties it is still difficult, and perhaps rightfully so, to have new and untreated early-stage patients entered on experimental protocols utilizing rather toxic cancer chemotherapeutic drugs with unknown but hoped-for benefits in the control of human prostatic cancer. And yet this choice may be necessary if any real progress is to be made in the future against this common and stubborn form of cancer. In these cases it would be most helpful in making such difficult clinical decisions if we had experimental evidence that a proposed regimen showed promise in a well-controlled and appropriate animal model. Emphasis should be placed on controls because many important factors which can be controlled properly in the laboratory are difficult or almost impossible to control adequately in similar clinical studies. These factors include 1) uniformity of genetic strain and age of host, 2) controlled onset of tumor growth, 3) uniformity of tumor type, 4) precise knowledge of tumor load and growth rates, 5) regulation of dietary elements and physical stress, 6) total compliance to drug intake and timing, 7) complete follow-up, 8) uniform control over onset and termination of the study and subject, with all subjects available for autopsy, 9) large numbers in each study group, all monitored at the same time, and 10) one physician or observer making all evaluations. Other important variables could be listed which can best be controlled in the laboratory, and the fact that many of these variables are not or cannot be regulated within a clinical setting further emphasizes some of the difficulties that we must face in a realistic manner in resolving differences in human studies. Pioneering efforts are presently under way by the National Prostatic Cancer Project to provide the best rational basis for establishing clinical criteria for the evaluation of cancer chemotherapeutic drugs in a nationwide cooperative study. Furthermore, effort is being expended to evaluate animal models for prostatic cancer and to characterize their properties and determine if these models can be helpful in providing new leads to the control of prostatic cancer.

In summary, animal models are not sufficient within themselves to assess the full clinical importance of a therapeutic approach. However, they do provide a unique opportunity to develop new concepts that are most difficult to obtain through available clinical studies and within reasonable cost, time, and ethical restraints. Appropriate animal studies and careful clinical trials must work in concert to assist the search for new and more effective management of prostatic cancer, a disease which at present still kills over 18,000 men per year in the United States alone.

REQUIRED PROPERTIES AND LIMITATIONS OF ANIMAL MODELS

Selecting a single animal model for prostatic cancer may not be realistic because the human cancer counterpart is itself a variable and multifaceted disease. Each type of human tumor is often characterized by a wide spectrum of diversity in relation to pathology, state and variability of cellular differentiation, uniformity of growth rate, and differences in therapeutic responsiveness to hormonal, nonhormonal, and radiation treatment. Indeed, many of these variations can sometimes be observed in one patient. Because of this variability in the types of human prostatic cancer it is possible that more than one animal model may be required to correspond to these different states of human cancer. Even though we are aware of these variations within human and animal prostatic cancer we can refer to the more typical clinical picture and strive toward an animal model with similar properties and response. These idealized properties for an animal model of prostatic cancer are summarized as follows:

1) spontaneous in origin
2) developed in aged animals
3) proven origin from prostatic tissue
4) adenocarcinoma, slow-growing tumor
5) histologic similarity to human prostatic cancer
6) biochemical profile similar to prostate
7) malignant and metastatic patterns to bone and lymph nodes
8) elevates serum prostatic acid phosphatase levels
9) hormone-sensitive
10) capable of responding to castration and estrogen therapy followed by relapse to hormone-insensitive state
11) immunological parameters
    A) developed in syngeneic animals
    B) transplantable or easily induced
    C) contains tumor specific antigens
12) large numbers of animals available for statistical considerations
13) similar therapeutic response to human prostatic cancer
    A) correlates with past therapy
        (1) hormonal therapy
        (2) nonhormonal therapy
        (3) radiation sensitivity
    B) accurately predicts response to future modalities of human therapy
14) wide diversity of tumor types (differentiation, hormonal response, etc.) corresponding to human tumor variability

Species and Origin

The etiology of human prostatic cancer is still unknown, and while external factors such as carcinogens and viruses are possible causative factors, they have nevertheless failed to be proven as direct etiologic agents. Efforts must continue to resolve the roles of these potentially important factors, but as yet they still remain very speculative. The only firm evidence is that prostatic cancer develops spontaneously in aged males who were not castrated before puberty; therefore, this should be a prime prerequisite for the animal model. The dog develops spontaneous prostatic cancer with age and a few old rats have likewise produced prostatic adenocarcinomas which can be propagated by transplantation.[6] The most popular include the rat prostatic adenocarcinoma of Dunning R-3327 and the Pollard tumors.[7-11] For a more complete list, see Table 1.

Older primates have not been adequately studied in large numbers to determine the true spontaneous incidence of either prostatic cancer or spontaneous benign prostatic hyperplasia. This is due in part to the great expense of maintaining large numbers of aged primates and to the difficulty in permitting them to age sufficiently in captivity to develop these diseases. It is also very difficult to capture large numbers of older males for study. Because of evolutionary considerations the ideal animal models for prostatic cancer might be the higher primates, and it is anticipated that increasing interest in animal models for abnormal prostatic growth will soon involve these important species.

Organ

In animal models it is essential to establish the organ of tumor origin. In the human, prostatic cancer develops primarily in the outer regions of the prostate. The dog and human have no clearly defined prostatic lobes and it is difficult to draw clear analogies to homologous lobes in rats and other species, although it is obvious that the histology of the dorsal lobe of the rat is more similar to the overall normal human prostate than is the larger ventral lobe which is almost devoid of stromal elements. Although the dog and human have no clearly defined anatomical lobes, they may nevertheless have different functional zones or areas of different embryologic origins. This has not been established but is the basis of several active studies. It is important to know why prostatic cancer in humans is primarily limited to specific areas of the prostate and why the aged prostates of other species are devoid of these tumors.

Histology

Many carcinogen-induced animal prostatic tumors are squamous carcinomas and therefore are not similar to the human prostatic adenocarcinomas. In contrast, the spontaneous canine and rat tumors, both Dunning R-3327 and Pollard, are adenocarcinomas. Therefore the epithelial nature of the animal tumor must be established by both light and electron microscopic analysis and should be substantiated by appropriate histochemical similarities to the prostate epithelium. The presence of microvilli and secretory granules help establish the epithelial nature. Nuclear analysis should indicate the pleomorphic nature of a cancer nucleus, and karyotyping is required for species identity and continued identification of the transplanted cells.

Biochemical Studies

Several biochemical markers have been used in concert to identify cells of prostatic origin and while no single test is completely definitive, when taken together they do provide an overall biochemical profile of tumor and prostate. In addition, many markers are decreased or lost as cells become malignant or dedifferentiated to a more anaplastic nature. In all cases monitoring of the biochemical profile usually provides an identity of the state of the tumor. There are many biochemical factors associated with prostatic tissue and some of the more important include:

Enzymes and isozyme patterns
acid and alkaline phosphatase
leucine aminopeptidase
β-glucuronidase
arginase, lactic dehydrogenase
fibrinolysin
5 α-reductase
3 α and 3 β hydroxy steroid dehydrogenase
7 α-steroid hydroxylase
Small molecules
high ratio of dihydrotestosterone to testosterone
pattern of steroid conjugate
zinc, cadmium
spermine and spermidine
citric acid
Receptors, cytoplasmic and nuclear
dihydrotestosterone (DHT)
17 β-estradiol
nuclear uptake of DHT
Tissue-specific and secretory proteins
electrophoretic profiles
tissue and tumor-specific antigens

Elevated serum acid phosphatase levels have provided one of the useful biomarkers of metastatic human prostatic cancer. This is primarily due to the extremely high tissue levels of acid phosphatase that under normal conditions enter the secretions of the prostate; however, from metastatic prostatic adenocarcinoma cells the enzyme enters directly into the general circulation, raising the serum levels and providing an enzymatic marker. The prostatic tissue levels of acid phosphatase are highest in humans and decrease in other species. For example, the level per unit of tissue in the mouse prostate is only 1/6,000 of that of the human prostate. Relative prostatic tissue levels of acid phosphatase activity are man, 1200; baboon, 1100; rhesus monkey, 130; dog, 60; rat, 1.0; and mouse, 0.20. Therefore the extent of elevation of the serum levels of prostatic acid phosphatase in animal tumor models would be dependent on five factors: 1) the levels of acid phosphatase in the animal prostate from which the tumor was derived, 2) the state of maintained differentiation of the tumor, 3) the location of the tumor implant and metastasis, 4) the overall tumor load in the animal, and 5) the specificity of the assay and the stability of the enzyme in serum. Thus all animal tumor models may not exhibit elevation in serum prostatic acid phosphatase.

Metastatic Pattern

Factors controlling the extent and route of metastasis of human tumors are still poorly understood. Human prostatic cancer invades locally and metastasizes primarily to the lymph drainage and bone. Spontaneous tumors in the prostates of animals such as the dog follow similar patterns of metastasis and also produce elevated serum acid phosphatase values.[6] Many other animal tumors such as the Dunning R-3327 and Pollard tumors are transplanted subcutaneously and would by necessity follow different routes of metastasis from that of spontaneous prostatic tumor, although the end result may be nearly the same. Site of injection of the tumors (subcutaneous, intraperitoneal, intraprostatic), number of cells and state (free-cell suspension or small tumor tissue implants), hormonal treatment, and drug therapy can have marked effects on metastasis.[12]

Hormonal Response

The tumor should be hormonally sensitive requiring the presence of androgens for full growth, and demonstrate growth inhibition following castration, estrogen, or antiandrogen treatment. Most prostatic cancers in humans respond to androgen deprivation (castration or estrogen therapy), but it is generally concluded that hormonal therapy is not curative and subsequent relapse occurs in essentially all cases to a hormone-insensitive state. There are very few exceptions and therefore this feature should be one of the most important requirements of an appropriate animal model for prostatic cancer since the model should mimic the most consistent and important clinical response seen with the human cancer.[13] At present the treatment of prostatic cancer is limited severely by the hormonal-insensitive state that almost invariably follows favorable response to hormonal treatment. At present we have no insight into the mechanism of induction of hormone insensitivity in humans. The mechanism of the development of this hormonal insensitivity appears to have been resolved for the first time for prostatic cancer in an animal model.[13] The mechanism appears to be a phenomenon of preexisting resistant cell selection (clone selection) as opposed to a conversion or induction of hormone-sensitive cells to an insensitive state. There is some reason to believe that human prostatic cancer may also be multifocal in nature.[14]

Immunologic Parameters

Tumor immunology is increasing in importance as a consideration in cancer biology, etiology, and immunotherapy. Although many easy expectations for immunotherapy of cancer have not been realized, there is still great potential for immunological approaches as we increase our basic understanding of immunology. Tumor-associated antigens have been detected in membrane extracts from human prostatic cancer.[15,16] Similar tumor membrane antigens have also been detected in the Dunning R-3327 rat prostatic adenocarcinoma.[17] These studies emphasize the need for further immunologic investigations into prostatic cancer and they can best be carried out in tumor models in syngeneic animals. Syngeneic animals are essentially immunologically identical and will accept transplants from other animals of the group.

It is important to remember that many of the transplantable animal tumors could conceivably have picked up viral particles or foreign elements during the years of continuous transplantation. These foreign factors could complicate immunological studies since they may appear as tumor-associated antigens not common to the host.

Growth Rate and Cell Kinetics

Human prostatic cancer is a relatively slow growing tumor although the time necessary for one cell to double has not been determined. It is estimated that the tumor-doubling time may be greater than one month, which is not uncommon for many human solid tumor adenocarcinomas. Preliminary DNA-labeling studies indicate a small fraction of the prostate cancer cells in active DNA synthesis, which indicates a low ^{3}H-thymidine-labeling index. One individual tumor cell must divide or double approximately 30 times to grow to a number of tumor cells of one billion (10^9) which is a total tumor volume of one cc and is about the minimal size for early clinical detection. For example, a single original tumor cell doubling each month would require a minimum of 2½ years to grow to a tumor volume of one cc (1 division/month × 30 divisions = 30 months). These cell kinetic considerations have been discussed for prostatic cancer.[18]

Most animal tumors are rapidly growing with division times in hours or days. These systems would not mimic the very slow-growing human prostatic cancer. The Dunning R-3327 rat prostatic adenocarcinoma is the only slow-growing model available at this time and has a tumor-doubling time of 20 days.[13,9]

While slow-growing animal tumor models may be more similar to the human situation they nevertheless limit the number of investigations because they require long times for inoculated tumors to grow out to detectable sizes and another long period of time before the cancers terminate the animals. This limitation requires large colonies of animals under study for an extended period of time.

Tumor Stability, Diversity, and Characterization

Many tumors change properties with growth and diversity can develop; while this also appears to occur with human prostatic cancer, it can nevertheless cause difficulties in transplantable tumors where tumor type, growth rate, and histology can often change. It is therefore easy to lose a transplantable tumor line through irreversible changes or to develop multiple sublines, which has occurred with the Dunning and Pollard rat prostatic tumors. This diversity can be helpful in developing a broad range of cancer types with specific properties that more closely mimic a specific type of grade of human prostatic cancer. *Since tumor lines do not always remain stable with time, it is therefore essential to monitor the histology, growth rate, hormone sensitivity, and some biochemical markers and to report these tumor characteristics with each published study.*

In summary, a rose does not always remain a rose. Nomenclature of many of these transplantable animal tumors refers to an inherited or earlier designated tumor line number which may now have changed properties with continued transplantation. This is why standardization of reporting and identity is essential, but as of now has not been realized. Very few of these animal tumor lines have been properly characterized and reported. Continuing this policy will only cause added and unnecessary confusion.

Availability

Canine prostatic cancer would probably be an excellent animal model, but unfortunately low incidence makes it difficult to obtain sufficient numbers of animals for statistical study. The Dunning rat prostatic tumor (R-3327) has been made available to interested investigators through the National Prostatic Cancer Project. Other models such as the Pollard tumor are being distributed on individual bases but must be carried in a Lobund-Wistar rat line in order to propagate properly. Unfortunately the Fortner hamster tumor has been lost and is not available. Individual centers have the aged AXC rat tumor under study as well as the Mastomy tumors (see Table 1).

In order to preserve many valuable prostatic tumor lines, the National Prostatic Cancer Project has established a tissue bank at the University of Miami School of Medicine under the direction of Dr Theodore I. Malinin. This bank will serve as a safe depository for these animal tumors and not as a distribution center. It is important to note that cryopreserved tumor samples require several cycles of transplantation before they stabilize their properties.

Table 1
Spontaneous Prostatic Ad enocarcinomas in Animals

Species	Year	Investigators	Tumor
Rat	1961	W. F. Dunning	From dorsal prostate of aged (22 months) Copenhagen rat; syngeneic; androgen-dependent; transplantable
	1973	M. Pollard P. H. Luckert	Aged, germ-free Lobund Wistar; ?lobe prostate; hormone-sensitive; transplantable
	1975	S. A. Shain B. McCullough A. Segaloff	Aged AXC rats; ventral prostate; no metastases; not transplanted
Hamster	1960	J. G. Fortner J. W. Funkhauser M. R. Cullen	Aged Syrian golden hamster; transplantable; tumor has been lost
Dog	1968	I. Leav G. V. Ling	Aged (>8 yrs) mongrels; metastases; no occult tumor
Mastomy	1965	K. C. Snell H. L. Stewart	Aged female African rodent prostate
	1970	J. Holland	
Monkey	1940	E. T. Engel A. P. Stout	Aged Macaca mulatta

TRANSPLANTABLE DUNNING RAT PROSTATIC ADENOCARCINOMAS R-3327 SERIES (R-3327 A, B, C, D, E, F, G, H, HI, and AT)

Source and History

In August 1961, Dr W. F. Dunning of the University of Florida observed a spontaneous tumor of the prostate which occurred at necropsy in a Copenhagen male rat from the 54th brother x sister generation of line 2331. The rat was a 22-month-old retired breeder, and the tumor occupied a large portion of the lower abdominal cavity and appeared to involve primarily the dorsal prostate gland. This primary tumor was classified as a papillary adenocarcinoma and no metastases were identified. Ten-milligram grafts of the soft tumor tissue were transplanted to 10 rats, four of the same inbred line as the host of the primary tumor and six F_1 hybrids from a male Copenhagen x Fischer female cross. The transplanted tumors grew very slowly and became palpable on the 60th day. Histologic analysis of this transplanted tumor on the 245th day indicated glandular formation and cellular material corresponding to a normal dorsal-type gland of the rat prostate. The tumor was positive to periodic acid-Schiff (PAS) stain and negative to the dithizone stain, typical of dorsal-type glands. Samples of heart blood from the rat did not indicate an elevated serum acid phosphatase level. These findings were reported by Dunning in 1963. The tumor has been transplanted subcutaneously for 17 years in over 20 passages. The mean animal survival in a 13-year period (1961 to 1974) was reported by Dunning to be 356 days (maximum 670 days, minimum 141 days). Survival did not change significantly over the 13-year period. These survival data were obtained after transplanting one cubic millimeter of solid tumor subcutaneously.

This R-3327 tumor remains histologically a well-differentiated adenocarcinoma. In 1974 Voigt and Dunning reported on hormone sensitivity and metabolism of testosterone in the tumor line. In an in vivo study they were able to demonstrate the 5 α-reduction pathway in this tumor line. In addition, they observed differences in the growth rate between males and castrates, thus establishing the hormone dependency of the R-3327 tumor.

Dunning isolated eight different tumors which she designated A through H. In 1975 Voigt, Feldman, and Dunning reported on the development of R-3327A line which is an androgen-insensitive *squamous* cell carcinoma derived from the established line R-3327. This androgen-insensitive tumor, R-3327A, has a growth rate approximately 10 times that of R-3327. The tumor developed in the fifth transfer generation in 1965 and has now been transferred over 60 times. The androgen-insensitive squamous cell carcinoma grows well in castrates, females, and males.

This tumor did not have the ability to metabolize testosterone by the 5 α-reduction pathway. In addition it appeared that the R-3327 had the androgen receptor in the cytoplasm while this receptor was absent from the hormone-insensitive line (R-3327A).

Dunning has not reported the characteristics of the other R-3327 lines B through H. Following her retirement, R-3327 lines designated D through H are now maintained in the laboratory of Dr Alice Claflin of the University of Miami.[17] The G tumor has been reported to be a rapidly growing undifferentiated carcinoma which is hormone dependent. Transplanting 2×10^7 cells of the G tumor into intact males produces a palpable tumor within 3 weeks.[19] The H tumor line is a well differentiated adenocarcinoma which grows much more slowly.

In 1976 an anaplastic line developed from the R-3327H which is hormone-insensitive and grows at a very rapid rate, doubling in volume approximately every 48 hours. This line has been designated R-3327AT.[9]

In 1977 the hormone-sensitive R-3327H was placed in a castrate and a small fraction of cells grew, thus establishing a new line which was hormone-insensitive, a differentiated adenocarcinoma which was slow-growing.

In summary, the following nomenclature exists for the Dunning R-3327 tumor:

R-3327A a rapidly growing, hormone-insensitive, squamous cell carcinoma.

R-3327B through F five sublines not fully described or characterized.

R-3327G rapidly growing, undifferentiated, hormone-dependent line.

R-3327H slow-growing, well differentiated adenocarcinoma with active acini, hormone-dependent, well characterized (see Table 2).

R-3327HI hormone-insensitive (HI), slow growing adenocarcinoma. This line was established in 1977 from hormone-insensitive clones of cell which were present originally in the R-3327H. These are the fraction of cells that grew out when the R-3327H was grown in a castrate animal for a long period.[9,13,20] This tumor tissue contains micro-acini which are lined by inactive epithelial cells.

R-3327AT rapidly growing, hormone-insensitive, anaplastic tumor developed in 1976[9,13,18] (See Table 2).

Characterization of the Dunning R-3327 Tumors

Only the Dunning R-3327H (hormone-sensitive) and R-3327AT (anaplastic tumor) have been well characterized.[9,13,18] The essential features of these tumors are summarized in Table 2 and refer to the original papers for specific details.

Table 2
Summary of Properties of a Transplantable Dunning Rat Prostatic Adenocarcinoma and an Anaplastic Tumor

	R-3327H	R-3327AT
Source	Spontaneous in 22-month-old male Copenhagen rat. Appeared in dorsal prostate. Carried by transplantation for 17 years.	Developed spontaneously in 1976 as a subline from a transplant of the R-3327H.
Histology	Well differentiated prostatic adenocarcinoma. Columnar epithelial cells with microvilli lining numerous well developed acini containing PAS-positive secretory material. Minimal stroma and connective tissue. No cystic formations. Histochemistry similar to epithelial cells.	Very anaplastic. No acini formation or columnar epithelial structure. No cystic formation. Not a squamous cell tumor.
Biochemistry	Enzyme profile of tumor similar to dorsal lateral prostate tissue. Moderate activity of 5α-reductase. Androgen and estrogen cytoplasmic receptors present. Large tumor mass reduces size of accessory sex tissue and elevates serum acid phosphatase levels.	Low biochemical correlation to normal lobes of rat prostate. Low in 5α-reductase activity. Androgen receptor absent. No effect of tumor mass on accessory sex tissue; no increase in serum acid phosphatase levels.
Hormone Dependency	Androgens required for maximal growth. Grows best in intact mature males.	Does not require androgens for growth. Tumor grows equally well in castrates, females, or males.
Cell Kinetics and Growth Rates	Slow-growing. Tumor volume doubles every 15 to 20 days. Approximately 80% of the total tumor cells require androgens for maintenance and growth; 20% of tumor cells are androgen insensitive. Both hormone-sensitive and -insensitive cell types have same growth rate.	Rapid-growing, doubles volume every two days. Tumor established as constant line and transplants true. No return to hormone sensitivity has been observed.
Metastasis	Very low rate $< 1\%$.	Not present.
Therapy	Tumor undergoes partial involution with castration, antiandrogen, or estrogen therapy; however, the smaller number (20%) of hormone-insensitive cells continue to grow unabated and tumor relapses to a hormone-insensitive state.	Tumor growth not affected by androgen deprivation.

For details of characterization, see Smolev et al,[13,9] Weissman et al.[18] Original tumor described by Dunning.[7]

R-3327H The histology of this well differentiated adenocarcinoma indicates abundant acini with secretions, and the histologic changes are almost identical at the light and electron microscopic level to a well differentiated human prostatic adenocarcinoma.[9,13] The tumor epithelial cell plasma membranes contain microvilli and secretory granules. The cell and nuclei shapes appear malignant. A selection of 20 histochemical stains indicates a graded activity similar to the epithelial cells of the rat prostate (Table 3).

Cell kinetic and growth rate studies indicate that 93% of the inoculated tumor cells grow subcutaneously in an adult intact male; the doubling time of the tumor is approximately 20 days (Table 4). The absence of androgen obtained by castration, estrogen, or antiandrogen therapy reduced the size of the tumor growth by 84% to 92%.

While the R-3327H tumor attains a larger size when grown for six months in the presence of androgens, it was nevertheless noted that some growth was observed even in the castrate animals (Table 4). When the growth of the tumor in the castrate was monitored for a period of time and the log of tumor volume plotted against time, a straight line was obtained which did not extrapolate to the origin.[9] These cell kinetic studies indicated clearly that a specific fraction or clone (8% to 29%) of the total original tumor cells inoculated were *hormone-insensitive* cells that were capable of growing in the absence of androgens. These hormone-insensitive cells doubled every 20 days in a manner similar to that of hormone-sensitive cells (Table 4). The cells growing in the castrate for 180 days in the absence of hormone yielded a different histologic appearance. The cellular morphology of hormone-insensitive cells was compared to that obtained in the same experiment using the identical R-3327H inoculum but grown for 180 days in intact male rats or with androgens. Tumor cells grown in the absence of androgens produce micro-acini devoid of secretion, and the epithelial cells appear much smaller.[9] This hormone-insensitive tumor tissue has been removed, transplanted, and carried in castrate animals as a new slow-growing hormone-insensitive prostatic adenocarcinoma line termed R-3327HI. The importance of this new line (R-3327HI) is that it represents the type of cells which grow out following relapse to hormonal therapy and as such are the types of cells requiring nonhormonal or special therapeutic considerations. As with human prostatic adenocarcinomas, castration and estrogen therapy will not cure animals carrying the R-3327H tumor because of the small clone of these hormone-insensitive cells which continue to grow.

Markland and Lee reported that the R-3327 tumor contained androgen and estrogen cytoplasmic receptors.[21] This has been confirmed by Heston, Menon, Tananis et al. and they have compared the hormone-sensitive (R-3327H) and -insensitive cells R-3327HI.[22] The insensitive R-3327HI has a 68% reduction in cytoplasmic androgen-binding protein but the level is still higher than the normal dorsal-lateral prostate tissue (Table 5). In contrast, the cytoplasmic estrogen receptor level does not change and remains in both tumors almost 10-fold higher than the normal prostate. Small levels of the progesterone receptor appear in the hormone-insensitive lines (Table 5).

Therapy Several preliminary therapeutic studies have been performed with the Dunning tumors, including castration, estrogen, Estracyt, chemotherapeutic agents, immunopotentiation, and combination and adjuvant therapy.[13,19,18,20,23] It appears that Dunning tumor will be an interesting model for studying the biology and control of prostatic cancer. The major limitation with this model concerns the low rate of metastasis which is very different from human prostatic cancer. The reason for this has not been elucidated and may pertain to the state of the cells and sites of injection.

Table 3
Comparable Histochemical Properties of the Rat Prostate and the R3327H Adenocarcinoma

	Prostate			Dunning Tumor R3327H
Enzyme	Dorsal	Lateral	Ventral	adenocarcinoma
Acid phosphatase	+ + +	+ +	+ + +	+ + +
Alkaline phosphatase	+	+	+ +	+ +
Acetylcholinesterase	−	−	−	+
5′-Nucleotidase	−	+ +	± +	+ + +
ATPase	+	+	+	+ + +
α-Glycerol phosphate DH	+ + + + + +	+ + + +	+ + + + +	+ + +
β-OH butyric DH	+ + +	+ + + +	+ +	+ + +
Butyryl cholinesterase	−	−	−	+ +
Cytochrome oxidase	+	+/−	+	+ +
NAD diaphorase	+ + + + +	+ + + +	+ + + + +	+ + + +
Glucose-6-phosphate DH	+ +	+ + +	+ + +	+ +
β-Glucuronidase	+ +	+/−	+	+ +
Isopropyl alcohol DH	+	+	+ + +	+ +
Leucine aminopeptidase	+	+ + + +	+ +	+
Monoamine oxidase	−	+/−	−	+ + +
Propyl alcohol DH	+ + +	+	+ +	+ +
Nonspecific esterase	+ + + + + +	+ + + + +	+ + + + +	+ + + +
NADP diaphorase	+ +	+ + +	+ + + +	+ +
Isocitric acid DH	+	+ +	+ + +	+ +
Succinic acid DH	+ + +	+ + + + +	+ + + + +	+ + + +

Table 4
Effects of Hormone Manipulation on the Six-Month Growth of 1.5 X 10^6 Tumor Cell Inoculation of the Dunning R3327H Tumor Line

Hormonal Status		Tumor Weight		Total Cell Number		Fold Increase In Initial Cell Inoculum	% of Inoculated Cells Growing	Cell Doubling Time
Animal	Six Month Treatment	Absolute (Grams)	Relative	Absolute (10^8)	Relative			
Intact	None	3.47 ± 1.48	100	6.48 ± 2.7	100	432	93	20.9
Intact	Androgen (TP)	4.25 ± 1.10	122	6.40 ± 1.7	99	427	74	18.7
Intact	Estrogen (DES)	0.41 ± 0.06	12	0.65 ± 0.21	10	43	8	20.2
Intact	Antiandrogen (Flutamide)	0.60 ± 0.19	16	1.20 ± 0.32	18	80	16	20.3
Castrate	None	0.31 ± 0.07	8	0.68 ± 0.16	10	45	29	24.8
Castrate	Androgen (TP)	5.26 ± 1.69	151	8.73 ± 3.0	134	582	83	19.8

All animals injected with identical subcutaneous inoculations containing 1.5 × 10^6 viable tumor cells. Animals treated daily as indicated with testosterone propionate (TP), 20 mg/day; diethylstilbestrol (DES), 100 μg/kg/day; flutamide, 50 mg/kg/day.
For details, see Smolev et al.[9,13]

Table 5
Steroid Cytoplasmic Receptors in the Normal Prostate and in the Dunning Prostatic Tumor

	Androgen Receptor (R-1881)		Estrogen Receptor (Estradiol)		Progesterone (R-5020)	
	Affinity (10^{-10} M)	Capacity (femtomoles/g)	Affinity (10^{-10} M)	Capacity (femtomoles/g)	Affinity (10^{-10} M)	Capacity (femtomoles/g)
Dorsal-Lateral Prostate	7	1660	10	130	Not Detected	
Dunning Tumor Androgen Sensitive R3327H	7	4550	5	1,880	Not Detected	
Dunning Tumor After Relapse To Castration R3327HI	7	1730	4	1,400	10	690

From the studies of Heston, Menon, Tananis and Walsh[22]
Assays by sucrose density gradient and Scatchard plots

POLLARD PROSTATIC ADENOCARCINOMAS IN LOBUND-WISTAR RATS

In 1973 Dr Morris Pollard at the University of Notre Dame reported that spontaneous tumors were observed in germ-free, random-bred Lobund-Wistar rats in increasing frequencies and numbers as the rats advanced in age beyond 24 months. Most of these tumors involved endocrine organs and/or their target organs.[24,11,25,12] The tumors were predominantly benign, but some with malignant characteristics were noted in individual animals over age 30 months. Among 80 germ-free male Lobund-Wistar rats over 30 months of age there were nine with prostate adenocarcinomas. He does not believe that the germ-free status of the animals was an important consideration, but only permitted the animals to survive to the old age without the complications of bacterial infection. All of the animals also had benign liver tumors of unknown etiology. The tumors were free of virus particles and possibly could represent a carcinogenic effect, although this has not been established. The prostate tumors retained their original structural characteristics of combined epithelial and connective tissue cells. In addition, a few animals who were treated with estrogens for eight weeks had a decrease in the tumor size by about 50%. Three of the spontaneous prostate carcinomas were transplanted subcutaneously and propagated in a series of conventionally random-bred Lobund-Wistar rats. These animals also developed lymph node and pulmonary metastases.

Three Pollard tumor lines (I, II, and III) have been established in Lobund-Wistar strain. The cells have been grown in vitro as cell monolayers and when inoculated back into either males or females grew extremely rapidly, forming back the histologic appearance of the original adenocarcinoma. A special feature of these tumors is their ability to metastasize rapidly to the lung and other sites, primarily through the route of lymph drainage. In addition the tumors can metastasize through the blood vascular system. The extent of metastasis could be monitored by tumor foci in the lung; this could be reduced markedly by either cyclophosphamide, aspirin, or *Corynebacterium parvum* treatment. This appears to be a primary effect on the mechanism of metastasis because the primary subcutaneous lesions were not reduced in size. In contrast, anesthetic agents increased the extent of metastasis. In addition, the tumors do not appear to be antigenic. They can be controlled, but not cured, with cyclophosphamide (Cytoxan) therapy.

These tumors may be good models for studying metastasis; furthermore, they can be grown easily in culture which is an asset for metabolic studies. The disadvantages of these models are that they are not hormone-sensitive nor well differentiated, and they grow very rapidly (doubling time of 18 to 20 hours in vitro).

PROSTATIC ADENOCARCINOMAS IN THE AGED AXC RAT

Spontaneous prostatic adenocarcinomas were detected in the ventral lobes of 7 of 41 virgin, male AXC rats whose ages exceeded 34 months.[26,27] No tumors were observed in the dorsolateral prostate. These adenocarcinomas form proliferating epithelial cells that build up into cribiform patterns which in some cases form secretory products. Treating a group of 33 aged AXC rats with exogenous testosterone increased the incidence of prostatic adenocarcinomas to 70%.

At present three tumors have been successfully transplanted.[27]

It is too early to assess the advantages and limitations of these tumor lines. They do, however, represent another case of a high incidence of spontaneous prostatic tumors in rats, a species that has often been assumed to be free of this disease.

OTHER SPONTANEOUS PROSTATIC ADENOCARCINOMAS

Dog

Spontaneous tumors of the prostate gland have been observed in other species. In 1968 Leav and Ling made a comprehensive study of the pathology of adenocarcinoma of the canine prostate.[6] In an 11-year period between 1956 and 1967 they reported on 20 cases of prostatic adenocarcinoma in the dog and compared their finding with 761 cases in an age-matched, (no tumor) control series. In this study 90% of the 20 cases of canine prostatic adenocarcinoma occurred in dogs eight years of age or older. Similarities of this neoplasm to the one in man were demonstrated. These included morphologic similarities, a frequency of the tumor in older animals, skeletal metastases, histochemical demonstration of acid phosphatase, lipids in neoplastic cells, and routes of metastasis similar to those thought to exist in man. The main differences between the neoplasm in man and dog were 1) the reported absence of latent carcinoma in the canine prostate, and 2) the apparent low frequency of prostatic tumors in dogs, probably less than 1%. In addition, no specific anatomic regions of the canine prostate have been associated with the development of adenocarcinoma.

Mastomy

Snell and Stewart in 1965 reported the observation of an adenocarcinoma of the prostate gland in one female Mastomy (*Rattus natalensis,* a small African rodent) and proliferative hyperplasia in four others among a group of 55 untreated virgins.[28] Holland has also reported on spontaneous prostatic adenocarcinomas in two untreated, 26-month-old female Mastomys.[29]

Hamster

Dr Joseph G. Fortner reported that a 21-month-old hamster of an untreated group died on August 10, 1960. On autopsy a large tumor was observed in the pelvic region in the area of the prostate gland. There was invasion of the abdominal wall and bony pelvis. Metastasis was also present on the serosa of the colon and in the lungs. The tumor was a moderately undifferentiated prostatic adenocarcinoma with foci of papillary formation. The tumor was transplanted and grew well in both male and female animals and did not appear to be hormone-sensitive. After 67 generations the tumor retained the morphology similar to the original tumor. Hosts bearing the transplantable tumor developed lymph node and pulmonary metastases. Details of these findings were reported by Fortner, Funkhaueser, and Cullen in 1963.[30] Karyotype studies indicated that this tumor was composed of several cell lines. It has been reported that this hamster prostatic tumor line was later lost due to a freezer storage failure.

INDUCED TUMORS

Hormone Induction

Dr R. L. Noble has reported the development of adenocarcinomas of the dorsal prostate of Nb rats following prolonged treatment with testosterone propionate alone or in combination with estrone.[31,32] A few transplantable tumors were obtained and were hormone-independent, but one required estrogens for growth. Following withdrawal of the required estrogen the tumor involuted, and when subsequently treated with androgens became androgen-sensitive. These experiments were more complex than described here; however, Noble believes he has produced tumor progression which is apparently directed by switching from exogenous androgens to estrogens. These are most interesting observations that require further study and elucidation.

Carcinogens

This review has emphasized spontaneous prostatic tumors. Much work with carcinogens has produced primarily squamous carcinomas and sarcomas of the prostate. Carcinogen-induced tumors of the prostate have been reviewed.[33] At present there are no reliable carcinogenic models for prostatic adenocarcinomas that have the advantages of the spontaneous tumors.

CONCLUSION

At present there are several promising animal models of prostatic adenocarcinoma. Better characterization and careful study will soon reveal the advantages and disadvantages of each system. The old statements that prostatic cancer occurs only in man and dog do not appear to be correct. It will also be interesting to monitor the occurrence of abnormal prostatic growth in the higher primates.

REFERENCES

1. Handlesman, H. The limitations of model systems in prostatic cancer. *Oncology.* 34:96-9, 1977.

2. White, J. W. The results of double castration in hypertrophy of the prostate. *Ann Surg.* 22:1-80, 1895.

3. Cabot, A. T. The question of castration for enlarged prostate. *Ann Surg.* 24:265-309, 1896.

4. Scott, W. W., and Coffey, D. S. Nonsurgical treatment of human benign prostatic hyperplasia. *Vitam Horm.* 33:439-65, 1975.

5. Coffey, D. S., DeKlerk, D. P., and Walsh, P. C. Benign prostatic hyperplasia: current concepts. In *V International Congress of Endocrinology.* Vol. II, p. 495. Amsterdam: Excerpta Medica, 1976.

6. Leav, J., and Ling, G. V. Adenocarcinoma of the canine prostate. *Cancer.* 22:1329-45, 1968.

7. Dunning, W. F. Prostate cancer in the rat. *Nat Cancer Inst Monogr.* 12:351-70, 1963.

8. Voigt, W., and Dunning, W. F. In vivo metabolism of testosterone-^{3}H in R-3327, an androgen-sensitive rat prostatic adenocarcinoma. *Cancer Res.* 34:1447-50, 1974.

9. Smolev, J., Heston, W., Scott, W. et al. Characterization of the Dunning R-3327H prostatic adenocarcinoma: an appropriate animal model for prostatic cancer. *Cancer Treat Rep.* 61:273-87, 1977b.

10. Pollard, M. Spontaneous prostate adenocarcinoma in aged germfree Wistar rats. *J Natl Cancer Inst.* 51:1235-41, 1973.

11. Pollard, M., and Luckert, P. H. Transplantable metastasized prostate adenocarcinomas in rats. *J Natl Cancer Inst.* 54:643-9, 1975.

12. Pollard, M., Chang, C. F., and Luckert, P. H. Investigations on prostatic adenocarcinomas in rats. *Oncology.* 34:129-32, 1977.

13. Smolev, J. K., Coffey, D. S., and Scott, W. W. Experimental models for the study of prostatic adenocarcinoma. *J Urol.* 118:216-20, 1977a.

14. Byar, D., and Mostofi, F. Carcinoma of the prostate: prognostic evaluation of certain pathologic features in 208 radical prostatectomies. Examination of the step-section technique. *Cancer.* 30:5-13, 1972.

15. Brannen, G., Gomolka, D., and Coffey, D. S. Specificity of cell membrane antigens in prostatic cancer. *Cancer Chemother Reports.* 59:127-30, 1975.

16. Brannen, G., and Coffey, D. S. Tumor-specific immunity in patients with prostatic adenocarcinoma or benign prostatic hyperplasia. *Cancer Treat Rep.* 61:211-16, 1977.

17. Claflin, A. J., McKinney, F. C., and Fletcher, M. A. The Dunning R3327 prostate adenocarcinoma in the Fisher-Copenhagen F_1 rat; a useful model for immunological studies. *Oncology.* 34:105-9, 1977.

18. Weisman, R. M., Coffey, D. S., and Scott, W. W. Cell kinetics studies of prostatic cancer: adjuvant therapy in animal models. *Oncology.* 34:133-7, 1977.

19. Block, N. L., Canuzzi, F., Denefrio, J. et al. Chemotherapy of the transplantable adenocarcinoma (R-3327) of the Copenhagen rat. *Oncology.* 34:110-13, 1977.

20. Isaacs, J., Weisman, R. M., and Coffey, D. S. Animal models for prostatic cancer: properties of the Dunning R-3327 tumor lines. *Cancer Res.* (In press)

21. Markland, F., and Lee, L. Estrogen receptor characterization of the R3327 transplantable prostatic adenocarcinoma. *Fed Proc.* 36:513, 1977.

22. Heston, W.D.W., Menon, M., Tananis, C. et al. Androgen, estrogen, and progesterone receptors of the R-3327 Copenhagen rat prostatic tumor. *Cancer Letters.* (In press)

23. Muntzing, J., Kirdani, R., Saroff, J. et al. Inhibitory effects of Estracyt on R-3327 rat prostatic carcinoma. *Urology.* 10:439-45, 1977.

24. Pollard, M. Prostate adenocarcinomas in Wistar rats. *Rush-Presbyterian St Luke's Med Bull.* 14:12-22, 1975.

25. Pollard, M., and Luckert, P. H. Chemotherapy of metastatic prostate adenocarcinoma in germfree rats. *Cancer Treat Rep.* 60:619-21, 1976.

26. Shain, S., McCullough, B., and Segaloff, A. Spontaneous adenocarcinomas of the ventral prostate of aged AXC rats. *J Natl Cancer Inst.* 55:177-80, 1975.

27. Shain, S., McCullough, B., Nitchuk, M. et al. Prostatic carcinogenesis in the AXC rat. *Oncology.* 34:114-22, 1977.

28. Snell, K. C., and Stewart, H. Adenocarcinoma and proliferative hyperplasia of the prostate gland in female *Rattus natalensis* (Mastomys). *J Natl Cancer Inst.* 35:7-14, 1965.

29. Holland, J. Prostatic hyperplasia and neoplasia in female Praomys (Mastomys) natalensis. *J Natl Cancer Inst.* 45:1229-36, 1970.

30. Fortner, J., Funkhauser, J., and Cullen, M. A transplantable spontaneous adenocarcinoma of the prostate in Syrian (golden) hamster. *Nat Cancer Inst Monogr.* 12:371-9, 1963.

31. Noble, R., and Hoover, L. A classification of transplantable tumors in Nb rats controlled by estrogen from dormancy to autonomy. *Cancer Res.* 35:2935-41, 1975.

32. Noble, R. Sex steroids as a cause of adenocarcinoma of the dorsal prostate in Nb rats, and their influence on the growth of the transplants. *Oncology.* 34:138-41, 1977.

33. Fraley, E., and Paulson, D. Experimental carcinogenesis of the prostate. Edited by David Brandes. In *Male Accessory Sex Organs: Structure and Function.* New York: Academic Press, 1974.

Detection and Diagnosis of Prostatic Cancer

8

Zew Wajsman and T. M. Chu

The malignant potential of prostatic cancer still seems to be underestimated by many. It is true that in about 50% of autopsies a prostatic cancer will be "incidentally" found.[1-4] These "incidental" tumors are thought to be latent and most of the efforts are directed only to those patients who have an active prostatic cancer. It is still not generally realized that prostatic cancer is indeed a very malignant tumor and will be responsible for 57,000 new cases in the year 1977 with a predicted mortality of 20,000. It is the second most common cause of death from malignancy in males in the United States. It is a very serious problem among black men in whom there is a markedly increasing rate of incidence of prostatic carcinoma: 55% for black, and only 22.8% for whites between the years 1947 to 1969.[5]

During the last 50 years rectal examination remained the best method for early diagnosis of prostatic cancer. Unfortunately, even in highly selected groups who underwent careful annual checkups, only 20% of detected cases of prostatic cancer were in the early stage, ie, stage B. The great majority were in advanced stages when first detected.[6] There is an urgent need for the early detection of this malignant disease, by finding a biologic marker which could be used in mass screening of males above the age of 45.

METHODS OF DIAGNOSIS

Patients with prostatic cancer are diagnosed when they develop obstructive symptoms similar to those produced by prostatitis or benign prostatic enlargement.[7,8] Any such symptoms which cannot be otherwise explained should lead to prostatic biopsy even if the consistency of the prostate is not suspicious.[6]

This work has been supported in part by Grant #CA 15126 from the National Cancer Institute through the National Prostatic Cancer Project.

Needle Biopsy

Although needle biopsy can be done on an outpatient basis, we suggest the following procedures to decrease the incidence of clinical understaging of the disease.

Spinal, epidural, or general anesthesia will permit a rectal examination in complete relaxation. In many cases additional nodules may be detected. A careful palpation of the prostate is possible, and extension of disease to the seminal vesicle will be easier to detect. Bimanual examination may reveal pelvic masses or infiltration of the base of the bladder. It is our opinion that this type of evaluation may decrease the percentage of so-called stage A cases when unsuspected cancer is found on pathologic examination of the prostate removed for apparently benign disease.

While the patient is under anesthesia, a needle biopsy is performed and three or four tissue specimens may be obtained from the suspicious as well as randomly selected areas. The needle used most widely is the Franklin modification of the Silverman needle. We found that the Travenol "Tru-Cut" needle yields larger specimens, and is easier and more accurate to use. The biopsy is performed either transperineally or transrectally. The latter is more accurate in directing the tip of the needle into suspicious areas, especially when dealing with small nodules.

The procedure is completed with thorough cystoscopic examination. Complications of this approach are rare when an accepted technique is used.

The accuracy of needle biopsy is high, but the pathology report should provide an explanation for abnormality felt on rectal examination. There is only a 50% chance that a palpable nodule is neoplastic in nature.[9] It may be a stone (to be demonstrated by x-ray), benign hyperplasia, granulomatous prostatitis, or tuberculosis. A normal prostatic gland found on histologic examination should alert the clinician to the fact he may have missed the suspicious area, and he should consider repeating the biopsy procedure.

Aspiration Fine-Needle Biopsy

In 1960 a cytologic diagnosis of prostatic tumors by aspiration biopsy was described.[10] A cytologic accuracy of 93.35% with this technique was recently reported.[11] The advantage of using a fine-needle biopsy is obvious as it can be carried out frequently and may provide preliminary information on the success of hormonal, radio-, or chemotherapy. Obviously this method can be used only in very specialized centers, which is the great disadvantage of aspiration prostatic biopsies.

Transurethral Biopsy

Transurethral resection to obtain suitable tissue usually is sufficient only in advanced prostatic carcinoma. The tissue thus obtained is generally available only indirectly, as this procedure has been designed primarily to relieve the symptoms of prostatism. It is uncommon for prostatic carcinoma in its early stages to be revealed by this means.[12]

Perineal Biopsy

Open perineal biopsy was widely used before the availability of biopsy needles and before staging lymphadenectomy and total retropubic prostatectomy had gained popularity. Today this particular approach is being used less and less frequently in most centers.

In rare cases it is difficult to distinguish between carcinoma of prostatic origin and carcinoma of the urethral glands extending into the prostate. The clinician should keep in mind that unfixed tissue can be treated for acid phosphatase staining, an aid to the pathologist in the diagnosis of these particularly perplexing cases.

In spite of all precautions, 8% carcinoma will be entirely unsuspected before surgery.[13] The pathologist is not only expected to diagnose a prostatic cancer, but often is pressed by the clinician to provide a prognosis based on cytologic and other criteria. This is a very important and debatable issue: to predict or detect the malignant potential of each specimen. It is a goal of the National Prostatic Cancer Project to combine the efforts of the pathologist and clinician in analyzing all possible factors to arrive at meaningful decisions with regard to treatment.

Clinical Staging

The commonly used Whitmore system divides all cases of prostatic cancer into four stages (Figure 1).[14]

Stage A A focus of prostatic cancer is found incidentally by the pathologist in tissue removed by transurethral resection or open prostatectomy for benign disease. Rectal examination does not reveal any suspicious lesion before surgery. Stage A disease may be present in only one or two small areas, or may be multifocal. The prognosis of such lesions depends on grading of the tumor and the number of foci found. To achieve maximal accuracy of staging in case of a focal involvement a repeat transurethral resection is indicated to detect or rule out multifocal disease.

CLINICAL STAGING OF
PROSTATIC CANCER

STAGE A
(? OCCULT
INCIDENTAL)

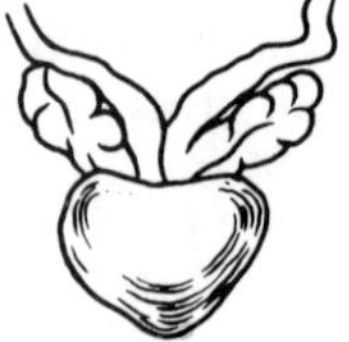

STAGE B
(NODULAR OR LIMITED
WITHIN THE GLAND)

STAGE C
(LOCALIZED TO THE
PERIPROSTATIC AREA)

STAGE D
(D_1 REGIONAL METASTASES
D_2 DISTANT METASTASES)

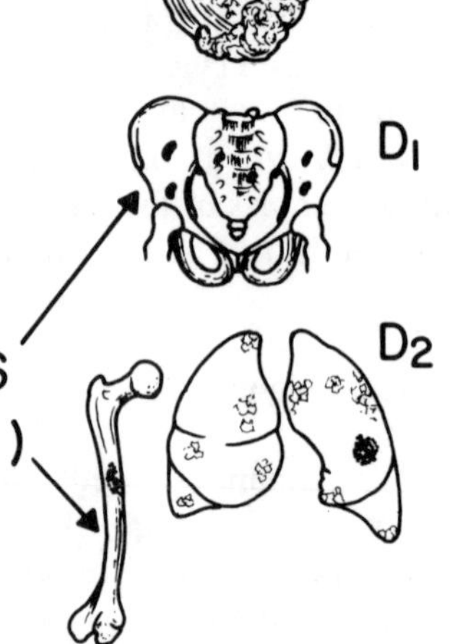

Figure 1. Commonly used method of clinical staging of prostatic cancer.

Recently clinicians recognized that clinically localized cancer should be subdivided on the basis of the extent of microscopic foci or the extent of induration.[15] Stage A_1 is essentially a focal carcinoma with lesions in only a few small areas. Stage A_2 consists of lesions throughout the resected tissue and is suggestive of increased risk of metastatic disease.

Stage B The disease is localized as a single nodule inside the prostatic lobe. In Stage B_1 the nodule is localized to a 1.0 to 1.5 cm portion of the lobe. In Stage B_2 there is a more extensive lesion involving the entire lobe, or it may be found in both lobes.

Stage C This consists of local spread of the cancer to most of the gland, extending to the capsule, and/or invading the seminal vesicle or bladder neck. This is the stage which commonly brings the patient to the physician with symptoms of lower urinary tract irritation and prostatism. Signs associated with hematuria are also frequently encountered.

Stage D This is divided into two classes and is frequently associated with metastases to bone or soft tissue in the area of the true pelvis.

Lymphatic spread confined to pelvic nodes below the aortic bifurcation is usually classified into subgroup D_1. Presenting symptoms range from those that are inapparent in Stages A and B to those associated with perineal discomfort and back pain, evidence of weight loss, anemia, and hematuria as seen in varying degree in Stage C or Stage D prostatic cancer.

Metastatic disease involving lymph nodes beyond the pelvis and/or soft tissue and bones is classified as Stage D_2.

Clinical staging of the prostate, however, is not entirely accurate. Further evaluation of this particular classification depends upon the effectiveness of other techniques.

Bone Scan

Radioisotope bone imaging is a rapid, easily performed, noninvasive method for evaluation of bone metastases. Introduction of a phosphate compound labelled with ^{99m}Tc has clearly improved the accuracy of this method. It has been demonstrated that 19% to 30% of patients with positive bone scan for metastatic prostatic cancer have normal bone radiographs.[16] It is now acceptable to evaluate the skeletal system for metastases with a bone scan and omit x-rays if the scan is negative.

There is, of course, a possibility of false-positive findings with this sensitive method. In doubtful cases bone scan followed by x-ray tomography of the suspicious area will confirm the diagnosis. If the diagnosis is still in doubt, a biopsy of the bone lesion may provide a definitive answer before radical surgery or radiotherapy is decided upon.

Much effort has been placed in the past on the direct identification of tumor cells in bone marrow of patients with prostatic cancer as a trial for improvement of the staging and in early detection of metastatic disease.[17,18] In some patients positive cytologic findings in bone marrow aspirates were the only evidence for distant metastases.

In reviewing 556 bone marrow aspirations performed during a 10-year period, Nelson and his coworkers found that 7.6% of the cases had positive cytologic findings.[19] Most of the positive cases were in late stages of the disease.

Because of the low incidence of positive cytology and high false-positive results in bone marrow acid phosphatase determination, it appears that this technique has little value in evaluating and staging patients with carcinoma of the prostate.[20]

Lymphangiography

The use of lymphadenectomy revealed that 20% of clinical stage B and about 50% of Stage C patients have positive nodes.[21] The preoperative evaluation of pelvic and paraaortic lymph nodes is made possible by pedal lymphography, which is a useful diagnostic aid in bladder cancer, and has been shown to have a high degree of accuracy in prostatic cancer.[22,23]

Castellino et al. reported an accuracy of 89% for lymphangiography.[24] The limitation of this procedure is in the evaluation of medially located lymph nodes which are at high risk for metastases. These nodes are not always opacified.[24] Other abnormalities of lymph nodes such as fibrosis, fatty replacement, and reactive hyperplasia may lead to false-positive reports. False-negative results occur when the tumor is confined to microscopic foci without change in the appearance of the opacified nodes. This diagnostic procedure requires considerable expertise and rigid criteria for interpretation to reduce the number of false-positives. However, when lymphangiographic findings are positive in the case of pelvic or paraaortic lymph nodes, the surgical approach and planning for radiotherapy are greatly facilitated.

Surgical Staging

Pelvic lymphadenectomy has been demonstrated to be a safe and valuable method in staging of patients with prostatic cancer.[21,25] An incidence of 35% of clinically unsuspected lymph node involvement was found in a prospective study. The frequency of nodal involvement was 21% in Stage B_1, 30% in stage B_2, and 50% in Stage C. In 24% of the cases the lymph nodes contained micrometastases only, and appeared normal on palpation. It appears that meticulous lymph node dissection rather than random sampling of pelvic nodes is necessary to achieve a high rate of detection of unsuspected metastases.

The new, recently described methods of percutaneous biopsy of retroperitoneal lymph nodes has yet to be proven to be of value in staging of prostatic cancer.

Growing experience with the CAT scanner may help in the evaluation of pelvic and paraaortic lymph nodes and improve the accuracy of clinical staging of prostatic malignancy.

BIOLOGIC MARKERS IN DIAGNOSIS AND STAGING

Acid Phosphatase

The acid phosphatases are a group of phosphohydrolases which hydrolyze phosphoric monoesters at an acidic pH. They may also be called orthophosphoric monoester phosphohydrolases. Acid phosphatase was first found in erythrocytes in 1924.[26] In 1935 Dmochowski and Assenhajm, while investigating phosphatase activity in human urine, noted a sporadic increase of acid phosphatase activity.[27] Kutscher and Wolbergs found an elevation of the enzyme activity only in adult males, indicating the male genital tract as a possible source of the enzyme.[28] The hypothesis was later confirmed when the ejaculate was found to contain an abundance of acid phosphatase.[29] They also found that the normal human prostate gland was very rich in acid phosphatase. These observations were confirmed and later extended by Gutman and his associates, who contributed greatly to the study of acid phosphatase.[30,31]

In addition to prostate, numerous tissues such as bone, spleen, kidney, and liver were found to have acid phosphatase activity.[32] The human prostate had the highest enzyme activity of all tissues, up to 1000 times more; although this high level appears only after puberty. The caudal lobe of the prostate gland of the Rhesus monkey was also found to have a very high activity of this enzyme.[33]

Gutman and his associates were the first to establish the significance of acid phosphatase in human disease.[31] An increase in serum acid phosphatase levels has been reported in 70% to 90% of patients with carcinoma of the prostate with bone metastases.[34,35] The enzyme activity was also increased in 5% to 30% of patients with nondemonstrable metastases.[36-38] Serum acid phosphatase may also be somewhat elevated in benign prostatic hypertrophy, prostatic infarction, and after prostatic massage.[39-41]

Although human erythrocytes are rich in acid phosphatase, Gutman showed the erythrocytic acid phosphatase is resistant to sodium fluoride and different from that of prostatic origin.[42] Acid phosphatase, because it hydrolyzes a wide spectrum of phosphate esters, is distinct from other enzymes, such as hexophosphatase, which are highly substrate-specific.

Acid phosphatase has been shown to exist as more than one isoenzyme. Sur, Moss and King demonstrated 13 active isoenzymes after starch gel electrophoresis of aqueous extract of human prostate.[43] These isoenzymes have the same pH optimum of 5.5 and the same Michaelis constant. Similar findings have been confirmed by other investigators; with gel electrophoresis, as many as 20 bands could be observed.[44] Recently, we have studied the acid phosphatase isoenzymes from prostatic tissues by isoelectric focusing technique.[45] A purified sample of prostatic acid phosphatase exhibited at least eight isoenzymes with pH of 4.5 to 5.5. Sera from patients with cancer of the prostate showed similar isoenzyme patterns of acid phosphatase.[46] The level of serum acid phosphatase activity depends upon the substrates used. Because the acid phosphatase has a broad spectrum of actions on a variety of phosphoric esters, elevation of acid phosphatase activity may be detected in patients with nonneoplastic disease.

In an attempt to determine a specific prostatic function of acid phosphatase, various inhibitors such as ethanol, formaldehyde, L-tartrate, and heat have been applied to alter or destroy the activity of other fractions of the enzyme.[47-49] It was observed more than two decades ago that sodium fluoride had only a slight (8%) inhibitory effect on erythrocytic acid phosphatase, but possessed a marked (96%) inhibition on prostatic acid phosphatase. Similarly, L-tartrate had a high (94%) inhibitory effect on prostatic acid phosphatase activity and none on erythrocytic acid phosphatase.[48] Fishman and Lerner advocated the use of tartrate-inhibited fractions of serum acid phosphatase as a specific index for the enzyme activity of prostatic origin.[49] However, the ability of this technique to differentiate prostatic acid phosphatase from total serum acid phosphatase has been disputed.[38,50]

Most recently the human prostatic acid phosphatase was characterized biochemically.[51] It has a molecular weight of 100,000 daltons, and biochemical analysis showed that the prostatic acid phosphatase was a glycoprotein consisting of 7% carbohydrates and 93% protein. The composition of the carbohydrates and amino acids is shown in Tables 1 and 2.

The elevation of serum acid phosphatase in patients with prostatic carcinoma has been reported to correlate more with the extent rather than the site of metastases. As noted above, about 10% to 30% of patients with carcinoma of the prostate, have normal enzyme activity levels in spite of bone metastases. This may be due to instability or inhibition of enzyme activity or because, when tumor cells are poorly differentiated, little acid phosphatase is produced.[52] The difficulties in measuring serum prostatic acid phosphatase activity, in addition to its instability, are most probably due to the use of a nonphysiologic pH environment (5.0 to 6.2), as well as the fact that it is an artificial substrate. The data of enzyme activity, therefore, may present the true activity of the enzyme in vitro.

An entirely different approach, primarily the use of immunochemical techniques, has been employed in the last few years for the detection of prostate-specific acid phosphatase. Cooper and Foti reported a radioimmunoassay for acid phosphatase.[53] They used acid phosphatase isolated from prostatic fluid of young males for production of an antiserum in rabbits, thereby developing a solid phase radioimmunoassay. Normal serum was found to have 39.9 ng/ml of prostatic acid phosphatase with a standard deviation of 24.0. Although the assay still presents a 13.5%

Table 1
Carbohydrate Analysis of Purified Human Prostatic Acid Phosphatase

Carbohydrate		Content (g/mol)
Fucose		346.2
Galactose		628.0
Mannose		1728.5
Sialic Acid		1985.0
N-Acetylglucosamine		2280.0
	Total	6967.7

The total carbohydrate content of 1 mole of acid phosphatase is approximately 7% of its total molecular weight.

Table 2
Amino Acid Composition of Purified Human Prostatic Acid Phosphatase Molecular Weight: 102,000

Amino Acids	Residues/ Molecule	Amino Acids	Residues/ Molecule
Aspartic Acid	54	Leucine	93
Threonine	50	Tyrosine	43
Serine	54	Phenylalanine	32
Glutamic Acid	100	Lysine	45
Proline	50	Histidine	26
Glycine	42	Arginine	33
Alanine	27	Tryptophan	18
Valine	34	Cysteine	16
Methionine	20		
Isoleucine	27	Total	764

The amino acid content of 1 mole of acid phosphatase is approximately 90% of its total molecular weight.

false-positive rate for male nonprostatic cancer patients, the test detected the elevation of serum prostatic acid phosphatase in seven untreated, Stage A prostatic cancers (mean 84 ng/ml, range 50 to 110) which were missed by conventional spectrophotometric methods.[54] A similar, double-antibody radioimmunoassay has also been developed by others.[55]

We have developed another immunochemical technique for the detection of prostatic acid phosphatase.[51] The purified acid phosphatase was obtained from cancerous human prostates and produced a specific antiserum in rabbits. This antiserum did not cross-react with acid phosphatase originating in other tissues. A counterimmunoelectrophoretic method, utilizing the specific antiserum and a sensitive chemical staining technique, has been developed (Figure 2). Sera from patients with prostatic cancer (6/20 of Stage B, 24/49 of Stage C and 98/125 of Stage D) gave positive results. The specificity of the method was tested with prostatic sera of 19 patients with benign hypertrophy, 89 males with other

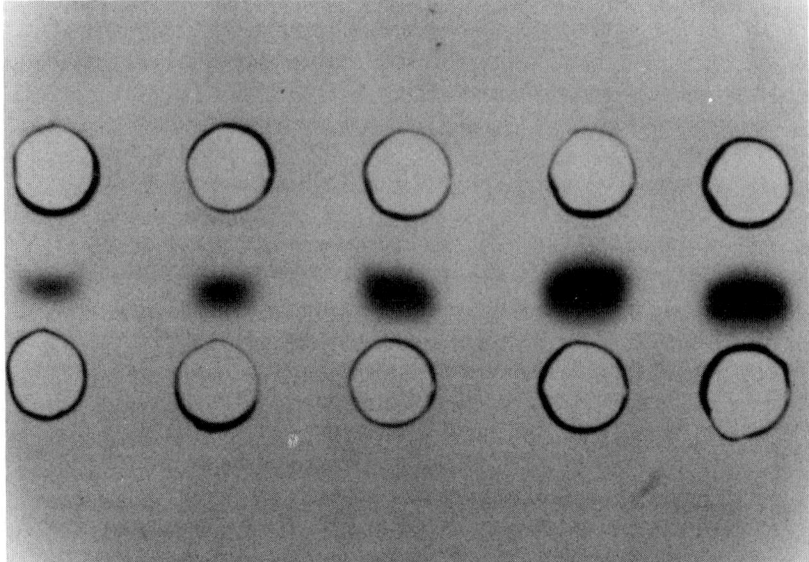

Figure 2. Serum prostatic acid phosphatase as detected by counterimmunoelectrophoresis. The wells at the cathodic (left) side, from top to bottom, contained 1.60, 0.80, 0.40 and 0.20 ng per 10 μl of the enzyme, respectively. Ten μl of diluted rabbit antiserum against purified prostatic acid phosphatase were placed in each well at the anodic (right) side. After electrophoresis at pH 6.5 for two hours, enzyme activity was detected by incubating gel with α-naphthyl phosphate and fast Garnet GBC salt.

cancer, 107 healthy volunteers, and 50 normal age-matched men. All exhibited negative results. The sensitivity of this method was 20 ng/ml of prostatic acid phosphatase protein, which was comparable to that of the radioimmunoassay.[54] A comparison of the new method with the conventional is shown in Table 3.

It is still questionable if this extremely sensitive method for human prostate-specific acid phosphatase is actually detecting an early microscopic metastatic spread, or if the enzyme level is elevated in localized disease and if so, if it could be used in mass screening of patients at high risk. The National Prostatic Cancer Project together with the American Cancer Society is testing this method in depth in many medical institutions, and final results should be available soon.

Bone Marrow Acid Phosphatase

Bone marrow acid phosphatase activity was described as a reliable and sensitive parameter for staging of prostatic carcinoma.[56] The determination of bone marrow acid phosphatase activity was found to be a more sensitive parameter for bone metastases than serum acid phosphatase, bone scanning, or routine skeletal survey. For instance, 5 of 16 patients

Table 3
Comparison of Conventional and New Method of Acid Phosphatase Determination

Conventional	National Prostatic Cancer Project Method
1. Not specific	1. Specific to prostatic acid phosphatase
2. Indirect activity only	2. Direct measurement of amount produced
3. 10% false-positives	3. No false positives
4. Usually not elevated in early cancer	4. Elevated in 30% of Stage B patients
5. Elevated in 30% with Stage C	5. Elevated in 55% of Stage C patients

with negative skeletal survey, negative bone scan, but elevated bone marrow acid phosphatase, died of disseminated prostatic cancer. In some patients initial elevation of bone marrow acid phosphatase was followed only later by positive bone scanning and subsequent radiologic signs of metastases. Some other investigators have recently advocated the use of bone marrow acid phosphatase for the staging of patients with carcinoma of the prostate as well as detecting bone metastases.[57-60] However, more recent reports have indicated that a significant number of false positive results were noted.[61,62] In our own study elevated levels of bone marrow acid phosphatase were detected in patients with prostatic cancer; however, false-positive results occurred at a 50% rate using a common spectrophotometric method; they were eliminated when acid phosphatase was measured by the immunologic technique.[63] Therefore, it is reasonable to conclude that the practical usefulness of bone marrow acid phosphatase as measured by conventional spectrophotometric methods is limited because of its poor specificity, and should not be used as the sole laboratory test for decisions concerning the management of patients. On the other hand, the high specificity and sensitivity of the counterimmunoelectrophoretic method for serum acid phosphatase and its high correlation with bone marrow assays usually eliminates the needs for the latter.[20]

Alkaline Phosphatase Isoenzyme

Serum alkaline phosphatase has been reported to be of value as an aid in diagnosis and evaluation of effectiveness of therapy in patients with cancer of the prostate.[64] In general, serum alkaline phosphatase activity was markedly elevated in patients with Stage D (greater than 80% of cases) carcinoma of the prostate. This is due to metastases from the prostatic tumor to bone, involving an osteoblastic process.[65] This is different from osteolytic metastases from breast tumor in which serum alkaline phosphatase is only slightly elevated.

Bone isoenzyme of serum alkaline phosphatase has been shown to be a more sensitive indicator of bone metastases than total alkaline phosphatase. In a study of 180 consecutive patients with Stage D cancer, 80% were found to have an abnormal activity of serum alkaline phosphatase, and 91% had elevated bone alkaline phosphatase.[66] Furthermore, the bone isoenzyme of alkaline phosphatase was shown to be of prognostic value, as patients with higher pretreatment levels generally showed a poorer response to therapy.[66] Bone alkaline phosphatase isoenzyme was found to be elevated in some cases in the presence of blastic metastases, while the total alkaline phosphatase was normal. It is suggested, therefore, that in staging of prostatic cancer determination of bone alkaline phosphatase isoenzyme may be used as a marker for early bone metastases.

In a significant number of patients (greater than 80%) with advanced stage of prostatic cancer, a "tumor" alkaline phosphatase isoenzyme (Regan or placental alkaline phosphatase), as measured by inactivating serum at 65°C for five minutes, was detected. It remains to be determined whether this "tumor" isoenzyme can be detected in the early stages of cancer.

Lactate Dehydrogenase Isoenzyme

The utilization of tissue lactate dehydrogenase isoenzyme has been reported in the diagnosis of prostatic carcinoma. In 1970 Oliver et al[67] reported a ratio of tissue LDH-V to LDH-I greater than one in 78% of instances of pathologically malignant lesions, and a ratio of less than 1 in 86% of the pathologically benign glands. However, this practice has not been widely accepted, as data regarding a negative aspect of LDH and LDH isoenzymes in prostatic cancer were subsequently reported.[68,69]

In a very recent study, Hein, Grayhack and Goldberg[70] measured the LDH isoenzyme patterns in prostatic fluid. Fluid from 12 (80%) of the 15 patients with prostatic cancer showed an LDH-V/LDH-I ratio of more than 3. This ratio was exceeded in only 6 (12%) of 57 and 14 (15%) of 97 patients in whom the diagnosis of benign prostatic hyperplasia without evidence of infection was established histologically or clinically. Therefore, they suggested that an LDH-V/LDH-I ratio of greater than 3 in the prostatic fluid, in the absence of a history of infection, should be regarded as an indication of a high risk for the presence or development of a malignancy in the prostate gland.

Urinary Cholesterol and Ketosteroids

Urinary excretion of nonesterified cholesterol has been reported to be useful in diagnosis of prostatic neoplasm.[71] In 32 patients with adenocarcinoma of the prostate, 29 (91%) had elevation of nonesterified (free) cholesterol in their urine. However, care should be taken in interpreting the relationship of urinary-free cholesterol and cancer of the prostate. Approximately 25% of the control patients older than 45 years, without histologically proven prostatic cancer, also exhibited an elevation of urinary nonesterified cholesterol. Further, patients with metastases demonstrated an elevation of this steroid even after the primary tumor had been resected. Individuals with cancer of the breast, testes, and other sites have been reported to have hyperexcretion of this steroid.[72]

Murphy et al. have reported that in a significant number of patients with prostatic cancer, the ratio of 11-deoxy to 11-oxy-ketosteroids in urine can be used as a laboratory parameter for the diagnosis of prostatic cancer.[73]

Multiple Biochemical Markers

It is apparent that no single test has been found to be satisfactory for the diagnosis and prognosis of prostatic carcinoma. An improved assay of a combination of tests which could be more sensitive in early detection of cancer and could monitor more accurately the course of disease would be most desirable and valuable. Chu et al. employed the simultaneous measurement of serum acid phosphatase activity, urinary total cholesterol, and ratio of urinary 11-deoxy to 11-oxy 17-ketosteroids in a group of 14 age-matched healthy individuals as controls.[72] The purpose was to evaluate whether or not the simultaneous determination of these three tests would increase the rate of detection obtained by a single assay alone. It was shown that the detection rate was 67% for serum acid phosphatase activity alone, 62% for urinary total cholesterol, and 22% for ratio of 17-ketosteroids. A significant increase in detection rate was observed when simultaneous determination of two assays was performed, 85% for serum acid phosphatase and ratio of 17-ketosteroids, and 74% for total urinary cholesterol and ratio of 17-ketosteroids. A much higher detection rate of 88% was obtained when all three assays were performed.

In another report Chu et al. compared serum ribonuclease and acid phosphatase.[74] Serum ribonuclease activities from patients with advanced prostatic carcinoma were significantly higher ($p<0.01$) than those from normal healthy men. In patients with prostatic tumor, no positive correlation was observed between serum ribonuclease and acid phosphatase activities. In some patients, where acid phosphatase activities were within the normal ranges, ribonuclease activities were elevated. Again, a combined positive detection rate increased to 85% when both tests were simultaneously determined, and the rate declined to 71% and 78% respectively when either assay was used alone. Therefore, it can be concluded that the use of multiple-markers testing may be of potential value in the diagnosis of prostatic cancer.

FUTURE PROGRESS

Computerized axial tomography ("whole body" scanners) can produce images from all parts of the body. This exciting major advance in radiology is gaining wide acceptance in detection of intraabdominal and intrathoracic masses.[75,76] It has also been used with success in precise biopsy localization, and has great potential value in early detection of prostatic cancer and accurate staging of this disease.[77] The recently described immunoassays for specific prostatic acid phosphatase are being tested on a national basis by the National Prostatic Cancer Project and the preliminary results are showing great promise for early detection and better staging of prostatic cancer.

REFERENCES

1. Rich, A. R. On the frequency of occurrence of occult carcinoma of the prostate. *J Urol.* 33:215-23, 1935.

2. Halpert, B., and Schmalhorst, W. R. Carcinoma of the prostate in patients 70 to 79 years old. *Cancer.* 19:695-8, 1966.

3. Schmalhorst, W. R., and Halpert, B. Carcinoma of the prostate gland in patients more than 80 years old. *Am J Clin Path.* 42:170-3, 1964.

4. Scott, R., Jr., Mutchnik, D. L., Laskowski, T. Z. et al. Carcinoma of the prostate in elderly men: incidence, growth characteristics, and clinical significance. *J Urol.* 101:602-7, 1969.

5. Cancer Statistics, 1976. American Cancer Society Professional Education Publications, Am. Cancer Society, Inc., New York.

6. Gittes, R. F., and Chu, T. M. Detection and diagnosis of prostate cancer. *Semin Oncol.* 3:123-30, 1976.

7. Bumpus, H. C. Carcinoma of the prostate: a clinical study of one thousand cases. *Surg Gynecol and Obstet.* 43:150-5, 1926.

8. Anderson, R. Carcinoma of the prostate: clinical observations and treatment. *Acta Chir Scand.* 246 (suppl):1-74, 1959.

9. Jewett, H. J. Significance of palpable prostatic nodule. *JAMA.* 160:838-9, 1956.

10. Franzen, S., Giertz, G., and Zajicek, Y. Cytological diagnosis of prostatic tumors by transrectal aspiration biopsy: a preliminary report. *Br J Urol.* 32:193-6, 1960.

11. Sonnenschein, R. The effectiveness of transrectal aspiration cytology in the diagnosis of prostatic cancer. *Eur Urol.* 1:189-92, 1975.

12. Hudson, P. B., Finkle, A. L., Trifilio, A. et al. Prostatic cancer: IX. Value of transurethral biopsy in search of early prostatic carcinoma. *Surgery.* 35:897-900, 1954.

13. Young, H. H., and Davis, D. M. *Young's Practice of Urology.* Philadelphia, W. B. Saunders Co., 1926.

14. Whitmore, W. F., Jr. Symposium on hormones and cancer therapy; hormone therapy in prostatic cancer. *Am J Med.* 21:697-713, 1956.

15. Grayhack, J. T., and Wendel, E. F. Carcinoma of the prostate. Edited by Lester Karafin, and A. Richard Wendel. In *Lewis' Practice of Surgery. Urology.* Vol. 2. New York: Harper & Row, 1977, pp. 1-25.

16. Marks, D. S., and Eyler, W. R. Radionuclide bone imaging in the evaluation of prostatic cancer. *Henry Ford Hosp Med J.* 23:161-8, 1975.

17. Clifton, J. A., Phillip, R. J., Ludovic, E. et al. Bone marrow and carcinoma of the prostate. *Am J Med Sci.* 224:121-30, 1952.

18. Flocks, R. H. Combination therapy for localized prostatic cancer. *J Urol.* 89:889-94, 1963.

19. Nelson, C.M.K., Boatman, D. L., and Flocks, R. H. Bone marrow examination in carcinoma of the prostate. *J Urol.* 109:667-70, 1973.

20. Catane, R., Wajsman, Z., Chu, T. M. et al. Simultaneous measurement of acid phosphatase activity in bone marrow and peripheral blood serum. *Surg Forum.* 28:128-30, 1977.

21. Whitmore, W. F., Jr., Hilaris, B., and Grabstald, H. Retropubic implantation of ^{125}Iodine in treatment of prostatic cancer. *J Urol.* 108:918-20, 1972.

22. Wajsman, Z., Baumgartner, G., Murphy, G. P. et al. Evaluation of lymphangiography for the clinical staging of bladder tumors. *J Urol.* 114:712-14, 1975.

23. Cerny, J. C., and Wechstein, M. Lymphangiography in staging carcinoma of the prostate. A comparison with operative findings. *Henry Ford Hosp Med J.* 23:169-74, 1975.

24. Castellino, R. A., Ray, G., Blank, N. et al. Lymphangiography in prostatic carcinoma. Preliminary observations. *JAMA.* 223:877-81, 1973.

25. McLoughlin, A. P., Saltzstein, S. L., McCullough, D. L. et al. Prostatic carcinoma: incidence and location of unsuspected lymphatic metastases. *J Urol.* 115:89-94, 1976.

26. Martland, M., Hansman, F. S., and Robinson, R. The phosphoric-esterase of blood. *Biochem J.* 18:1152-60, 1924.

27. Dmochowski, A., and Assenhajm, D. Urine and blood phosphatase. *Naturwissenschaften.* 23:501, 1935.

28. Kutscher, W., and Wolbergs, H. Prostatic phosphatase I. *Z Physiol Chem.* 236:237-40, 1935.

29. Kutscher, W., and Worner, A. Prostatic phosphatase II. *Z Physiol Chem.* 239:109-26, 1936.

30. Gutman, E. B., Sproul, E. E., and Gutman, A. B. Significance of increased phosphatase activity of bone at the site of osteoplastic metastases secondary to carcinoma of prostate gland. *Am J Cancer.* 28:485-95, 1936.

31. Gutman, A. B., and Gutman, E. B. An "acid" phosphatase occurring in the serum of patients with metastasizing carcinoma of the prostate gland. *J Clin Invest.* 17:473-8, 1938.

32. Woodward, H. G. Acid and alkaline glycerophosphatase in tissue and serum. *Cancer Res.* 2:497-508, 1942.

33. Gutman, A. B., and Gutman, E. B. "Adult" phosphatase levels in prepubertal Rhesus prostate tissue after testosterone propionate. *Proc Soc Exp Biol Med.* 41:277-81, 1939.

34. Robinson, J. N., Gutman, E. B., and Gutman, A. B. Clinical significance of increased serum "acid" phosphatase in patients with bone metastases secondary to prostatic carcinoma. *J Urol.* 42:602-18, 1939.

35. Bensley, E. H., Wood, P., Mitchell, S. et al. Estimation of serum acid phosphatase in the diagnosis of metastasizing carcinoma of the prostate. *Can Med Assoc J.* 58:261-4, 1948.

36. Herbert, F. K. The estimation of prostatic phosphatase in serum and its use in the diagnosis of prostatic carcinoma. *Quart J Med.* 59:221-41, 1942.

37. Kurtz, C. W., and Valk, W. L. Limitation of prostatic acid phosphatase determination in carcinoma of prostate. *J Urol.* 83:74-9, 1960.

38. Murphy, G. P., Reynoso, G., Kenny, G. M. et al. Comparison of total and prostatic fraction serum acid phosphatase levels in patients with differentiated and undifferentiated prostatic carcinoma. *Cancer.* 23:1309-14, 1969.

39. Nesbit, R. M., and Baum, W. C. Serum phosphatase determinations in diagnosis of prostatic cancer. A review of 1150 cases. *JAMA.* 145:1321-4, 1951.

40. Prout, G. R. Chemical tests in the diagnosis of prostatic carcinoma. *JAMA.* 209:1699-1700, 1969.

41. Schwartz, M. K., Fleisher, M., and Bodansky, O. Clinical application of phosphohydrolase measurement in cancer. *Ann NY Acad Sci.* 166:775-93, 1969.

42. Gutman, A. B. The development of the acid phosphatase test for prostatic carcinoma. *Bull NY Acad Med.* 44:63-76, 1968.

43. Sur, B. K., Moss, D. W., and King, E. J. Apparent heterogeneity of prostatic acid phosphatase. *Biochem J.* 84:55, 1962.

44. Lundin, L. G., and Allison, A. C. Acid phosphatases from different organs and animal forms compared by starch-gel electrophoresis. *Acta Chem Scand.* 20:2579-92, 1966.

45. Chu, T. M., Wang, M. C., Kuciel, L. et al. Enzyme markers in human prostatic carcinoma. *Cancer Treat Rep.* 61:193-200, 1977.

46. Chu, T. M., Bhargava, A., Barnard, E. A. et al. Tumor antigen and acid phosphatase isoenzymes in prostatic cancer. *Cancer Chemother Rep.* 59:97-103, 1975.

47. Delory, G. E., Sweetser, T. H., and White, T. A. The use of formalin and alcohol in the estimation of prostatic phosphatase. *J Urol.* 66:724-33, 1951.

48. Abul-Fadl, M.A.M., and King, E. J. Properties of acid phosphatases of erythrocytes and of the human prostatic gland. *Biochem J.* 45:51-60, 1949.

49. Fishman, W. H., and Lerner, F. A method of estimating serum acid phosphatase of prostatic origin. *J Biol Chem.* 200:89-97, 1953.

50. Ishibe, T., Usui, T., and Nihira, H. Prognostic usefulness of serum acid phosphatase levels in carcinoma of the prostate. *J Urol.* 112:237-40, 1974.

51. Chu, T. M., Wang, M. C., Scott, W. W. et al. Immunochemical detection of serum prostatic acid phosphatase methodology and clinical evaluation. *Invest Urol.* (In press)

52. Yam, L. T. Clinical significance of the human acid phosphatase. A review. *Am J Med.* 56:604-16, 1974.

53. Cooper, J. F., and Foti, A. A radioimmunoassay for prostatic acid phosphatase. I. Methodology and range of normal male serum values. *Invest Urol.* 12:98-102, 1974.

54. Foti, A. G., Herschman, H., and Cooper, J. F. A solid phase radioimmunoassay for human prostatic acid phosphatase. *Cancer Res.* 35:2446-52, 1975.

55. Choe, B. K., Pontes, E. J., Morrison, M. K. et al. Human prostatic acid phosphatase: II. A double-antibody radioimmunoassay. *Arch Androl.* 1:227-33, 1978.

56. Gursel, E. O., Rezvan, M., Sy, F. A. et al. Comparative evaluation of bone marrow acid phosphatase and bone scanning in staging of prostatic cancer. *J Urol.* 111:53-7, 1974.

57. Reynolds, R. D., Greenberg, B. R., Martin, N. D. et al. Usefulness of bone marrow serum acid phosphatase in staging carcinoma of the prostate. *Cancer.* 32:181-4, 1975.

58. Pontes, J. E., Alcorn, S. W., Thomas, A. J. et al. Bone marrow acid phosphatase in staging prostatic carcinoma. *J Urol.* 114:422-4, 1975.

59. Yarrison, G., Mertens, B. F., and Mathies, J. C. New diagnostic use of bone marrow acid and alkaline phosphatase. *Am J Clin Path.* 66:667-71, 1976.

60. Veenema, R. J., Gursel, E. O., Romas, N. et al. Bone marrow acid phosphatase: prognostic value in patients undergoing radical prostatectomy. *J Urol.* 117:81-2, 1977.

61. Khan, R., Turner, B., Edson, M. et al. Bone marrow acid phosphatase: another look. *J Urol.* 117:79-80, 1977.

62. Dias, S. M., and Barnett, R. N. Elevated bone marrow acid phosphatase. The problem of false positives. *J Urol.* 117:749-51, 1977.

63. Wang, M. C., Killian, C. S., Murphy, G. P. et al. Acid phosphatase activity in bone marrow and serum measured by spectrophotometric vs immunologic methods. Presented at Tenth International Congress of Clinical Chemistry, Mexico City, 1978.

64. Killian, C. S. Serum alkaline phosphatase isoenzymes as quantitative markers of bone and liver metastases in prostatic cancer. M. A. Thesis, State University of New York at Buffalo, NY, 1977.

65. Bodansky, O. *Biochemistry of Human Cancer.* New York: Academic Press, 1975.

66. Wajsman, Z., Chu, T. M., Bross, D. et al. Clinical significance of serum alkaline phosphatase isoenzyme levels in advanced prostatic cancer. *J Urol.* (In press)

67. Oliver, J. A., El Hilari, M. M., Belitsky, P. et al. LDH isoenzymes in benign and malignant prostate tissue. The LDH V/I ratio as an index of malignancy. *Cancer.* 25:863-6, 1970.

68. King, L. R., and Holland, J. M. Serum lactic acid dehydrogenase (LDH) level in patients with prostatic cancer. *J Urol.* 89:472-4, 1963.

69. Clark, S. S., and Srinivasan, V. Correlation of lactic dehydrogenase isoenzymes in prostatic tissue with serum acid phosphatase, digital examination, and histological diagnosis. *J Urol.* 109:444-5, 1973.

70. Hein, R. C., Grayhack, J. T., and Goldberg, E. Prostatic fluid lactic dehydrogenase isoenzyme patterns of prostatic cancer and hyperplasia. *J Urol.* 113:511-16, 1975.

71. Acevedo, H. F., Campbell, E. A., Saier, E. L. et al. Urinary cholesterol. V. Its excretion in men with testicular and prostatic neoplasms. *Cancer.* 32:196-205, 1973.

72. Chu, T. M., Shukla, S. K., Mittelman, A. A. et al. Comparative evaluation of serum acid phosphatase, urinary cholesterol, and androgens in diagnosis of prostatic cancer. *Urology.* 6:291-4, 1975.

73. Murphy, G. P., Reynoso, G., Schoonees, R. et al. Hypophysectomy and adrenalectomy for disseminated prostatic carcinoma. *J Urol.* 105:817-25, 1971.

74. Chu, T. M. Serum acid phosphohydrolase (phosphatase) and ribonuclease in diagnosis of prostatic cancer. *Antibiot Chemother.* 22:121-7, 1977.

75. Stephens, D. H., Hattery, R. R., and Sheedy, P. F., II. Computed tomography of the abdomen. *Radiology.* 119:331-6, 1976.

76. Stanley, R. J., Sagel, S. S., and Levitt, R. G. Computed tomography

of the body: early trends in application and accuracy of the method. *Am J Roentgenol.* 127:53-67, 1976.

77. Haaga, J. R., and Alfidi, R. J. Precise biopsy localization by computed tomography. *Radiology.* 118:603-7, 1976.

Surgical Management of Prostatic Cancer

9

Joseph D. Schmidt and Jeffrey J. Pollen

Adenocarcinoma of the prostate is the second most common cause of death from malignancy in males in the United States. The disease occurs in older age groups, generally between 60 and 75 years. Only one percent of cases occurs in men under 50 years of age. The glandular elements of the prostate are arranged into a narrow periurethral zone and a broader outer zone mainly situated posteriorly. Benign adenomas develop from the central glands whereas adenocarcinoma arises most commonly from the peripheral subcapsular zone.[1] Pathologically differentiated tumors reproduce well-defined glandular elements whereas undifferentiated tumors do not. Prognosis for survival correlates directly with histologic grade in addition to clinical stage of the tumor.[2]

Except in unusual circumstances, a definite histologic diagnosis of carcinoma should be obtained before specific treatment is instituted. Transperineal or transrectal needle biopsy has greatly facilitated diagnosis and pretreatment planning. Biopsy of a suspicious area, repeated if necessary, will yield the correct positive or negative diagnosis in over 90% of cases. Open perineal exposure with incisional biopsy of the lesion is still the most accurate diagnostic technique. It is frequently performed with frozen-section control so that definitive treatment can be instituted immediately if desired.

Cancer of the prostate is potentially curable at an early stage. Unfortunately, about 80% of patients present when the tumor has spread beyond the confines of the prostatic capsule. Comparison of the effectiveness of different therapeutic modalities is difficult because of lack of controlled studies and the necessity for prolonged follow-up.

Surgery has a well-established role in the staging, cure, and palliative treatment of cancer of the prostate (Table 1). Pelvic lymphadenectomy with histologic control is widely recognized as an important staging procedure. Prostatovesiculectomy remains the most definitive method for cure of the early lesion. Since Huggins and Hodges investigated the hormonal dependence of cancer of the prostate in 1941, bilateral orchiectomy has frequently been employed for the palliation of symptoms produced by cancer of the prostate.[3] The contribution of palliative surgery for the relief of obstructive uropathy in promoting quality of life and survival should not be underestimated.

CLINICAL STAGING

Accurate staging of the extent of the tumor is essential before rational treatment can be applied. A clinical staging classification, modified from Whitmore, Jewett, and Prout is presented in Table 2.[4-6]

Stage A (incidental) cancer of the prostate is clinically unsuspected. It is discovered on histologic study of the specimen obtained by transurethral resection or enucleation for apparently benign disease. The A-1 lesion consists of only isolated microscopic foci of well-differentiated adenocarcinoma present within a large proportion of benign adenomatous hyperplasia. If microscopy reveals the lesion to be any more extensive or the cells show any degree of dedifferentiation, the tumor should be classified as A-2. When cancer of the prostate presents with metastases in the presence of a clinically benign gland, the primary tumor is referred to as occult.

Stage B cancer of the prostate is palpably confined within the true capsule. The early B-1 lesion consists of an area of induration less than 1.5 cm within one lobe. Included in this stage is the discrete nodule less than 1.5 cm in diameter with normal compressible prostate on at least two sides. Any lesion greater than 1.5 cm in diameter or occupying both prostatic lobes is considered as Stage B-2.

Stage C cancer of the prostate has spread through the prostatic capsule but remains localized to the periprostatic area. The C-1 lesion is smaller and has an estimated weight of less than 70 grams. When the tumor is larger than this, or invasion of the bladder neck, trigone, or seminal vesicles is evident, the lesion is classed as C-2.

Stage D (advanced) cancer of the prostate can also be subdivided. The D-1 lesion is locally extensive, invading the bladder, ureters, or rectum. Lateral extension to the pelvic wall or metastases below the common iliac vessels are also included in this category. When nodal involvement at or above the common iliacs or distant metastases outside the pelvis are demonstrated, the lesion is classified as D-2.

Techniques of Staging

The extent of the primary lesion can be determined only by skillful rectal palpation and bimanual examination. The opportunity to examine the patient under general anesthesia should not be missed. Involvement of the bladder neck and trigone is best assessed by careful cystourethroscopy. Evidence of obstructive uropathy or deviation of the collecting systems is searched for on an excretory urogram. The total body technetium^{99m} pyrophosphate or diphosphonate bone scan is a sensitive technique for the detection of osseous metastases. Suspicious areas

Table 1
Surgery of Cancer of the Prostate

Diagnosis	Staging	Treatment			
		Definitive	Palliative		
Closed needle biopsy	Pelvic lymphadenectomy	Total prostatectomy	Bilateral orchiectomy	Ureteral Reimplantation	Laminectomy
Open perineal biopsy	Supraclavicular node biopsy	Radical prostatectomy	Bilateral adrenalectomy	Transuretero-ureterostomy	Rhizotomy
Fine-needle aspiration	Bone marrow aspiration and biopsy	Cystoprostatectomy	Hypophysectomy	Cutaneous Ureterostomy	Cordotomy
		Pelvic exenteration	Transurethral resection	Intestinal Conduit	Leukotomy
		Extended prostatectomy with Au^{198}	Nephrostomy	Nephrectomy	
		Pelvic lymphadenectomy with I^{125}	Ureterostomy in situ	Colostomy	
		Cryosurgery	Ureteral intubation	Internal fixation of fractures	

Table 2
Clinical Staging of Cancer of the Prostate

Incidental (Clinically undetectable)	Confined (Within the prostatic capsule)	Localized (Extracapsular extension)	Advanced (Extensive or widespread)
A-1 Focal and well-differentiated A-2 Diffuse or undifferentiated	B-1 Less than 1.5 cm in one lobe B-2 More than 1.5 cm or more than one lobe	C-1 Less than 70 grams C-2 More than 70 grams or involving bladder neck, trigone, seminal vesicles	D-1 Invasion of bladder, ureters, rectum or lymph nodes below common iliacs D-2 Nodal involvement at or above common iliacs or distant metastases

should be confirmed on conventional radiographs. The skeletal survey is relatively insensitive for the detection of early metastases. More than 80% of metastases visualized on x-ray are of the osteoblastic variety. Osteolytic lesions alone are unusual. If osseous metastases are not demonstrated, aspiration and biopsy of the iliac crest are suggested to help exclude involvement of the bone marrow. An x-ray of the chest should be obtained routinely, as well as brain and liver scans when clinically indicated. A raised serum acid phosphatase level generally means the tumor has spread beyond the prostatic capsule. It is most likely to be raised when distant metastases are present. Prout has indicated that when curative treatment is elected for a local lesion, the serum acid phosphatase should be within normal limits.[6]

The incidence of pelvic lymph node metastases related to the clinical stage, when routine studies for distant metastases are negative, is shown in Table 3. High stage, large size, and poor histologic differentiation are associated with a significantly higher probability of lymph node metastases.[14] Lymphangiography is too inaccurate for routine use.[13] Both false-negative and false-positive results account for errors in interpretation. The lymphangiogram is more likely to be interpreted as positive and correct in patients with advanced disease and involvement of the paraaortic group of nodes. Micrometastases cannot be detected and furthermore, the obturator and hypogastric group of glands, which are the earliest to become involved, are not outlined on a routine bipedal lymphangiogram.

Table 3
Incidence of Lymph Node Metastases
Related to the Clinical Stage of Prostate Cancer

Clinical Stage	Positive Lymph Nodes
A-1	0%
A-2	20%
B-1	15%
B-2	35%
C-1	50%
C-2	85%

Adapted from Arduino and Glucksman,[7] McCullough, Prout, and Daly,[8] McLaughlin et al.,[9] Wilson, Dahl, and Middleton,[10] Nicholson and Richie,[11] Donohue et al,[12] and Loening et al.[13]

Surgical pelvic lymphadenectomy is an accurate and safe method for the assessment of early metastases to the regional lymph nodes. It should be performed prior to any definitive treatment directed at cure of A-2, B, or C lesions. Pelvic lymphadenectomy is performed extraperitoneally through a lower abdominal midline or transverse incision, or separate oblique groin incisions. On each side the dissection clears the fibroareolar and lymphatic tissue around the common iliac, external iliac, and hypogastric vessels in a pyramidal area bounded laterally by the genitofemoral nerve, posteriorly by the obturator nerve, and medially by the ureter and bladder. The obturator space specifically is cleared of all lymphatic tissue. The surgical specimens should be carefully oriented by side and position to help the pathologist in interpretation. Suspicious or random nodes may be examined by frozen section. If positive, the surgery is generally terminated; if negative, the operator may choose to proceed with definitive treatment through the same retropubic approach or through a separate perineal incision. An obvious pitfall here is the not infrequent reporting of nodal metastases on permanent sections of the entire specimen. For this reason pelvic lymphadenectomy is best performed as an independent procedure, and definitive treatment postponed until the permanent sections are available. In general, definitive treatment of the primary lesion is not advised in the presence of nodal metastases.

There is no mortality associated with pelvic lymphadenectomy. Lymphocele formation complicates 10% of operations. Pelvic hematoma, transient obturator nerve palsy, edema of the genitalia or extremities, and thrombophlebitis with pulmonary embolism have all been reported.[9,15]

Although paraaortic lymph node biopsy theoretically can improve the staging of patients with no other evidence of metastatic disease, increased morbidity of this extended procedure, usually transperitoneal, lessens its practicality. A newer technique combining pedal lymphangiography and percutaneous transperitoneal needle biopsy may play a role in assessing the status of the paraaortic nodes.[16]

MANAGEMENT

Stage A

Latent cancer of the prostate is a frequent finding at autopsy, incidence rising progressively from 40% to 80% between the eighth and tenth decades.[17,18] The microscopic focal pattern occurs with greater frequency than the diffuse variety.

In the clinical situation Stage A or incidental cancer of the prostate is detected histologically in 7% to 14% of specimens removed for clinically benign disease.[19] Most incidental tumors are found in men over the age of 80. Approximately 70% of A lesions belong to the focal, well-differentiated A-1 group. Most of these tumors remain biologically inactive as evidenced by the fact that less than 10% show progression and are rarely the cause of death.[20] The prognosis for survival in these patients equals that of the general population of the same age group.[21] It is possible for the original transurethral resection or open enucleation of the prostate to have removed the entire cancer cell population.[22] This incidental "cure" accounts in part for the good prognosis in Stage A-1 lesions.[23] Our usual program of management for the A-1 lesion includes follow-up transurethral and transperineal prostatic biopsies at three months and again at six months to distinguish those patients with biologically more active and more widespread local disease. Those with positive follow-up biopsies are then considered as A-2 lesions. Those with negative biopsies are followed at six- to twelve-month intervals.

About 30% of incidental lesions are either diffuse or show cellular dedifferentiation (Stage A-2). Sixty percent of A-2 cancers show progression and 25% of patients may die of their disease. For this reason further treatment is indicated. At time of diagnosis, about 20% of patients with A-2 cancer of the prostate already have regional lymph node metastases.[12] If the metastatic work-up is negative, staging lymphadenectomy is recommended prior to definitive treatment.

Goodwin and Lehman et al. have emphasized the difficulty of total perineal or retropubic prostatectomy after previous prostatic surgery.[19,24] The hazards are much greater following open enucleation, there being less difficulty in carrying out a total prostatectomy following transurethral resection. Nichols, Barry, and Hodges reported on 33 patients who underwent secondary total prostatectomy following diagnosis of multifocal cancer of the prostate.[25] Pelvic recurrence, rectal injury, and anastomotic stricture occurred with an equal frequency of 9%. More than half the patients had some form of incontinence, and there was one operative death. Importantly, however, excellent five- and ten-year survivals of 75% and 60% respectively were obtained. It is of interest that residual cancer was present in 80% of the specimens.

Secondary total prostatectomy for A-2 cancer of the prostate should probably be restricted to patients who have previously undergone transurethral resection rather than open enucleation. Emphasizing the difficulties associated with secondary prostatectomy, Jewett recommends external megavoltage irradiation as the treatment of choice for clinical A-2 lesions.[5]

If incidental carcinoma is detected on routine needle biopsy for clinically benign disease, then transurethral resection of the prostate should be performed to document further the grade and extent of the lesion before deciding on additional treatment. Estrogens or castration do not influence the course or prognosis of early cancer of the prostate and should not be used at this stage.

Stage B

The B-1 lesion is the clinical tumor most likely to be truly confined within the capsule of the prostate. Patients with single nodules managed with endocrine treatment alone have a mean survival of 5.4 years.[26] Total prostatectomy is the most definitive and best documented treatment of the B-1 lesion.

Total prostatectomy is defined here as the surgical removal of the prostate gland, seminal vesicles, proximal vasa deferentia, and investing fascia, as shown in Figure 1. Radical prostatectomy implies concomitant removal of regional pelvic lymph nodes with total prostatovesiculectomy generally performed by the retropubic approach. In 1905 Young described the technique of total perineal prostatectomy for the cure of cancer of the prostate.[27] Further excellent descriptions of the procedure were presented by Chute, Belt and Parry.[28-30] This approach is fairly bloodless, allows accurate vesicourethral anastomosis under vision, and is well-tolerated by most patients. The retropubic approach to the prostate was popularized by Millin and the technique of total retropubic prostatectomy was well-described by Memmelaar and Parry.[30-32] This approach is preferred by many urologic surgeons because of greater familiarity with the anatomy. Although blood loss is greater than with the perineal approach, an advantage is the wide access to the regional lymph nodes through the same incision.

The operative mortality of total or radical prostatectomy should not exceed one percent. A variety of postoperative complications occurs in 50% of patients. Specific complications including local recurrence and stricture of the vesicourethral anastomosis occur in less than 10% of cases. Incontinence, either stress or total, is common in the immediate postoperative period; however, within six months only 10% have less

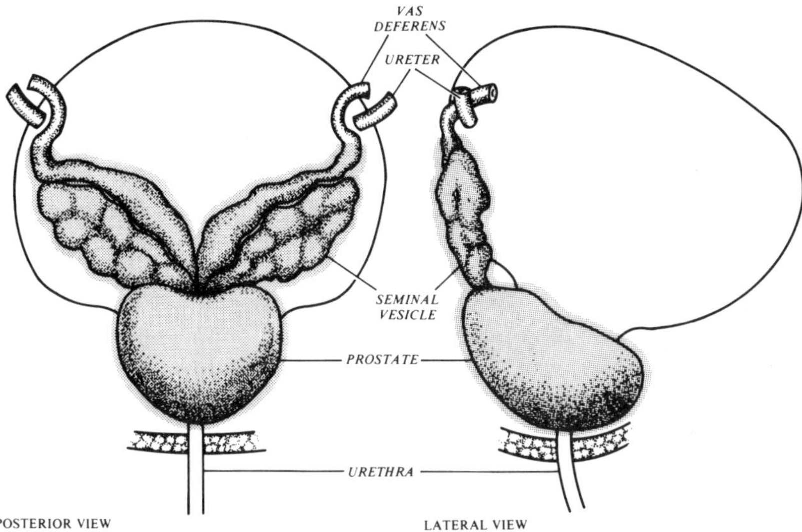

Figure 1. Shaded areas designate structures removed during total prostatectomy.

than perfect control. The nearly 100% incidence of postoperative impotence occurs whether the prostatectomy is performed by the perineal or retropubic route.

Strict criteria are necessary for the selection of patients to be cured by total prostatectomy alone. The tumor must be no more than 1.5 cm in diameter and be well-differentiated histologically. Routine staging procedures for distant metastases must be negative and there should be no increase in the prostatic fraction of serum acid phosphatase level. The patient should be no more than 70 years of age, be free of severe associated disease, and have an expected natural lifespan of at least 10 years. In addition, he must be prepared to accept almost inevitable impotence and a modest risk of urinary incontinence.

It has been suggested that for rigidly defined B-1 lesions, prior staging lymphadenectomy is unnecessary as the regional nodes will be involved in less than 10% of these cases.[11] Others have shown an incidence of lymph node metastases of more than 20% in patients with clinical B-1 disease.[9] We recommend staging lymphadenectomy for early cancer of the prostate. If metastases are demonstrated, then prostatectomy is generally not carried out. Currently, pelvic lymphadenectomy must be considered a diagnostic rather than therapeutic modality since there is no objective evidence that it improves survival.[23] McLaughlin et al. are more optimistic. When the lymphadenectomy specimen reveals micrometastases less than 2 mm in diameter in less than three nodes, they proceed with total prostatectomy and suggest that the survival rates may thus be improved. Supplementary use of estrogens or bilateral orchiectomy to total prostatectomy does not improve survival statistics and is not recommended.[33]

The surgical management of clinical B-2 cancer of the prostate is less well-documented. Up to 50% of B-2 lesions have extended microscopically beyond the prostate locally.[34] For this reason it has been suggested that Stage B-2 lesions be managed as clinical Stage C disease. Unquestionably some B-2 tumors can be cured by prostatovesiculectomy. Whatever definitive treatment is finally employed, a 35% incidence of regional lymph node metastases makes prior staging lymphadenectomy mandatory.

The survival data following total prostatectomy for clinical Stage B cancer of the prostate is presented in Table 4. Approximately 50% of patients with B-1 lesions survive 10 years and 30% survive 15 years without evidence of cancer. The 15-year, tumor-free survival rate of 18% for B-2 lesions is substantially lower. Kopecky, Laskowski and Scott performed preliminary pelvic node biopsy and examination with frozen section.[39] They proceeded with retropubic prostatectomy only if this was negative. Their 10-year survival rate of 50% in 73 patients with clinical Stages A-2 and B cancer of the prostate was attributed to improved selection of cases.

Table 4
Results of Total Prostatectomy for Clinical Stage B Cancer of the Prostate: Survival without Evidence of Cancer

Authors	Clinical Stage	Number Followed	10-Year Survival	Number Followed	15-Year Survival
Turner and Belt[35]	B	35	34%	—	—
Vickery and Kerr[36]	B	148	32%	—	—
Jewett et al[37]	B-2	79	37%	79	18%
	B-1	103	50%	103	27%
Culp and Meyer[5,38]	B-1	115	57%	74	34%

Several workers have reported their survival statistics after post-operative rearrangement to include only those patients whose tumors were histologically confined to the prostate. The expected improved survival statistics are shown in Table 5. The figures presented by Berlin et al.[40] and Belt and Schroeder[41] represent calculated actuarial survivals. It should be noted also that the survival data presented in Table 5 include patients who may be alive with cancer. In Jewett's series (Table 6) 8% of the survivors have recurrent cancer.

Table 5
Overall Survival Following Total Prostatectomy for Histologic Stage B Cancer of the Prostate

Authors	Number Followed	5-Year Survival	Number Followed	10-Year Survival	Number Followed	15-Year Survival
Turner and Belt[35]	42	76%	17	47%	—	—
Berlin et al[40]	116	81%	116	57%	116	38%
Belt and Schroeder[41]	185	78%	185	55%	185	31%
Jewett[5]	—	—	—	—	86	41%
Boxer[42]	129	86%	73	61%	—	—

Table 6
Results of Total Perineal Prostatectomy in 86 Patients with Histologic Stage B Cancer[5]

No Evidence of Cancer 15–32 Years Postoperatively	Living 15 Years with Cancer	Died with Cancer within 15 Years	Died without Cancer within 15 Years
33%	8%	16%	43%

In most of the above series the use of endocrine treatment is uncontrolled and not specified in detail. However, this aspect is not expected to influence survival figures to any great extent.

Reasons for Failure of Radical Prostatectomy to Cure the Early Lesion

The relationship of the status of pelvic lymph nodes to the presence of seminal vesicle invasion in clinical B lesions is indicated in Table 7. When regional lymph nodes contain tumor, invasion of seminal vesicles can be demonstrated in 80% of specimens. When regional lymph nodes are clear, only a small percentage of specimens will show invasion of seminal vesicles, and these patients are more likely to be cured with total prostatectomy. On the other hand, when seminal vesicles show microscopic invasion, metastases to pelvic nodes can be demonstrated in approximately 80% of patients. In Jewett, Eggleston, and Yawn's series, no patient with microscopic invasion of the vesicles survived 15 years following total prostatectomy for disease which seemed clinically confined to the prostate.[43]

In the absence of seminal vesicle invasion, Jewett et al. also related local recurrence and metastases to the presence and extent of microscopic invasion of the layers of the prostatic capsule.[43] The fact that capsular invasion could be demonstrated in about one-third of long-term survivors with histologic B lesions suggests that giving the prostate a wider berth at surgery can improve the survival rate and that capsular invasion alone does not have the same significance as involvement of the seminal vesicles.

Therapeutic failure is inevitable if unrecognized metastases exist at time of surgery. It is doubtful whether tumor emboli produced by operative manipulation of the prostate are important in establishing metastases. The prognosis for survival is closely related to the grade of the lesion. Up to 90% of patients with well-differentiated localized lesions may be expected to survive 10 years. Anaplastic tumors have a great propensity to metastasize and long-term survivals are rare even when the lesion is pathologically localized.

When considering survival results, it is important to understand that cancer of the prostate occurs in older age groups when other degenerative diseases are commonly present. After total prostatectomy 40% to 50% of patients can be expected to die of associated diseases within a 15-

Table 7
Incidence of Seminal Vesicle Invasion Related to Status of Pelvic Nodes in Clinical Stage B Cancer of the Prostate

Nodal Status	Invasion of Vesicles		
Negative	0% (B-1)		10% (B-2)
Positive		70% (B)	
Unknown	15% (B-1)		50% (B-2)

Adapted from Arduino and Glucksman,[7] Jewett, Eggleston, and Yawn,[43] and Wilson, Dahl, and Middleton.[10]

year follow-up period. Cardiovascular accidents account for one-half of associated deaths. Survival rates exceeding 50% in a 15-year period following total prostatectomy for early cancer will be difficult to achieve unless the degenerative diseases are simultaneously controlled. It has been stated that cancer of the prostate is more aggressive in younger men.[26,44] Others, however, do not agree.[45] Perhaps active prostatic cancer is equally aggressive in both the younger and older age groups, but the younger man is more likely to die of his cancer than from associated degenerative disease. Documentation of death directly attributable to cancer will therefore be more common in the younger age group.

Stage C

Stage C cancer of the prostate frequently responds to hormonal manipulation. However, in no way can this be curative. Staging lymphadenectomy followed by definitive external irradiation is a rational choice for the curative treatment of localized cancer.[46] The place of total prostatectomy for cure of Stage C disease is limited since more than 50% of patients already have metastases to the pelvic lymph nodes, and 10% have metastases to the bone marrow.[10,44] Schroeder and Belt reported actuarial survival rates of 35% and 20% at 10 and 15 years respectively in 213 patients with pathologic Stage C disease who underwent total perineal prostatectomy.[47] The implication is that selected patients with Stage C disease are in fact truly localized and potentially curable with total prostatectomy. When considered, prior staging lymphadenectomy would be mandatory.

Extended surgical procedures have been used to encompass increasingly large local lesions.[48] Prostatocystectomy with pelvic lymphadenectomy and urinary diversion has occasionally been employed for the eradication of a locally extensive lesion. As expected, there are only occasional reports of long-term, disease-free survivors following this procedure.[49] Pelvic exenteration with urinary and fecal stream diversion is unlikely to eradicate locally extensive lesions often enough to justify the morbidity and mortality associated with such a major procedure. In any case, once the rectum is invaded with tumor the prognosis is uniformly poor.

Transurethral cryosurgery was developed as a simple technique for the treatment of bladder neck obstruction.[50] Unfortunately it is not uniformly effective and is associated with a high rate of morbidity.[51,52] Cryosurgical destruction of the entire prostatic tumor as described by O'Donoghue et al. is performed by the open perineal route because the main tumor mass lies outside the prostatic urethra.[53] The rectum is displaced posteriorly to avoid injury and under direct vision the cryoprobe is applied to the surface of the prostate or a pointed probe is inserted to the desired depth in the tumor. Overlapping spheres of freezing are made to include the entire prostate and seminal vesicles, but care must be taken to avoid the ureters. Patients usually void well after a few weeks of catheter drainage. A perineal fistula may occur but heals with further catheter drainage. Incontinence is seldom a problem. Rectal examination within three months revealed no evidence of tumor in 86% of patients. Ten out of 12 patients with Stage C disease survived two years, some with endocrine support.

Combined therapy for localized prostatic cancer may offer many advantages over single therapeutic modalities. Following the experience of Colston and Brendler, other workers have taken advantage of the response of the local lesion to endocrine manipulation to expand their indications for total prostatectomy.[54] Scott and Boyd reported on 44 patients with C-1 lesions that showed marked regression with estrogens and castration and subsequently were treated by total prostatectomy.[55] Remarkably, of 31 patients followed for 15 years or more, 29% survived without evidence of cancer. It seems unlikely that endocrine treatment can convert an advanced lesion to a localized one. It may facilitate surgery, perhaps by reducing the size of the lesion.

Flocks et al. have reported on the value of extended surgery with adjuvant interstitial irradiation.[56] The prostatic tumor and seminal vesicles are removed as far as possible through a retropubic or perineal approach. Any remaining indurated tissue is thoroughly electrocoagulated. Thereafter 100 mc of ^{198}Au in a total volume of 2 ml is injected into the bladder base, the ligated ends of the vasa, and the area of the urogenital diaphragm. In a series of 69 patients treated with radical retropubic prostatectomy plus interstitial irradiation in the presence of negative pelvic lymphadenectomy, 66% survived 10 years and 27% survived 15 years without evidence of tumor. The only complication of note was delayed wound healing. The local recurrence rate of 4% is well below the 25% average which follows surgical removal alone for Stage C prostatic cancer.

Whitmore, Hilaris, and Grabstald have reported on lymphadenectomy combined with the retropubic implantation of ^{125}I for treatment of clinical Stages B and early Stage C cancer of the prostate.[57] When bladder outlet obstruction exists, a conservative transurethral resection is performed, leaving sufficient tissue to support radioactive seeds. Six weeks to three months are allowed for healing; thereafter, pelvic lymphadenectomy is performed through a lower abdominal incision, followed by the insertion of hollow steel needles at regular intervals into the prostate, using the bimanual technique. After estimating the volume of the gland, ^{125}I seeds at the required dosage are inserted through the needles to be distributed uniformly throughout the gland. Morbidity with this procedure was extremely low. However, as expected the most important factor determining the outcome was the presence of lymph node metastases.

This has prompted investigators to consider supplemental supervoltage radiation to the paraaortic and common iliac lymph nodes.[58]

Total perineal prostatectomy as a palliative procedure for Stage C cancer of the prostate has been reported by Tomlinson, Currie and Boyce.[59] When compared to a similar group of patients treated with transurethral resection or prostatic enucleation, they noted that complications such as urethral obstruction, ureteral obstruction, hematuria, and incontinence occurred some five to ten times more frequently in the conservatively treated group. The five-year survival in the aggressively treated group was 82% compared with 69% in the group treated conservatively. Prostatocystectomy with urinary diversion may be necessary in certain patients with more extensive local lesions that are unresponsive to hormonal treatment and require repeated transurethral procedures for control of bleeding and bladder neck obstruction.

Stage D

Management of Stage D cancer of the prostate is aimed at halting the progression of the disease and relief of symptoms. The mainstay of treatment is hormonal manipulation to create an antiandrogen environment. About 75% of patients with advanced cancer of the prostate show objective and subjective improvement with either estrogen administration or bilateral orchiectomy.[60] The prompt response to orchiectomy is best appreciated when faced with obstructive uropathy or when neurologic compression symptoms threaten. Orchiectomy also avoids the cardiovascular thromboembolic complications associated with the administration of estrogens.

Bilateral adrenalectomy and pituitary irradiation or hypophysectomy have been utilized for the treatment of patients with reactivation of symptoms following bilateral orchiectomy and estrogen treatment. Since both androgens and prolactin are required for prostatic growth, each procedure theoretically produces an equivalent effect. Short-lived objective and subjective remission rates of 35% and 70% respectively may be anticipated after either procedure, but the duration of survival remains limited. Potent antiandrogens like SCH-13521 (Flutamide) or inhibitors of prolactin secretion like L-dopa certainly offer many advantages over endocrine surgery.

Chemotherapy is playing an increasing role in the management of Stage D cancer of the prostate. This aspect of treatment is the subject of intensive investigation by the National Prostatic Cancer Project and other groups.

Total prostatectomy is generally not advised in patients with advanced tumor.[61] Rarely, persistent hematuria from a friable lesion does not respond to local or systemic treatment. In a patient who is otherwise in reasonably good condition, this life-threatening circumstance may dictate total prostatectomy or even cystoprostatectomy with urinary diversion.

Occasionally invasion of the rectum by tumor produces intestinal obstruction requiring diverting colostomy. Generally such tumors are extensive and require simultaneous urinary diversion.

Pathologic fracture of long bones presents a special problem. Treatment consists of internal fixation and local irradiation. Increasing pain, particularly at the site of a lytic metastasis and with marked thinning of the cortex, should raise suspicion of imminent fracture. Prophylactic internal fixation and irradiation should be considered.

Similarly, a patient may present with or develop symptoms and signs of spinal cord compression due to a metastasis. At the first indication of cord involvement the patient should receive dexamethasone combined with either estrogens or, preferably, bilateral orchiectomy. If no definite improvement occurs within 24 hours, a neurosurgical consultation should be obtained. Cord compression producing acute retention of urine or increasing paraparesis is an indication for immediate myelography and laminectomy to decompress the cord. Local irradiation of the lesion is also recommended.

Pain in cancer of the prostate is both common and disabling. When various forms of endocrine control fail, prostaglandin inhibitors such as acetylsalicylic acid or indomethacin may prove effective. Thereafter progressively more powerful analgesics are employed. Neurosurgical control of pain in cancer of the prostate is not commonly practiced but when required, bilateral procedures are performed because the pain generally arises from both sides of the body or from the midline. An open- or closed-radiofrequency sacral rhizotomy may be effective for pain localized to the pelvis. In most circumstances the pain is more diffuse and cordotomy of the lateral spinothalamic tracts will prove more useful. Intracranial procedures to relieve pain are not encouraged, but rarely saline or electrofrequency leukotomy of the frontal lobes has been performed in patients with diffuse metastases and uncontrollable pain.

CANCER OF THE PROSTATE AND OBSTRUCTIVE UROPATHY

The relationship of cancer of the prostate to the concomitant presence or absence of benign hyperplasia and obstructive uropathy is summarized in Figure 2. Stage A-1 disease demands concomitant benign hyperplasia for the production of bladder outflow obstruction, whereas subsequent stages do not. Unrelieved retention of urine is eventually followed by bilateral hydronephrosis and renal failure. Stages C and D cancer of the prostate can in addition produce obstruction to one or both lower ureters by direct invasion. In the presence of benign hyperplasia the response of bladder neck obstruction to treatment of the tumor may be less than optimal, and further surgical relief is usually necessary.

Bladder neck obstruction due to carcinoma may improve with endocrine manipulation, chemotherapy, or external beam irradiation (Figure 3). If symptoms are of only moderate severity, then response to treatment can be awaited before surgical intervention is considered. When the patient presents with acute or chronic retention of urine, urethral or occasionally suprapubic catheterization is necessary. The uremia of hydronephrosis associated with chronic retention of urine usually resolves fairly promptly with drainage of the bladder.

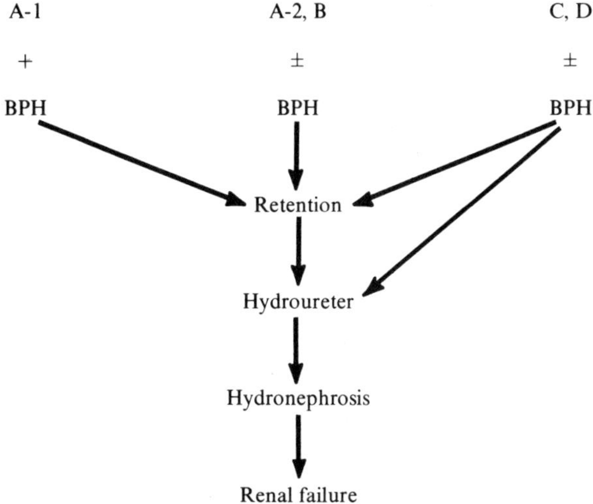

Figure 2. Obstructive uropathy: relationship between stage of prostatic cancer and presence or absence of benign prostatic hyperplasia.

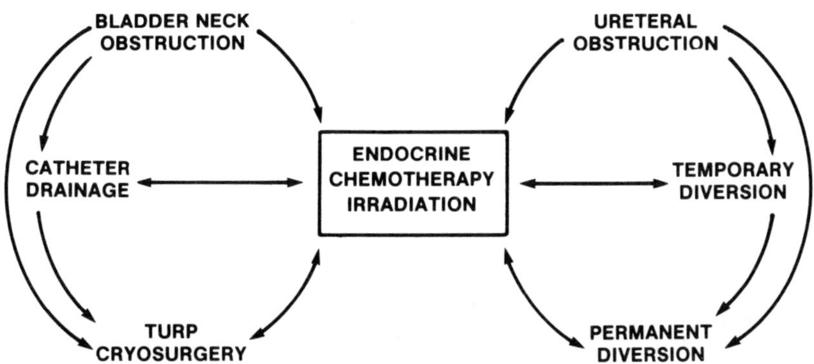

Figure 3. Management of obstructive uropathy due to cancer of the prostate.

Once acute or chronic retention of urine has supervened, we generally advise surgical relief of the bladder neck obstruction. Endoscopic transurethral resection of the prostate, repeated when necessary, is the most common procedure for the control of bladder outflow obstruction. An adequate channel is cleared through the obstructing cancer from the bladder neck down to the region of the verumontanum. No attempt is made to remove the entire local tumor. Bleeding is generally less of a problem than during resection of benign hyperplastic tissue. If the area of the external sphincter is invaded by cancer, there is a high risk of incontinence after the procedure.

A useful alternative to transurethral resection is transurethral or perineal cryodestruction of the obstructing lesion. A bonus of cryosurgery is that many patients with bone pain experience definite relief for periods ranging between one and 27 months.[62] In addition, metastases in different sites have been noted to regress after local cryosurgery.[63] If an immunologic mechanism is at work, its exact nature is unknown.[64]

Bilateral orchiectomy is usefully combined with the surgery for outflow obstruction. If indicated, estrogens, chemotherapy, or external beam irradiation may be employed after recovery.

Bilateral ureteral obstruction caused by direct invasion by cancer may respond to systemic treatment or local external beam irradiation. It will not resolve with catheter drainage of the bladder. If increasing hydronephrosis is documented or frank renal failure is present, urgent urinary diversion is indicated. Percutaneous nephrostomy on one or both sides under local anesthesia is a simple and safe technique for emergency upper urinary tract diversion. With the patient prone, fluoroscopic localization of the dilated collecting system is achieved with intravenous infusion of contrast medium. Alternatively, an ultrasound probe is used as a guide for the introduction of a suitable catheter into the dilated pelvis.[65] If for any reason urinary drainage is inadequate, surgical placement of a tube or preferably loop nephrostomy should be done on one or both sides.

Ureterostomy in situ, as described by Walsh is employed less often.[66] One or both ureters are exposed extraperitoneally. A polythene tube is directed through a small ureterotomy to the pelvis of the kidney and secured to the skin. A soft Silastic T-tube is less likely to become dislodged accidentally.

Another option available for emergency drainage of the upper urinary tracts is endoscopic insertion of ureteral catheters. The ureteral tubes emerging from the urethra are taped to a self-retaining balloon catheter in the bladder, and all the tubes drain into a urine collecting bag. The use of internal drainage by means of Gibbons' ureteral stents is of great value. These tubes drain the urine from the renal pelvis to the bladder. They have a larger internal diameter and thus are less prone to become obstructed with debris or blood clots. The small projecting wings prevent expulsion by ureteral peristalsis. Temporary or even long-term upper tract drainage may be achieved without the need for an external urine-collecting device. Sometimes it is impossible to negotiate the obstructing lesion with any form of ureteral catheter endoscopically. Under these circumstances, open cystotomy has been successfully employed for the insertion of Gibbons' stents. An indwelling foreign body is a potential source of serious infection at all times.

If dangerous electrolyte imbalances exist, preliminary dialysis will make any subsequent operative procedure much safer. Depending on the degree of renal damage, the uremic state gradually resolves with drainage of the upper tracts. Endocrine treatment, chemotherapy, or external beam irradiation may be instituted at this time. Antegrade pyelograms are performed at regular intervals to check patency of the lower ureters. If the ureters remain obstructed and the prognosis seems limited, one may elect to maintain tube diversion indefinitely.

Supravesical diversion should be considered in the patient whose performance status prior to the onset of renal failure was reasonable, has a good response to treatment, and has an expected survival of three months or more. Bladder neck obstruction must be completely controlled if reimplantation of the ureters into the dome of the bladder is considered. Transureteroureterostomy with a single ureteral reimplantation may be necessary. These forms of internal diversion, performed with frozen section control to exclude tumor-bearing ureter, are useful because they avoid the need for an external appliance.

Cutaneous transureteroureterostomy with a single stoma requires the use of only one collecting device. All forms of cutaneous ureterostomy, however, are prone to stenosis at the ureterocutaneous junction. An ileal conduit is probably the commonest form of supravesical diversion performed. When the pelvis has been subjected to intense irradiation, a transverse colon conduit offers several advantages.[67] The transverse colon and upper ureters are generally outside the usual field of pelvic irradiation. Fewer complications related to poor wound healing and fistula formation are encountered.

Provided the opposite moiety is anatomically and functionally normal, no surgical treatment is advised for the asymptomatic unilaterally obstructed kidney. Loin pain may prompt consideration of unilateral reimplantation, transureteroureterostomy, or simple nephrectomy. The procedure chosen will depend on the functional status of the involved kidney and the condition of the patient. Superimposed infection in an obstructed system is a potentially lethal situation. If percutaneous nephrostomy does not effect prompt resolution, there should be no delay in exploring the kidney. Nephrectomy may be carried out at this time if the surgery seems simple and the patient's condition permits. Otherwise, adequate drainage with a tube or preferably loop nephrostomy is all that should be done. When the crisis is over, the unilaterally obstructed kidney may be managed as described above.

PROPHYLAXIS

The peripheral zone of prostatic tissue posteriorly is unusually susceptible to the development of carcinoma. Since benign nodular hyperplasia arises from the periurethral glands located centrally, it follows that routine prostatectomy, performed by transurethral resection or enucleation, would not be expected to provide complete prophylaxis against the subsequent development of cancer. Six percent of patients with carcinoma of the prostate have previously had a simple prostatectomy for benign hyperplasia.[68]

As previously mentioned, prostatectomy might cure many A-1 lesions. In a similar fashion simple prostatectomy might prevent the small percentage of cancers that arise primarily in the periurethral zone.

Total prostatectomy without removal of the seminal vesicles has been suggested by Smith and Woodruff as treatment for benign hyperplasia with obstructive symptoms.[68] This would remove the organ at risk, but increased morbidity and inevitable impotence make the procedure unacceptable as routine. Turner-Warwick recommends that the entire posterior surgical capsule be routinely excised at the time of open prostatectomy for benign hyperplasia.[69] This simple procedure removes a high-risk area for the subsequent development of cancer and probably should be practiced more widely to determine its possible benefit in prevention of prostatic cancer.

CONCLUSION

At the present time only 15% to 30% of patients with cancer of the prostate are detected at a stage early enough to be considered for curative treatment. The presence of symptoms at the time of diagnosis is associated with a poor prognosis.[70] Routine annual rectal examinations of all males over the age of 40 years will detect many more patients with early cancer of the prostate.[71] Transrectal fine-needle aspiration biopsy should enhance the value of any screening program.[72] It is hoped that in the future newer gray scale ultrasound techniques and computerized axial tomography will facilitate the staging of the primary lesion.[73,74] Estimation of bone marrow acid phosphatase holds promise as a sensitive method for the early detection of blood-borne metastases.[75] Adjuvant chemotherapy to control undetected micrometastases at the time of total prostatectomy will be subjected to a critical clinical trial. It is hoped this treatment will further improve survival following curative surgery for localized cancer of the prostate.

REFERENCES

1. McNeal, J. E. Regional morphology and pathology of the prostate. *Am J Clin Pathol.* 49:347-57, 1968.

2. Gleason, D. F., Mellinger, G. T. and The Veterans Administration Cooperative Urological Research Group. Prediction of prognosis for prostatic adenocarcinoma by combined histological grading and clinical staging. *J Urol.* 111:58-64, 1974.

3. Huggins, C., and Hodges, C. V. Studies on prostatic cancer. I. The effect of castration, of estrogen, and of androgen injection on serum phosphatases in metastatic carcinoma of the prostate. *Cancer Res.* 1:293-7, 1941.

4. Whitmore, W. F., Jr. Hormone therapy in prostatic cancer. *Am J Med.* 21:697-713, 1956.

5. Jewett, H. J. The present status of radical prostatectomy for Stages A and B prostatic cancer. Edited by R. H. Flocks and W. W. Scott. In *The Urologic Clinics of North America. The Prostate.* Philadelphia: W. B. Saunders Co., 1975.

6. Prout, G. R., Jr. Diagnosis and staging of prostatic carcinoma. *Cancer.* 32:1096-1103, 1973.

7. Arduino, L. J., and Glucksman, M. A. Lymph node metastases in early carcinoma of the prostate. *J Urol.* 88:91-3, 1962.

8. McCullough, D. L., Prout, G. R., Jr., and Daly, J. J. Carcinoma of the prostate and lymphatic metastases. *J Urol.* 111:65-71, 1974.

9. McLoughlin, A. P., Saltzstein, S. L., McCullough, D. L. et al. Prostatic carcinoma: incidence and location of unsuspected lymphatic metastases. *J Urol.* 115:89-94, 1976.

10. Wilson, C. S., Dahl, D. S., and Middleton, R. G. Pelvic lymphadenectomy for the staging of apparently localized prostatic cancer. *J Urol.* 117:197-8, 1977.

11. Nicholson, T. C., and Richie, J. P. Pelvic lymphadenectomy for stage B-1 adenocarcinoma of the prostate: justified or not? *J Urol.* 117:199-201, 1977.

12. Donohue, R. E., Pfister, R. R., Weigel, J. W. et al. Pelvic lymphadenectomy in stage A prostatic cancer. *Urology* 9:273-275, 1977.

13. Loening, S. A., Schmidt, J. D., Brown, R. C. et al. A comparison between lymphangiography and pelvic node dissection in the staging of prostatic cancer. *J Urol.* 117:752-6, 1977.

14. Barzell, W., Bean, M. A., Hilaris, B. S. et al. Prostatic adenocarcinoma: relationship of grade and local extent to the pattern of metastases. *J Urol.* 118:278-82, 1977.

15. McCullough, D. L., McLaughlin, A. P., and Gittes, R. F. Morbidity of pelvic lymphadenectomy and radical prostatectomy for prostatic cancer. *J Urol.* 117:206-7, 1977.

16. Zornoza, J., Wallace, S., Goldstein, H. M. et al. Transperitoneal percutaneous retroperitoneal lymph node aspiration biopsy. *Radiology.* 122:111-15, 1977.

17. Hirst, A. E., and Bergman, R. T. Carcinoma of the prostate in men 80 or more years old. *Cancer.* 7:136-41, 1954.

18. Halpert, B., and Schmalhorst, W. R. Carcinoma of the prostate in patients 70 to 79 years old. *Cancer.* 19:695-8, 1966.

19. Lehman, T. H., Kirchheim, D., Braun, E. et al. An evaluation of radical prostatectomy for incidentally diagnosed carcinoma of the prostate. *J Urol.* 99:646-50, 1968.

20. Correa, R. J., Jr., Anderson, R. G., Gibbons, R. P. et al. Latent carcinoma of the prostate—why the controversy? *J Urol.* 111:644-6, 1974.

21. Hanash, K. A., Utz, D. C., Cook, E. N. et al. Carcinoma of the prostate: a 15-year followup. *J Urol.* 107:450-3, 1972.

22. Barnes, R. W., Bergman, R. T., Hadley, H. L. et al. Early prostatic cancer: long-term results with conservative treatment. *J Urol.* 102:88-90, 1969.

23. Whitmore, W. F., Jr. The rationale and results of ablative surgery for prostatic cancer. *Cancer.* 16:1119-32, 1963.

24. Goodwin, W. E. Radical prostatectomy after previous prostatic surgery. Technical problems encountered in treatment of occult prostatic carcinoma. *JAMA.* 148:799-803, 1952.

25. Nichols, R. T., Barry, J. M., and Hodges, C. V. The morbidity of radical prostatectomy for multifocal stage I prostatic adenocarcinoma. *J Urol.* 117:83-4, 1977.

26. Cook, G. B., and Watson, F. R. A comparison by age of death rates due to prostate cancer alone. *J Urol.* 100:669-71, 1968.

27. Young, H. H. The early diagnosis and radical cure of carcinoma of the prostate. *Bull Johns Hopkins Hosp.* 16:315-21, 1905.

28. Chute, R. Radical retropubic prostatectomy for cancer. *J Urol.* 71:347-72, 1954.

29. Belt, E. Radical perineal prostatectomy in early carcinoma of the prostate. *J Urol.* 48:287-99, 1942.

30. Parry, W. L. Prostate malignancies. Edited by J. F. Glenn and W. H. Boyce. In *Urologic Surgery.* 2nd Ed. Hagerstown, Md.: Harper & Row, 1975.

31. Millin, T. Retropubic prostatectomy. A new extravesical technique. *Lancet.* 2:693-6, 1945.

32. Memmelaar, J. Total prostatovesiculectomy—retropubic approach. *J Urol.* 62:340-8, 1949.

33. Williams, J., Marshall, V. F., and Gray, G. F., Jr. Radical perineal prostatectomy with bilateral orchiectomy for carcinoma of the prostate. *J Urol.* 113:380-4, 1975.

34. Jewett, H. J. The case for radical perineal prostatectomy. *J Urol.* 103:195-9, 1970.

35. Turner, R. D., and Belt, E. A study of 229 consecutive cases of total perineal prostatectomy for cancer of the prostate. *J Urol.* 77:62-77, 1957.

36. Vickery, A. L., Jr., and Kerr, W. S., Jr. Carcinoma of the prostate treated by radical prostatectomy. A clinicopathological survey of 187 cases followed for 5 years and 148 cases followed for 10 years. *Cancer.* 16:1598-1608, 1963.

37. Jewett, H. J., Bridge, R. W., Gray, G. F., Jr. et al. The palpable nodule of prostatic cancer. Results 15 years after radical excision. *JAMA.* 203:403-6, 1968.

38. Culp, O. S., and Meyer, J. J. Radical prostatectomy in the treatment of prostatic cancer. *Cancer.* 32:1113-18, 1973.

39. Kopecky, A. A., Laskowski, T. Z., and Scott, R., Jr. Radical retropubic prostatectomy in the treatment of prostatic carcinoma. *J Urol.* 103:641-4, 1970.

40. Berlin, B. B., Cornwell, P. M., Connelly, R. R. et al. Radical perineal prostatectomy for carcinoma of the prostate: survival in 143 cases treated from 1935 to 1958. *J Urol.* 99:97-101, 1968.

41. Belt, E., and Schroeder, F. H. Total perineal prostatectomy for carcinoma of the prostate. *J Urol.* 107:91-6, 1972.

42. Boxer, R. J. Adenocarcinoma of the prostate gland. *Urol Survey.* 27:75-94, 1977.

43. Jewett, H. J., Eggleston, J. C., and Yawn, D. H. Radical prostatectomy in the management of carcinoma of the prostate: probable causes of some therapeutic failures. *J Urol.* 107:1034-40, 1972.

44. Flocks, R. H. Clinical cancer of the prostate. A study of 4,000 cases. *JAMA.* 193:89-92, 1965.

45. Silber, I., and McGavran, M. H. Adenocarcinoma of the prostate in men less than 56 years old: a study of 65 cases. *J Urol.* 105:283-5, 1971.

46. Bagshaw, M. A., Ray, G. R., Pistenma, D. A. et al. External beam radiation therapy of primary carcinoma of the prostate. *Cancer.* 36:723-8, 1975.

47. Schroeder, F. H., and Belt, E. Carcinoma of the prostate: a study of 213 patients with stage C tumors treated by total perineal prostatectomy. *J Urol.* 114:257-60, 1975.

48. Whitmore, W. F., Jr., and Mackenzie, A. R. Experiences with various operative procedures for the total excision of prostatic cancer. *Cancer.* 12:396-405, 1959.

49. McCullough, D. L., and Leadbetter, W. F. Radical pelvic surgery for locally extensive carcinoma of the prostate. *J Urol.* 108:939-43, 1972.

50. Gonder, M. J., Soanes, W. A., and Shulman, S. Cryosurgical treatment of the prostate. *Invest Urol.* 3:372-8, 1966.

51. Kishev, S. V., Coughlin, J. D., and Dow, J. A. Late results following cryosurgery of the prostate (a clinical and panendoscopic study of 80 patients). *J Urol.* 104:893-7, 1970.

52. Marshall, A., Brown, A. K., Jones, W. W. et al. An assessment of cryosurgery in the treatment of prostatic obstruction. *J Urol.* 109:1026-8, 1973.

53. O'Donoghue, E.P.N., Milleman, L. A., Flocks, R. H. et al. Cryosurgery for carcinoma of prostate. *Urology.* 5:308-16, 1975.

54. Colston, J.A.C., and Brendler, H. Endocrine therapy in carcinoma of the prostate. Preparation of patients for radical perineal prostatectomy. *JAMA.* 134:848-53, 1947.

55. Scott, W. W., and Boyd, H. L. Combined hormone control therapy and radical prostatectomy in the treatment of selected cases of advanced carcinoma of the prostate: a retrospective study based upon 25 years of experience. *J Urol.* 101:86-92, 1969.

56. Flocks, R. H., O'Donoghue, E.P.N., Milleman, L. A. et al. Surgery of prostatic carcinoma. *Cancer.* 36:705-17, 1975.

57. Whitmore, W. F., Jr., Hilaris, B. S., and Grabstald, H. Retropubic implantation of Iodine 125 in the treatment of prostatic cancer. *J Urol.* 108:918-20, 1972.

58. Hilaris, B. S., Whitmore, W. F., Jr., Batata, M. A. et al. Radiation therapy and pelvic node dissection in the management of cancer of the prostate. *Am J Roentgenol.* 121:832-8, 1974.

59. Tomlinson, R. L., Currie, D. P., and Boyce, W. H. Radical prostatectomy: palliation for stage C carcinoma of the prostate. *J Urol.* 117:85-7, 1977.

60. Resnick, M. I., and Grayhack, J. T. Treatment of stage IV carcinoma of the prostate. Edited by R. H. Flocks and W. W. Scott. In *The Urologic Clinics of North America. The Prostate.* Philadelphia, W. B. Saunders Co., 1975.

61. Hudson, H. C., and Howland, R. L., Jr. Radical retropubic prostatectomy for cancer of the prostate. *J Urol.* 108:944-7, 1972.

62. Gursel, E., Roberts, M., and Veenema, R. J. Regression of prostatic cancer following sequential cryotherapy to the prostate. *J Urol.* 108:928-32, 1972.

63. Ablin, R. J., Soanes, W. A., and Gonder, M. J. Prospects for cryo-immunotherapy in cases of metastasizing carcinoma of the prostate. *Cryobiology.* 8:271-9, 1971.

64. Schmidt, J. D. Cryosurgical prostatectomy. *Cancer.* 32:1141-3, 1973.

65. Harris, R. D., McCullough, D. L., and Talner, L. B. Percutaneous nephrostomy. *J Urol.* 115:628-31, 1976.

66. Walsh, A. Ureterostomy in situ. *Br J Urol.* 39:744-5, 1967.

67. Schmidt, J. D., Hawtrey, C. E., and Buchsbaum, H. J. Transverse colon conduit: a preferred method of urinary diversion for radiation-treated pelvic malignancies. *J Urol.* 113:308-13, 1975.

68. Smith, G. G., and Woodruff, L. M. The development of cancer of the prostate after subtotal prostatectomy. *J Urol.* 63:1077-80, 1950.

69. Wulfsohn, M. A. Retropubic prostatectomy. Edited by J. F. Glenn and W. H. Boyce. In *Urologic Surgery.* 2nd Ed. Hagerstown, Md.: Harper & Row, 1975.

70. Byar, D. P., and Mostofi, F. K. Cancer of the prostate in men less than 50 years old: an analysis of 51 cases. *J Urol.* 102:726-33, 1969.

71. Kimbrough, J. C. Carcinoma of the prostate: five-year followup of patients treated by radical surgery. *J Urol.* 76:287-91, 1956.

72. Nienhaus, H. Aspiration biopsy cytology of prostate carcinoma. *Recent Results Cancer Res.* 60:53-60, 1977.

73. Resnick, M. I., Willard, J. W., and Boyce, W. H. Recent progress in ultrasonography of the bladder and prostate. *J Urol.* 117:444-6, 1977.

74. Hattery, R. R. Computed tomography of the genitourinary tract. Edited by D. Norman, M. Korobkin, and T. H. Newton. In *Computed Tomography 1977.* St. Louis: The C. V. Mosby Company, 1977.

75. Bruce, A. W., O'Cleireachain, F., Morales, A. et al. Carcinoma of the prostate: a critical look at staging. *J Urol.* 117:319-22, 1977.

Perspectives on Radiation Treatment of Prostate Cancer: History and Current Focus

10

Malcolm A. Bagshaw

Carcinoma of the prostate stands second only to lung cancer among neoplasms in the male. The American Cancer Society estimated an incidence of 57,000 new cases (and 19,000 deaths) from prostate cancer in the United States in 1977. This neoplasm is now more common than the combined incidence of all neoplasms in the buccal cavity and pharynx, leukemia, and all lymphomas among males (41,000 cases).

EARLY USE OF BRACHYTHERAPY BY UROLOGISTS (1910–1942)

In 1910 Pachkis and Tittinger treated a few patients with carcinoma of the prostate using a specially designed radium applicator fitted to a cystoscope.[1] At about the same time Pasteau employed a radium capsule carried in a coudé catheter.[2] Hugh Young soon thereafter acquired a stock of radium sources and fabricated a set of applicators which could be placed intraurethrally, intrarectally, or transperineally.[3,4] By 1915 he had developed a sophisticated system for the local radiation of prostatic carcinoma. Through the 1920s and 1930s others, including Barringer at Memorial Hospital, Bumpus at the Mayo Clinic, and Smith and Peirson at the Massachusetts General Hospital reported the results of treatment of several hundred patients using various combinations of brachytherapy (intracavitary or interstitial), and occasionally even external orthovoltage irradiation.[5-7] This early era was dominated by urologists, and radium brachytherapy was employed almost exclusively. It closed with Barringer's report in 1942 in which he described the results of radium treatment in 352 consecutive cases of prostate cancer.[8] Two patients in this series survived six and seven years respectively, with no evidence of cancer in the prostate at autopsy. Barringer emphasized the contribution of Huggins and Hodges "on the remarkable effects of castration upon

The author's data presented herein has been generated under Public Health Service Grant CA-15455 and CA-05838 from the National Cancer Institute, National Institutes of Health, and the National Prostatic Cancer Project.

primary prostatic carcinoma, bone metastases, pain, and general health."[9] The widespread adoption of hormonal therapy followed, and early activities of urologists in radiation treatment of carcinoma of the prostate were interrupted for more than a decade.

Interstitial therapy was reintroduced by Flocks et al. with injection of radioactive colloidal gold suspension directly into the neoplasm.[10] Later, Carlton et al. successfully used combinations of interstitial gold grain implants, external beam therapy, and node resection.[11] More recently Hilaris et al. have employed ^{125}I implants coupled with pelvic node dissection.[12] Both groups have reported survival and local control rates comparable to those reported herein for external beam irradiation.

EXTERNAL BEAM RADIATION THERAPY (1932–1940)

Early History

Widman in 1932 achieved significant palliation with orthovoltage treatment in the 140 to 200 kV range in a number of patients with far advanced prostatic neoplasm.[13] Hultberg at the Radiumhemmet in Stockholm reported similar encouraging palliation in a retrospective review of 167 cases treated between 1929 and 1940 with both orthovoltage technique and external therapy with a high intensity radium source, the forerunner of the modern Cobalt 60 unit.[14] After 1940 there followed a 24-year period of lack of activity in the use of external beam therapy in this disease due to introduction of hormone therapy.

Recent Developments (1964–1977)

In 1964 Budhraja and Anderson, while recognizing that early experience with radiotherapy had not been notably successful, suggested that newly developed high-energy, megavoltage radiation equipment beyond 2 MeV in energy, and Cobalt 60 devices could be used in treatment of prostatic cancer.[15] They retrospectively compared a group of patients treated with a combination of surgery, stilbestrol, and radiotherapy with other patients treated with stilbestrol and surgery alone. Radiation doses up to 5,900 rads were achieved, with most patients receiving about 5,000 rads. At five years no difference in survival was observed between the two groups. It was concluded that radiotherapy did no harm and was beneficial in those patients who had relapsed after estrogen treatment. This series of patients had relatively advanced disease.

The status of subsequent external beam radiotherapy (between 1964 and 1974) was summarized in 1975 by Ray and Bagshaw in a detailed review of 16 published reports which included some 600 published cases.[16] The review demonstrated increasing widespread application of the new generation of high-energy radiotherapy machines in treatment of prostatic cancer, but because of short observation periods little could be said about long-term results.

Since 1974 a number of additional contributions have been published. Most of these more recent papers describe the use of external beam photon radiation obtainable from the ^{60}Co unit, linear accelerator, or betatron. Most investigators report on irradiation with curative intent limited to the prostatic region, although some describe treatment volumes which extend beyond the prostate region to include the pelvic and paraaortic lymph nodes. While there is some disagreement as to the optimal radiation dose for, and the efficacy of, extended field irradiation, there is a trend toward development of treatment programs more precisely tailored to fit the individual needs of the patient.

CURRENT FOCUS

In the next section the following aspects of current radiation therapy will be described: diagnosis, diagnosis and evaluation of the patient for therapy, technique of therapy employed at Stanford University (with updated results of the Stanford series), and relevant summaries of other series.

Controversial issues will be identified and use of radiation therapy for salvage of patients following inadequate resection will be discussed.

Diagnosis

Patients who present for treatment may be either asymptomatic or symptomatic. Currently about one-third of our patients present without symptoms (compared with only about one-fifth 10 years ago). Concern for early diagnosis and increased attention to diagnosis by routine rectal examination is thought to account for this improvement. The symptomatic patients complain of classical symptoms of prostatism which include, in decreasing order of frequency, nocturia, diminished urinary stream, frequency, hesitancy, frank obstruction, urgency, hematuria, dribbling, and occasionally hematospermia. Other less frequent symptoms include penile pain, perineal pain, sensation of mass, and bone pain.

Physical Examination and Laboratory Studies Prior to rectal examination, acid and alkaline phosphatase specimens should be obtained, as well as other significant blood studies including a complete blood count. It is beyond the scope of this chapter to discuss the significance of prostatic acid phosphatase determinations except to predict that with improvement of immunoassay techniques, this will play an increasing role in the initial and follow-up study of patients with this neoplasm.

Rectal examination of the gland should be performed to determine the size and extent of the neoplasm as accurately as possible. Prostatic cancer has a stony-hard texture and often can be distinguished from the surrounding more resilient prostatic tissue as a discreet nodule. The size of the nodule, if the tumor seems to be localized, should be carefully estimated. Extension outside the capsule, particularly superiorly into the seminal vesicles or laterally into the sulcus, should be noted. A diagram showing clinical impression of the degree of extension should be prepared at the initial examination. A clear understanding of the gross extent of disease is important in order to plan therapeutic strategy. For example, 22% of our patients with Disease Limited to the Prostate (DLP) (nominal Stage B) who have had surgical staging had involved lymph nodes, while 58% of those who had Extracapsular Extension (ECE) (nominal Stage C) had involved nodes found at surgical staging (Table 1). Similar lymph node involvement relative to stage has been noted by others (see Chapter 9, Table 3). The importance of the consideration of local or lymph node extension will be discussed later in connection with planning of radiation treatment.

Biopsy diagnosis is confirmed by transrectal needle biopsy, transperineal needle biopsy, or transurethral resection. Needle biopsy is used most frequently in the asymptomatic patient, whereas transurethral resection is employed in most symptomatic patients. Overall, about one-half of the Stanford series patients are diagnosed by transurethral resection specimens.

Diagnostic Imaging Procedures The presence or absence of bone metastases is determined primarily by radionuclide scintiscan confirmed by diagnostic x-rays or occasionally, biopsy with a Jamshidi needle if the scintiscan is equivocal. Pulmonary metastases, although rare in early prostate carcinoma, should be ruled out by chest films. Intravenous pyelograms for evaluation of ureteral obstruction should also be a part of the clinical evaluation.

Radiation Therapy Technique

Simulation, Treatment Planning, and Therapy Most radiotherapists today use a treatment planning simulator in order to prepare the proper positioning of the patient with respect to treatment beams. A simulator has geometric properties of the treatment machine, but it contains a diagnostic x-ray tube instead of a therapeutic radiation source. By employing the simulator precise positioning of the therapeutic beams can be determined in advance. The target volume, ie, the volume of tissue containing the primary neoplasm and, if desired, the regional lymphatics, can be well-defined relative to the therapeutic beam. During simula-

Table 1
Correlation of Clinical Stage of Primary Tumor and Lymph Node Biopsy Results (Protocol Series—90 Patients)

Stage		Lymph Node Biopsy Results				
Am. Urol.	UICC	No Tumor	+ Regional Nodes Only	+ PA Nodes Only	+ Regional and PA Nodes	Positive Total
A	T0	2	0	0	0	0/2 (0%)
B	T1,T2	39	9	0	2	11/50 (22%)
C	T3	16	10	0	12	22/38 (58%)
Total		57 (63%)	19 (21%)	0	14 (16%)	33/90 (37%)

tion, image intensification fluoroscopy or localization x-ray films may be used to document the therapeutic program. The majority of modern therapeutic sources are isocentrically-mounted Cobalt 60 units or small linear accelerators. Usually the patient lies in a recumbent position and the C-armed gantry which supports the primary beam source is rotated at a constant source-axis distance around the longitudinal axis of the patient. The point at which all of the therapeutic beams intersect is termed the isocenter (Figure 1).[17] By matching the isocenter of the treatment beam to the center of the tumor or the center of the target volume, accurate daily positioning of the patient is facilitated. More importantly, the patient may be treated in the supine position with the therapeutic

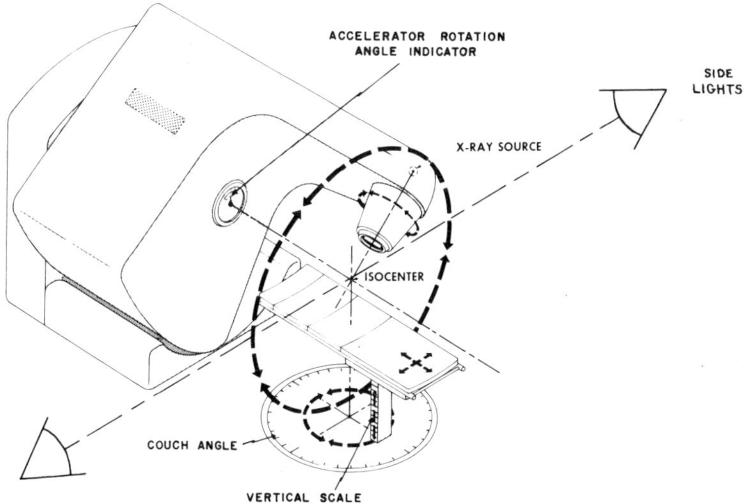

Figure 1. Location of the isocenter for 6 MeV Varian accelerator. The isocenter is defined by the horizontal (gantry) axis of rotation of the treatment unit and the central axis of the radiation beam. Note that side lights are used to locate the isocenter. (Reprinted from Gardner, A., Bagshaw, M. A., Page, V. et al. Tumor localization, dosimetry, simulation and treatment procedures in radiotherapy: the isocenter technique. *Am J Roentgenol.* 114:163-71, 1972, with permission from the publisher.)

beam penetrating from any angle without the necessity of turning the patient from side to side or from prone to supine, as would be the case with a more fixed beam arrangement. This isocentric technique is the most accurate and reproducible method for the treatment of prostatic cancer (Figures 2a & b). It is also important that the radiotherapist treat each field every day. This assumption is made in the isodose plans which are demonstrated in Figures 3 and 4. If shortcuts are taken, such as treating only with anterior and posterior fields rather than the four-field box technique, or treating with only two fields on one day and the two other fields the next day, the incidence of adverse radiation reactions mounts appreciably.

The isocentric technique is adaptable both to rotational and to arc therapy with a moving beam source. It will be noted by reference to Table 2 that we employ a booster dose to the prostate gland which is delivered by 120° lateral arc moving beams. This delivers a homogeneously applied 2,000 rad dose increment to the prostate and is well tolerated. If the patient is to be treated to the prostate only rather than to the prostate and the pelvic adenopathy, the left and right lateral arc technique is preferred and the entire dose is delivered in this manner. The calculations for treatment are computerized in most departments, and a resume of the treatment sequence is given in Table 2.

Table 2
Radiation Dose Regimens, Stanford Technique
Radiation Source–Clinac IV Linear Accelerator
Source-Axis Distance–80 cm

Target Volume	Technique	Dose (Rads Absorbed at Isocenter)	
		Subtotal	Total
Prostatic region only. 7×6 up to 9×8 cm Fig. 2a & b, rectangular field enclosing prostate only.	120° lateral arc moving beam.	7600	7600/7½ weeks
Prostatic region and pelvic lymph nodes. (Fig. 2a & b)	4-field "box" with corners trimmed.	2600/2½ wks	
Reduced to prostatic region only. (Prostatic boost) Fig. 2a & b, small rectangle.	120° lateral arc moving beam.	2000/2 wks	7000/7 weeks (Prostate)
Enlarged to original extent. Fig. 2a & b.	4-field "box" with corners trimmed.	2400/2½ wks	5000/7 weeks (Pelvis)
(1, 2, and 3 are performed in sequence)			
Paraaortic nodes.	Anterior-Posterior cross-fire.	4000/4 wks	
Paraaortic node boost.	Lateral cross-fire or shallow anterior oblique beams.	1000/1 wk	5000/5 weeks

The isocenter dose is 200 rads/day. All fields are treated each day to ensure homogeneous dose distribution to the respective target volumes. This plus the interposition of the prostatic boost midway through treatment of the pelvic volume has virtually eliminated significant radiation sequellae, either during therapy or later.

Treatment to the paraaortic region is usually carried out concomitantly with treatment to the pelvic region.

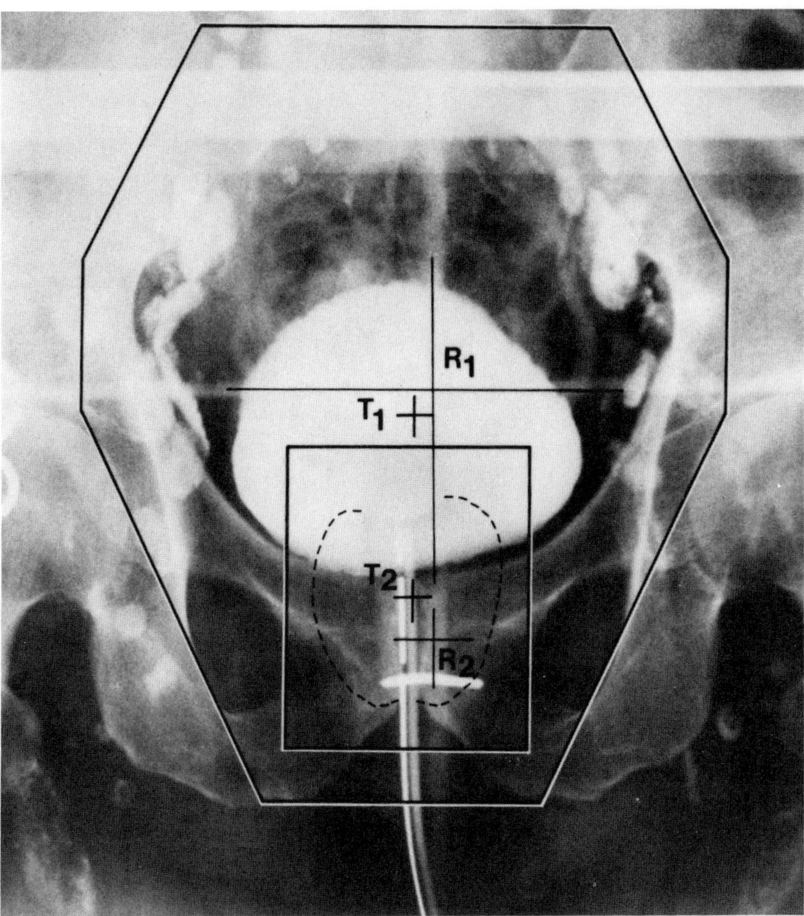

Figure 2A.

Results of External Beam Radiotherapy The treatment of prostatic carcinoma with external beam megavoltage irradiation was initiated at Stanford in 1956.[18-20] The series currently consists of 653 patients treated definitively with external beam megavoltage irradiation. Some have received concomitant hormone therapy (estrogenic treatment and/or castration). No patients who have had pretherapeutic definitive resection are included except those mentioned later in the discussion of surgical salvage, and no patients with second primary neoplasms or who had generalized tissue or bone metastases are included. Patients with regional adenopathy *are* included, but these are segregated according to the extent of lymphadenopathy insofar as it was known.

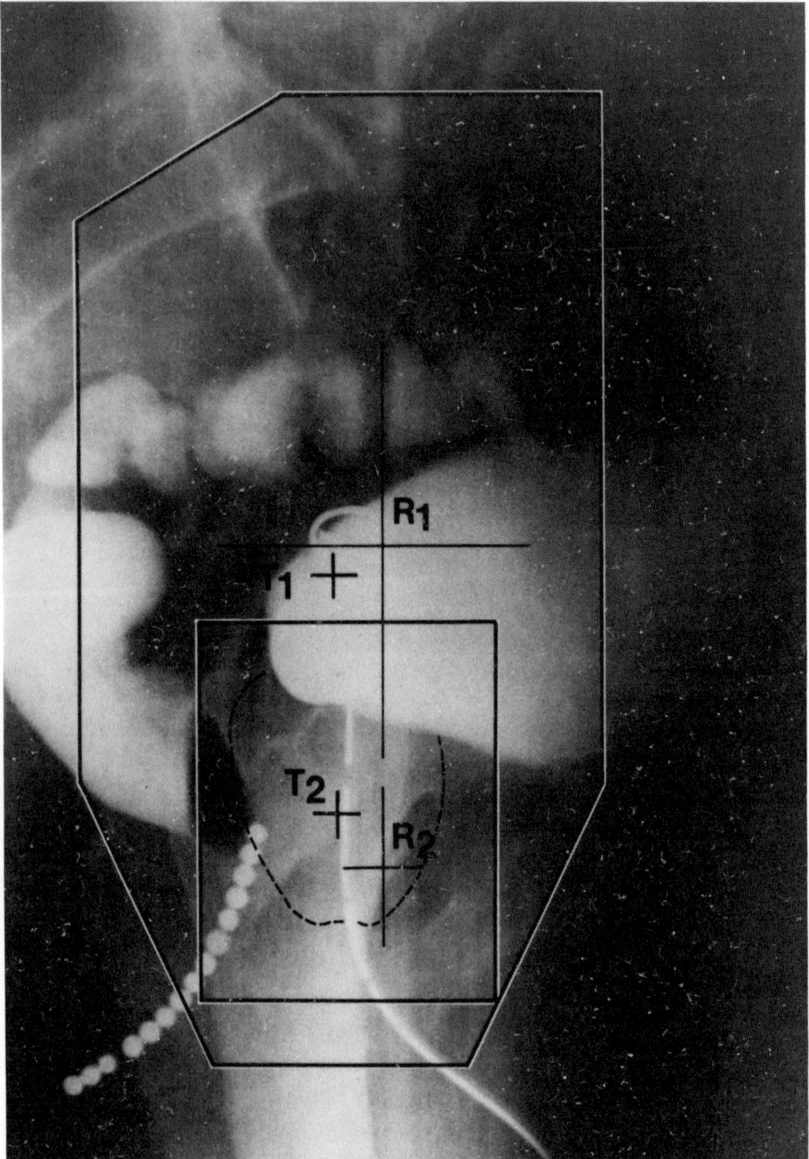

Figure 2B.

Figure 2. In the execution of the simulation procedure the radiotherapist needs 2 x-ray film exposures: one frontal, Figure 2a and one lateral, Figure 2b, exposed at exactly 90°. This must be accomplished without moving the patient between the exposures. In order to identify the target volume, it is best to have some opaque device which demonstrates the position of the prostate, and either lymphangiographic dye (as demonstrated) or surgical clips which demonstrate the position of the lymph nodes. For the demonstration of the prostate, we use a small caliber Foley catheter which is inserted through the urethra, well lubricated with 2% lidocaine jelly, into the bladder. The balloon is filled with mercury and the catheter pulled downward so it is in direct contact with the superior surface of the prostate gland. We also instill 30 ml of Hypaque (50%) into the bladder in order to appreciate better the position of the superior surface of the prostate in the lateral view. Mercury is the preferred contrast for the Foley catheter because it is dense enough to demonstrate the position of the prostatic urethra. About 100 ml of thin barium solution is instilled into the rectum and the position of the anus is marked with a soft rubber catheter which has been filled with lead shot. By using the landmarks described above, the radiotherapist may deduce the volume of tissue which is to be irradiated and mark these directly upon the localization films (black and white perimeter marks). In patients who proclaim sexual potency, the procedure is carried out with the testicles fitted within a specially designed heavy lead box (not shown). This reduces scattered radiation to the testicles, eliminates the possibility of an accidental exposure, and psychologically seems to be a great comfort to the patients. Thus an isocentric 4-field box technique is used for the treatment of the target volume which employs an anterior field, a posterior field, and left and right lateral fields. These fields are arranged so that the central rays always intersect at the isocenter point. The anterior-posterior fields extend from the ischial tuberosities to about either the superior or inferior surface of L5, depending upon whether there is to be an extended paraaortic field. The bony landmarks are only approximate. In practice, the condition and anatomy of the lymph nodes determine the upper extent of the pelvic field. The lateral margins are established at about 1½ cm lateral to the iliac nodes at the pelvic inlet. The corners are trimmed. This is done to minimize unnecessary irradiation of bone marrow in the innominate bone. The lateral fields have superior and inferior margins identical to the anterior and posterior fields. The posterior margin of the lateral fields are arbitrarily placed at the midplane of the rectal lumen and the anterior margin about 1½ cm anterior to the anterior most iliac lymph nodes. Again the corners are trimmed. Thus the field sizes are determined individually according to the anatomy of each patient. In practice the isocenter points for the localization films are designated R1 and R2 as indicated in the figure. After the actual field size and position have been designated by the radiotherapist, it is usually found that the central axis of the anterior and posterior and lateral beams must be moved slightly to accommodate for the modified geometry. The new points are designated T1 and T2, respectively, and these then become the points that are marked on the skin for the entry of the central ray of the actual treatment beam. It should be reemphasized that the patient always lies supine for the treatment, no matter which beam is being used. The patient's position is indexed by illuminated cross-hairs which coincide with the isocenter point and which project a bright cross onto a predetermined tatoo mark on the skin which is placed during the simulator session. These coincide with the projected image of the cross wires of the actual treatment fields which are shown as faint white lines in the figure. Thus in a normal treatment sequence, the patient is treated first with a vertical beam, then with a left lateral beam, then the accelerator is rotated beneath the table and the patient treated with a posterior beam which is directed through a mylar window in the treatment couch, and finally with a right lateral beam. Each time the position of the beam is changed, the radiation fields are trimmed according to the initial treatment plan. If the paraaortic lymph nodes are to be treated also, a similar isocentric technique is used. In addition, a booster dose is added to the prostatic region only. This is indicated by the black and white lines which enclose the prostate within a rectangle, usually 8×7 cm.

The series may be divided into the following groups:

The basic series: N=370 patients treated between 1956 and July 1971. These were patients with localized carcinoma which was in most cases too extensive for radical prostatectomy, or patients who might have been candidates for resection but either declined the operation or were rejected as poor surgical risks. The treatment volume was restricted to the prostate region only, and there was no attempt to evaluate regional adenopathy. The basic series includes 193 patients with disease limited to the prostate (DLP) (nominal Stage B) and 177 patients with extracapsular extension (ECE) (nominal Stage C).

The extended series: N=283 patients treated between July 1971 and January 1977 in whom increasing attention was given to the determination of lymphadenopathy. 249 have had lymphograms, 104 have had surgical staging of pelvic and, when possible, paraaortic lymph nodes, and 97 have had both lymphograms and surgical exploration. Among the patients explored 47 had pathologically proven adenopathy and 57 had benign lymph nodes. This series may also be subdivided into 143 patients with extracapsular extension (ECE) (nominal Stage C) and 140 patients with disease limited to the prostate (DLP) (nominal Stage B).

The protocol cohort: This is a subgroup in the extended series of 90 precisely-staged patients.[21] Although the period of follow-up is too short to report survival for this group separately, the data concerning lymphography, incidence of lymphadenopathy, and influence of pathologic grade on the incidence of lymphadenopathy are derived from this protocol group.

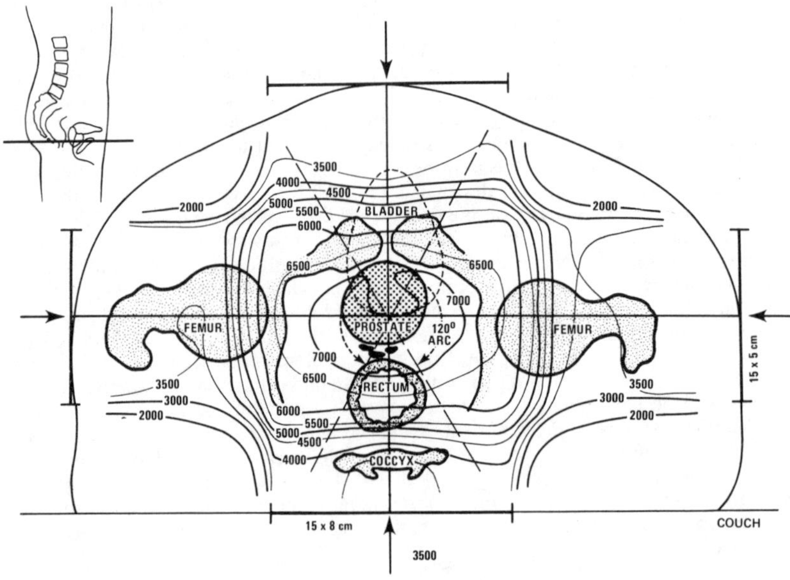

Figure 3. Transverse body section at the level indicated in figure insert through the mid-prostate. The position of the bladder indicated by the dotted line is at a somewhat more superior level. Note that the anterior portion of the bladder actually extends anterior to the pubic symphysis. This is clearly shown in Figure 2b. The three black ovoid structures between the prostate and rectum are the so-called intercalating lymph nodes of Rouvière. Other nodes which drain the prostate are at a more superior level. The isodose patterns are labeled with the total dose in rads delivered to each isodose line at the conclusion of the entire course of treatment. These isodose curves combine the 4-field technique and the prostatic boost in order to demonstrate the total dose distribution throughout the pelvis at this level. Boost dose is delivered as per the schedule indicated in Table 3 by 120° lateral arc therapy as indicated in the figure.

The overall survival and the disease-free survival for the Stanford patients is presented in Table 3. A tabulation of recently reported results of several other substantial series in which similar therapy was administered has been included for comparison.[22-27] The staging system described in Table 2, Chapter 9, is followed, although frequently the staging description in the various reports does not permit precise allocation into the subgroups of the basic A, B, C, and D categories. Considering allowances for probable standard errors, the results among the various series are remarkably consistent. They also demonstrate clearly that progressively more advanced clinical stage has an adverse influence on survival.

Hill et al. generally used larger radiation fields of 15×15 cm compared to the much smaller rotational radiation fields of from 6×6 cm to 8×8 cm used in the Stanford basic series.[22] Since the survival rates of the Hill series at five and 10 years are not significantly different from those reported for the same period for the Stanford basic series, they concluded that treatment of the primary echelon lymph nodes which might have been included in their patients and which were not included in the Stanford patients did not contribute to an improvement in survival rates. However, the 15×15 cm field probably is not sufficiently

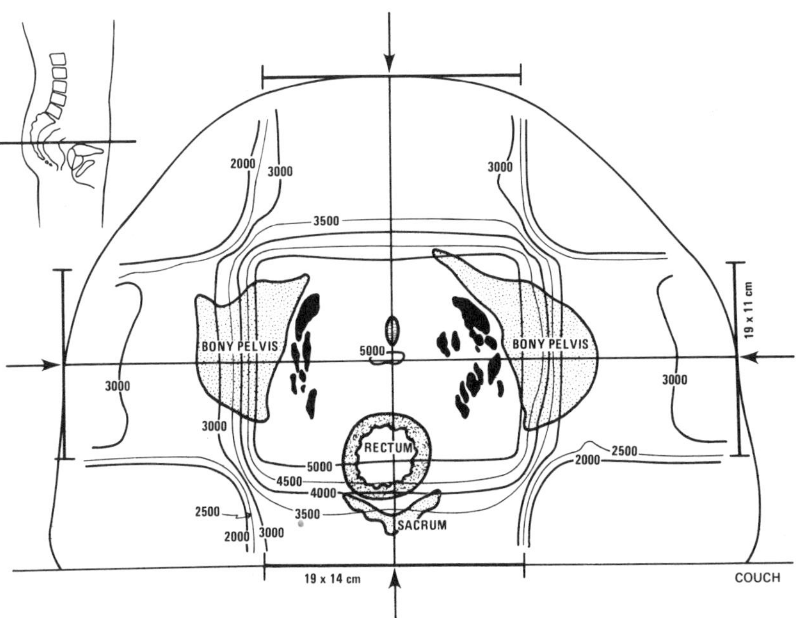

Figure 4. Isodose distribution throughout the mid-pelvis at the level indicated in the figure insert. This is superior to the level of the prostatic boost; therefore, the total dose is limited to 5000 rads. The position and number of external and internal iliac lymph nodes as actually determined in a patient by lymphography are also delineated.

Table 3
Percentage Survival After Radiation Therapy (Prostate Adenocarcinoma). Recently Reported Series. Total N = 1281

Authors	Total	Number Stage[1] A B	C	Radiation Therapy Equipment Used	Survival At 5 Years % Survival	At 5 Years % Disease-free Survival	At 10 Years % Survival	At 10 Years % Disease-free Survival
1a. Bagshaw* et al. (Basic Series) 1956-1971		A&B 193		4.7 MeV, LA	75	67	47	47
			177		52	44	28	33
	370				63		40	
1b. Bagshaw* et al. (Extended Series) 1971-1977		A&B 140		4 or 6 MeV LA	78			
			143		60			
	283				68			
2. Lipsett* et al. 1976		A&B 23		^{60}Co, or 4 or 6 MeV LA	95			
			56	25 MeV B	55			
	79							
3. Taylor et al. 1976†		0		^{60}Co or 4 MeV LA	—			
		12			75			
			96		54 ± 10%			
	108							

4. Hill et al. 1974† (1959-70)					^{60}Co			
	68					64		38
5. Neglia* et al. 1977		0	4	$97(C_1)$ $53(C_2)$	Most by 22 MeV B, some ^{60}Co.	— 100 ~ 70 ~ 45		
	154							
6. McGowan et al. 1977†					^{60}Co	A 88 B_1 90 B_2 66 C 39	84 61 43 37	
	107					74	58	
7. Perez et al. 1977†		0	15	97	25 MeV B	— 60 42		
	112							

LA = Linear Accelerator, b = Betatron, ^{60}Co = Cobalt 60, teletherapy
1 = American Urological Stage
* = Using Kaplan-Meier Survival Method
† = Using Cumulative Survival Curves (Presumed to be Berkson-Gage curves.)

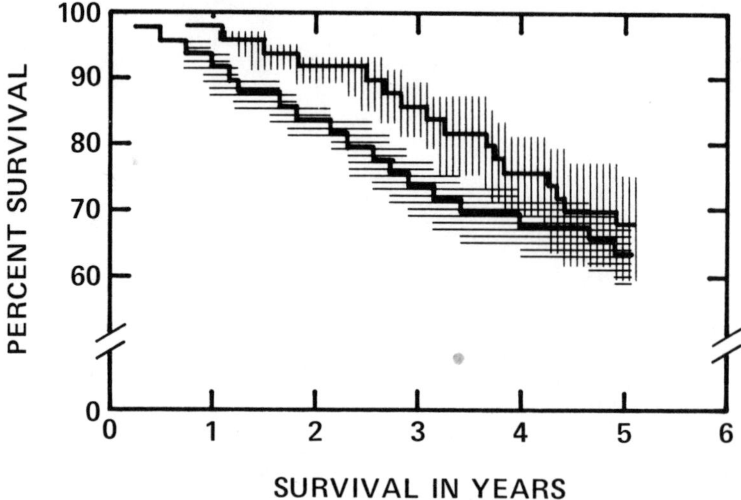

Figure 5. Kaplan-Meier survival curves for the extended series (upper curve) and the first 5-year interval of the basic series (lower curve). Two standard deviations above and below the mean are indicated for each curve. The survival is significantly improved in the overall for the extended series. The Gehan test is significant at p<.01 (p=.0022). The curves appear to be converging at 5 years, and whether a significant difference is maintained depends upon further follow-up. Most of the patients in the extended series received full pelvic irradiation, although some patients who were randomly allocated to treatment to the prostate only after negative lymphadenectomy are included.

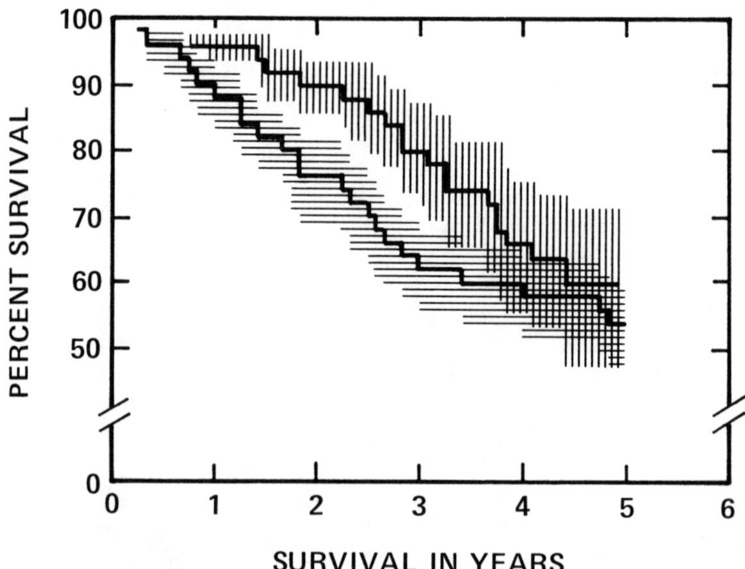

Figure 6. Kaplan-Meier survival curves for Stage C patients only. The extended series is represented by the upper curve; the lower curve represents the basic series. The Gehan test is significant at p<.01 (p=.0025). The curves indicate that for Stage C, survival is again improved for patients treated with full pelvic irradiation.

large to include the common iliac nodes which we have found involved in 17% of the Stanford cases examined (Table 4). Figure 5 also demonstrates the comparison for survival in the first five years between the Stanford basic series and the extended series. The survival is significantly improved (Gehan test p=.0022) in the extended series, although the curves appear to be converging at the fifth year. Figure 6 demonstrates that improvement in survival for the extended series is most significantly improved among patients classified as Stage C (Gehan test p=.0025). Figure 7, however, shows an unequivocal improvement in survival when 57 patients with surgically negative lymph nodes are compared to 47 with biopsy-proven adenopathy. Only one death has occurred in patients with uninvolved lymph nodes, whereas survival at five years is 58% for those with biopsy-proven adenopathy. When we add to this group 36 patients with unproven positive lymphograms, survival for all 83 remains essentially the same (60%) at five years. Therefore, the question of the efficacy of extended field treatment is likely related to inclusion of the primary echelon nodes of the prostate within the target volume, unless, of course, the mere presence of any lymph adenopathy presages

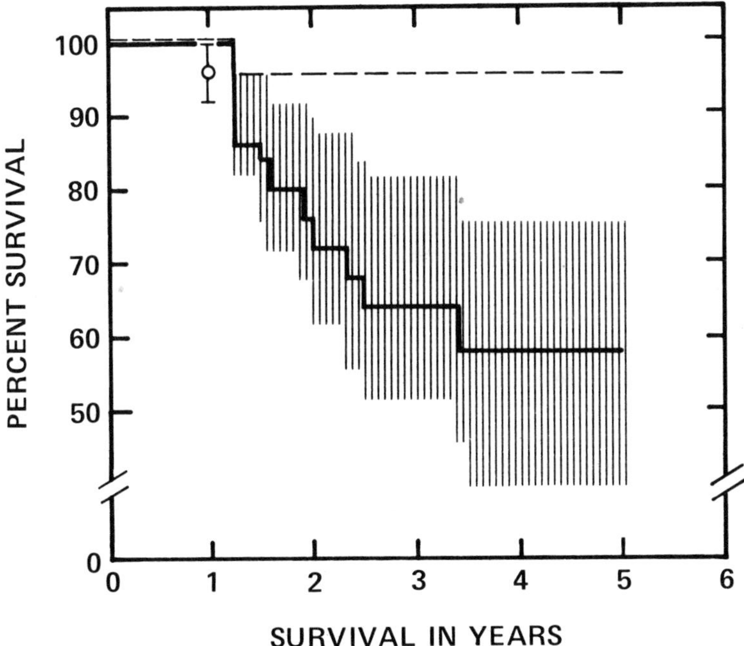

Figure 7. Comparative survival between 57 patients with negative lymphadenectomy and 47 patients with positive lymphadenectomy, as per upper and lower curves, respectively. Since only one death has occurred in the patients with no lymph node metastases, the presence of lymph node metastases appears to be the most significant factor influencing survival, at least for the first 5 years following treatment.

general dissemination of metastases. Rouvière defined the primary echelon nodes as follows: "the entire lymphoid girdle of the superior strait of the pelvis, viz, the external iliac, the hypogastric, and the lymph nodes of the promontory."[28] By lymph nodes of the promontory he meant the common iliac nodes. This distribution is consistent with the lymph node distribution presented in Table 4. It should be noted that Rouvière describes the obturator node as a satellite of the middle node of the internal chain of the *external iliac nodes.* It is located adjacent to the obturator nerve. This description of the obturator node has been confirmed in a comprehensive lymphographic study of the lymphatics of the pelvis by Herman et al.[29] Merrin et al. also were able to demonstrate radiopaque dye in all 50 samples of the obturator nodes removed during pelvic node dissection.[30]

The usefulness of lymphography, however, remains an open question. The correlation between lymphography and histology in 89 patients is shown in Table 5. An earlier analysis of this study was presented by Spellman et al.[31] False negative lymphograms occurred in 15 instances (when the lymphogram appeared negative but the histology was positive). On the other hand, a clearly positive lymphogram appears more reliable so that in spite of this high incidence of false-negative studies, we

Table 4
Incidence of Lymph Node Involvement by Tumor (90 Patients)

Paraaortic*	Common Iliac	External Iliac	Internal Iliac	Obturator
13/73 (18%)	13/75 (17%)	16/71 (23%)	15/62 (24%)	16/50 (32%)

Frequency of Opacification of Lymph Nodes by Pedal Lymphography (88 Patients)

Common Paraaortic	External Iliac	Internal Iliac	Iliac	Obturator
67/72 (93%)	67/71 (94%)	64/68 (94%)	50/58 (86%)	45/48 (94%)

*During the initial phase of this investigation when a transperitoneal surgical exposure was used, the incidence of paraaortic adenopathy was even higher. The incidence has dropped with the employment of a retroperitoneal exposure with which only the distal 2 to 4 cm of the aorta is explored.

Table 5
Lymphographic Histologic Correlation in 89 Patients With Prostatic Carcinoma*

Lymphogram	Histology	
	Positive	Negative
Positive	17	5
Negative	15	52
TOTAL	32	57

*Four additional patients who had lymph node biopsies are excluded. Two did not have lymphograms for medical reasons, and two did not have lymphographically abnormal nodes biopsied.

find lymphography useful in directing the surgeon toward potential disease at time of adenectomy or in preparation of the target volume for radiotherapy in patients in whom lymphadenectomy has not been performed.

Table 6 details the correlation of clinical stage of the primary tumor with histopathologic grade in a consecutive series of 93 protocol patients. Table 7 also demonstrates the powerful influence of the degree of differentiation of the primary tumor on the incidence of lymph node metastases.* The lowest proportion of well differentiated tumors and the highest proportion of poorly differentiated tumors occurred in Stage C. The incidence of positive node biopsies was one of nine patients (11.1%) with well-differentiated tumors; 16 (26.2%) of 61 patients with moderately differentiated tumors; and 16 (69.6%) of 23 patients with poorly differentiated tumors. Comparing all three grades for trend, the incidence of lymph node metastases increased significantly (Chi square=14.1, $p<.01$) as the tumors became less well differentiated.

In summary, this discussion of the potential value of lymph node irradiation indicates that its efficacy cannot be decided in the absence of detailed data concerning clinical stage, histopathologic grade, pathologic staging of lymph node extent, and long-term follow-up of patients after extended field irradiation. These studies are in progress.

---

* The histopathology of all patients in this series has been reviewed in depth by Richard L. Kempson, M.D. of the Stanford Department of Pathology.

Table 6
Distribution of Patients According to Clinical Stage and Differentiation of Primary Tumor

Stage		Primary Tumor Differentiation		
Patients	Am. Urol.	Well-Differentiated	Moderately Differentiated	Poorly Differentiated
2	A	0	1 (50%)	1 (50%)
52	B	8 (15%)	39 (75%)	5 (10%)
39	C	1 (3%)	21 (54%)	17 (44%)
Total 93		9 (10%)	61 (66%)	23 (25%)

Table 7
Distribution of Patients With Nodal Metastases According to Stage and Differentiation of Primary Tumor

Stage		Primary Tumor Differentiation			
No. of Patients	Am. Urol.	Well Differentiated	Moderately Differentiated	Poorly Differentiated	% Patients With Nodal Metastases
2	A	0	0/1*	0/1*	0
52	B	1/8 (12.5%)	8/39 (20.5%)	2/5 (40%)	21.1%
39	C	0/1	8/21 (38%)	14/17 (82.4%)	56.4%
Total 93		1/9 (11.1%)	16/61 (26.2%)	16/23 (69.6%)	35.4%

*Ratio denotes: $\frac{\text{Number of patients with nodal metastases}}{\text{Number in histopathologic group}}$

The issue of treatment of paraaortic node metastases cannot be dealt with in this chapter because no long-term data are available on treatment of lymph node involvement in this region, and it should be considered highly experimental. Reference to Table 4, however, discloses that approximately 20% of paraaortic lymph nodes may be expected to be involved in patients with Stage C neoplasms.

Hormones in Radiation Therapy

In a previous report it was found that survival was not improved by hormonal manipulation through castration or estrogen therapy in conjunction with radiation therapy.[19] Perez et al. also reported no difference in survival between a group of 41 patients treated with radiation alone and a group of 50 patients treated with a combination of radiation and hormone therapy.[26] Neglia et al. in a randomized prospective experiment found no improvement of survival due to the use of hormones combined with radiation.[25] Survival was 77.5% for 40 patients treated with radiotherapy alone and 65.8% for 38 patients treated with radiation therapy plus hormonal manipulation. Thus to date there is no statistically significant evidence to indicate that hormonal manipulation during irradiation increases survival.

On the other hand, hormonal therapy combined with radiation may have some merit in certain special situations. If there is impending obstruction of the urinary tract because of a large mass, several weeks of stilbestrol therapy prior to or during irradiation may reduce the size of the neoplasm sufficiently to prevent development of obstructive symptoms during radiation therapy. And when a patient has received estrogen before radiotherapy, it seems prudent to continue the hormone at least until the course of radiation has been completed.

Delay Between Diagnosis and Radiation Treatment

There are several studies which suggest that the earlier the radiotherapy is commenced following diagnosis the better the results. Ray et al. reported that a delay between diagnosis and treatment had an adverse effect on survival.[19] In this study, the actuarial survival at five years dropped from 61% to 39% when the delay between diagnosis and treatment exceeded one year ($p<0.05$). Cantril et al. noted that when the delay interval was reduced to less than three months the local failure rate was 12%, as opposed to 30% for those treated more than three months after diagnosis.[32] He also reported a five-year survival of 50% in the "no delay" (within three months) group as compared to only 28% for the "delayed" group. Perez et al. observed that 70.7% of 58 patients treated with radiation therapy at time of diagnosis were alive without evidence of disease at three years, compared with only 34.7% of 23 patients in whom radiation therapy was delayed.[26] Therefore early radiotherapy in the treatment of prostatic cancer seems to offer considerably improved survival rates, as is the case for most neoplasms treated by radiation.

Post-Treatment Biopsy

Bumpus in 1922 was the first to call attention to the difficulty in ascertaining the reproductive viability of prostatic cancer cells after subjection to high intensity radium applications.[6] In 1972 Rhamy, Wilson and Caldwell reopened the controversy as to whether or not prostatic neoplasm was sterilized by radiation.[33] In post-treatment biopsies he noted apparently viable prostatic neoplasm in 13 (87%) out of 15 specimens obtained 4 to 38 months following irradiation of the primary tumor. Sewell et al. extended this series to 17 patients performing serial biopsies for as long as 84 months post-therapy.[34] Six (35%) of the 17 became negative. Eight of the 17 patients were surviving, six with negative biopsies. Hill et al. obtained prostatic biopsies in 21 patients from six months to seven years following ^{60}Co radiation.[22] Sixteen of 17 patients who appeared negative by palpation were biopsy-negative, whereas four of four patients who appeared positive by palpation were biopsy-positive. Overall, 16 (76%) of the 21 patients were biopsy-negative one year or more post-therapy. In two patients biopsies were positive at six and eight months, respectively, but converted to negative at one and two years. Several other contributors have made similar observations.[26,35,36] Between 1970 and 1973 Cox and Stofel prospectively studied 38 consecutive patients with carcinoma of the prostate (Stage C-1) who were irradiated to 7,000 rads at the anatomic center of the prostate.[37] All patients completed treatment without interruption and in each case the palpable tumor regressed. There were 139 serial biopsies of the prostate obtained post-treatment. Of these, 49 were considered positive and 90 were negative. The percentage of positive biopsies correlated inversely with the interval after radiation. Thus, 60% were positive at six months, 37% at one year, 30% at 18 months, and 19% at 2½ years. The positive-biopsy rate did not correlate with radiation dose, previous hormonal therapy, or prognosis. The authors reported local control in 28 of 30 patients, or 93%. Twenty-three patients (61%) were surviving at a median interval of 48 months with no evidence of cancer. While this seems to be one of the most decisive contributions to date on the reproductive viability of irradiated prostatic carcinoma, one would like to see a larger group of patients and a somewhat longer follow-up.

Clearly it is difficult to determine whether residual neoplastic cells at the primary site are viable in terms of the cells being capable of sustained replication. Despite this, it is important to attempt to do so, especially in patients who appear on rectal examination to have a growing neoplasm post-therapy. We have demonstrated recently in 12 patients that it is possible to administer full treatment by employing interstitial insertion of ^{125}I seeds as reported by Hilaris et al.[12] Others, including Gill et al. have successfully carried out radical prostatectomy following aggressive radiation therapy.[38] Therefore, in view of the possibility of a second chance for definitive therapy in the face of failure of primary radiation, post-treatment biopsy of the gland offers a possibly useful albeit perplexing guide.

Radiation Salvage After Radical Resection

A patient may develop an apparently local recurrence in the prostatic bed at some interval after radical prostatectomy, or pathologic examination of the radical prostatectomy specimen may disclose neoplasm at the margins of the resected tissue. If there is no evidence of distal metastasis, a second attempt at definitive therapy may be carried out with external beam irradiation. Dykhuizen et al. presented four patients with extracapsular extension proven by examination of the surgical specimen following perineal prostatectomy successfully treated by ^{60}Co radiation.[39] Ray, Cassady, and Bagshaw described patients who were irradiated following surgical resection.[40] Their status at time of publication is presented in Table 8. Thus, 12 of this group of 21 patients were either alive without cancer (eight) or had died without cancer (four).

Table 8
Radiation Salvage of Failure Following Radical Resection

Prompt Treatment after Incomplete Surgical Resection			Later Treatment after Frank Recurrence (Biopsy Proven)		
Alive		9		8	17
With local disease	(3)		(6)		(9)
Without local disease	(6)		(2)		(8) (27 to 97 mos.)
Dead		2		2	4
Without local disease	(2)		(2)		
TOTAL		11		10	21

Taylor noted at least a five-year survival in seven out of seven patients treated for postoperative residual neoplasm, and one out of three who survived for five years following treatment for a postoperative recurrence.[27] Neglia et al. noted local control in six patients living without evident disease among nine treated patients who had prior radical resection.[25] Therefore, radiation therapy offers an opportunity for salvage among patients who either have had an incomplete radical resection or who have frankly recurred at the primary site.

SUMMARY

A group of 1281 patients with carcinoma of the prostate who have been treated definitively with external beam radiation therapy are reviewed. Forty others who have been irradiated after postsurgical recurrence or incomplete resection are summarized. In general, five-year survivals of between about 60% and 75%, and some 10-year survivals of over 40%, have been achieved. Disease-free survivals of between about 65% and 45% have been recorded at five and 10 years respectively. In some reports survivals approaching 100% for small numbers of patients with early neoplasms are described. Most patients have been clinically staged as either Stage B or Stage C, with higher survivals obtained in the lower stages. The variation in survival is undoubtedly influenced by, and probably can be attributed to variations in the distribution of histopathologic grade and the relative incidence of lymph node metastases. Survival is greater if there is no substantial delay between diagnosis and treatment. Hormone therapy concomitant with radiation appears to have no influence on survival. Hormone manipulation remains probably the most important palliative measure for symptomatic advancing, recurrent, or metastatic neoplasm.

Patients with incomplete radical resection or frank postsurgical recurrence may be salvaged by aggressive radiation therapy and, in some instances, isolated local recurrence after a potentially curative course of external beam irradiation can be safely implanted with ^{125}I seeds. However, interpretation of post-irradiation biopsies is difficult and may be an unreliable sole indicator of viable persistent disease.

Whether surgical staging of adenopathy should be considered mandatory prior to radiotherapy in all patients who are good surgical candidates is difficult to answer because of insufficient data and the relatively short follow-up of patients treated with extended-field irradiation after adequate staging. For some, the greater than 20% incidence of positive nodes in Stage B and the 60% or higher incidence in Stage C is sufficient evidence for recommendation of this procedure.[41,42] Clearly, a firm knowledge of the degree of lymph node involvement appears to be of prognostic value, and it is undoubtedly useful to remove bulky adenopathy prior to irradiation. However, microscopic metastases in regional lymph nodes which cannot be detected by lymphography might be treated just as effectively by irradiation alone, as has been found to be the case for occult cervical adenopathy in squamous carcinoma of the head and neck. Thus, lymphography, if clearly positive, might prove to be valuable in the selection for surgical staging and debulking of those patients who will be treated ultimately by irradiation.

REFERENCES

1. Pachkis, R., and Tittinger, W. Radiumbehandlung eines Prostatasarkoms. *Wiener klinische Wochenschrift.* Nr. 48, 1910.

2. Pasteau, O. Traitement du cancer de la prostate par le radium. *Revue des Maladies de la Nutrition.* p 363, 1911.

3. Young, H. H., and Fronz, W. A. Some new methods in the treatment of carcinoma of the lower genitourinary tract with radium. *J Urol.* 1:505-36, 1917.

4. Young, H. H. Technique of radium treatment of cancer of the prostate and seminal vesicles. *Surg Gynecol Obstet.* 34:93-8, 1922.

5. Barringer, B. S. Carcinoma of the prostate. *Surg Gynecol Obstet.* 34:168-76, 1922.

6. Bumpus, H. C. Roentgen rays and radium in the diagnosis and treatment of carcinoma of the prostate. *Am J Roentgenol.* 9:269-89, 1922.

7. Smith, G. G., and Peirson, E. L. The value of high voltage x-ray therapy in carcinoma of the prostate. *J Urol.* 23:331-41, 1930.

8. Barringer, B. S. Prostatic carcinoma. *J Urol.* 47:306-10, 1942.

9. Huggins, C., Stevens, R. E., and Hodges, C. V. Studies on prostatic cancer: effects of castration on advanced carcinoma of prostate gland. *Arch Surg.* 43:209-23, 1941.

10. Flocks, R. H., Kerr, H. D., Elkins, H. P. et al. Treatment of carcinoma of the prostate by interstitial radiation with radioactive gold (Au-198): a preliminary report. *J Urol.* 68:510-22, 1952.

11. Carlton, C. E., Jr., Hudgkins, P. T., Guerriero, W. G. et al. Radiotherapy in the management of stage C carcinoma of the prostate: 452 patients over 11 years. *J Urol.* 116:206-10, 1976.

12. Hilaris, B. S., Whitmore, W. F., Jr., Batata, M. A. et al. Radiation therapy and pelvic node dissection in the management of cancer of the prostate. *Am J Roentgenol.* 121:832-8, 1974.

13. Widman, G. Cancer of the prostate. The results of radium and roentgen-ray treatment. *Radiology.* 22:153-9, 1934.

14. Hultberg, S. Results of treatment with radiotherapy in carcinoma of the prostate. *Acta Radiol.* 27:339-49, 1946.

15. Budhraja, S. N., and Anderson, J. C. An assessment of the value of radiotherapy in the management of carcinoma of the prostate. *Br J Urol.* 36:535-40, 1964.

16. Ray, G. R., and Bagshaw, M. A. The role of radiation therapy in the definitive treatment of adenocarcinoma of the prostate. *Ann Rev Med.* 26:567-88, 1975.

17. Gardner, A., Bagshaw, M. A., Page, V. et al. Tumor localization, dosimetry, simulation and treatment procedures in radiotherapy: the isocenter technique. *Am J Roentgenol.* 114:163-71, 1972.

18. Bagshaw, M. A., Kaplan, H. S., and Sagerman, R. H. Linear accelerator supervoltage radiotherapy. VII. Carcinoma of the prostate. *Radiology.* 85:121-9, 1965.

19. Ray, G. R., Cassady, J. R., and Bagshaw, M. A. Definitive radiation therapy of carcinoma of the prostate. *Radiology.* 106:407-18, 1973.

20. Bagshaw, M. A., Ray, G. R., Salzman, J. R. et al. Extended-field radiation therapy for carcinoma of the prostate: a progress report. *Cancer Chemother Rep.* 59:165-73, 1975.

21. Ray, G. R., Pistenma, D. A., Castellino, R. A. et al. Operative staging of apparently localized adenocarcinoma of the prostate: results in fifty unselected patients. *Cancer.* 38:73-83, 1976.

22. Hill, D. R., Crews, Q. E., Jr., and Walsh, P. C. Prostate carcinoma:

radiation treatment of the primary and regional lymphatics. *Cancer.* 34:156-60, 1974.

23. Lipsett, J. A., Cosgrove, M. D., Green, N. et al. Factors influencing prognosis in the radiotherapeutic management of carcinoma of the prostate. *Int J Rad Oncol Biol Phys.* 1:1049-58, 1976.

24. McGowan, D. G. Radiation therapy in the management of localized carcinoma of the prostate. A preliminary report. *Cancer.* 39:98-103, 1977.

25. Neglia, W. J., Hussey, D. H., and Johnson, D. E. Megavoltage radiation therapy for carcinoma of the prostate. *Int J Rad Oncol Biol Phys.* 2:873-82, 1977.

26. Perez, C. A., Bauer, W., Garza, R. et al. Radiation therapy in the definitive treatment of localized carcinoma of the prostate. *Cancer.* 40:1425-33, 1977.

27. Taylor, W. J. Radiation oncology: cancer of the prostate. *Cancer.* 39:856-61, 1977.

28. Rouvière, H. Lymphatiques de la Prostate. Edited by Masson et Cie. In *Anatomie des Lymphatiques de l'Homme.* Paris: Libraires de l'academie de Medecine, 1932, 395-8.

29. Herman, P. G., Benninghoff, D. L., Nelson, J. H., Jr. et al. Roentgen anatomy of the ilio-pelvic-aortic lymphatic system. *Radiology.* 80:182-93, 1963.

30. Merrin, C., Wajsman, Z., Baumgartner, G. et al. The clinical value of lymphangiography: are the nodes surrounding the obturator nerve visualized? *J Urol.* 117:762-4, 1977.

31. Spellman, M. C., Castellino, R. A., Ray, G. R. et al. An evaluation of lymphography in localized carcinoma of the prostate. *Radiology.* 125:637-44, 1977.

32. Cantril, S. T., Vaeth, J. M., Green, J. P. et al. Radiation therapy for localized carcinoma of the prostate: correlation with histopathological grading. *Front Rad Ther Oncol.* 9:274-94, 1974.

33. Rhamy, R. K., Wilson, S. K., and Caldwell, W. L. Biopsy-proved tumor following definite irradiation for resectable carcinoma of the prostate. *J Urol.* 107:627-30, 1972.

34. Sewell, R. A., Braren, V., Wilson, S. K. et al. Extended biopsy follow-up after full course radiation for resectable prostatic carcinoma. *J Urol.* 113:371-3, 1975.

35. DeMuelenaere, G. F., Sandison, A. G., and Coetzee, F. C. Radiotherapie in Prostaatkarsinoom. *South Afr Med J.* 48:321-4, 1974.

36. Kagan, A. R., Gordon, J., Cooper, J. F. et al. A clinical appraisal of post-irradiation biopsy in prostatic cancer. *Cancer.* 39:637-41, 1977.

37. Cox, J. D., and Stoffel, T. J. The significance of needle biopsy after irradiation for stage C adenocarcinoma of the prostate. *Cancer.* 40:156-60, 1977.

38. Gill, W. B., Marks, J. E., Strauss, F. H. et al. Radical retropubic prostatectomy and retroperitoneal lymphadenectomy following radiotherapy conversion of stage C to stage B carcinoma of the prostate. *J Urol.* 111:656-61, 1974.

39. Dykhuizen, R. F., Sargent, C. R., George, F. W. et al. The use of Cobalt 60 teletherapy in the treatment of prostatic carcinoma. *J Urol.* 100:333-8, 1968.

40. Ray, G. R., Cassady, J. R., and Bagshaw, M. A. External-beam megavoltage radiation therapy in the treatment of post-radical prostatectomy residual or recurrent tumor: preliminary results. *J Urol.* 114:98-101, 1975.

41. McLaughlin, A. P., Saltzstein, S. L., McCullough, D. L. et al. Prostatic carcinoma: incidence and location of unsuspected lymphatic metastases. *J Urol.* 115:89-94, 1976.

42. McCullough, D. L., Prout, G. R., and Daly, J. J. Carcinoma of the prostate and lymphatic metastases. *J Urol.* 111:65-71, 1974.

Hormonal Therapy for Prostatic Cancer

11

Mani Menon and Patrick C. Walsh

For over 30 years, since the pioneering efforts of Huggins and Hodges, hormonal therapy has constituted the major modality of treatment for men with metastatic carcinoma of the prostate.[1] Endocrine manipulations have included castration, estrogen administration, hypophysectomy or adrenalectomy, and treatment with corticosteroids or antiandrogens. It is chastening to note that endocrine therapy is successful in palliating disease in only 60% to 70% of patients and that as yet no simple method of identifying responders or nonresponders has been developed. It is also sobering that after 35 years of work no consensus exists as to the timing or the preferred form of treatment. In this chapter we shall attempt to explain the physiologic rationale behind hormonal therapy, briefly review the existing clinical information, and propose a plan of management based on available data.

PHYSIOLOGY OF PROSTATIC GROWTH AND FUNCTION

Although it has been known for several years that the integrity of prostatic epithelium is dependent upon adequate levels of circulating androgen, the precise mechanism of androgenic action has been elucidated only recently.[2] In 1968 Bruchovsky and Wilson, and Anderson and Liao demonstrated that following the administration of testosterone to rats the major metabolite isolated from the nuclei of the ventral prostate was dihydrotestosterone.[3,4] Subsequent studies showed that when a wide variety of androgens was administered intravenously to rats, dihydrotestosterone was once again the major steroid isolated from the nucleus.[5] Furthermore a close correlation existed between the relative biologic potency of the steroid injected and the amount of dihydrotestosterone recovered from the nucleus (Table 1). These observations suggest strongly that dihydrotestosterone is the major androgen responsible for growth and functional integrity of the prostate.

A two-step mechanism for the nuclear uptake of testosterone has been proposed (Figure 1). Testosterone is initially converted to dihydrotestosterone by the membrane-bound enzyme, 5α-reductase (NADPH-dependent Δ^4-3 ketosteroid 5-α-oxidoreductase).[6] Dihydrotestosterone is then bound to a specific cytoplasmic macromolecular protein, the receptor. The steroid-receptor complex then undergoes a temperature-dependent physical change and is transported to the nucleus. There the complex is bound to acceptor substances on chromatin. By some as yet unidentified mechanism these events activate transcription and result in formation of messenger RNA and increased protein synthesis.[18]

Synthesis and Distribution of Androgens in the Body

Circulating androgens are of dual origin: testicular and adrenal.

Table 1
Evaluation of Five Natural Androgens: Correlation Between Biologic Potency and the Incorporation of Dihydrotestosterone-^{3}H into the Nucleus of the Ventral Prostate After Intravenous Injection into Castrated, Functionally Hepatectomized Rats.*

Hormone	Relative Potency (Ventral Prostate)	Amount Injected N Moles	Dihydrotestosterone Content of Nuclei
Dihydrotestosterone-^{3}H	268	2.0	19.0
Testosterone-^{3}H	100	2.4	24.2
Androstanediol-^{3}H	276, 187	1.7	25.5
Androstenedione-^{3}H	39	1.9	7.0
Dehydroepiandrosterone-^{3}H	15	4.0	0.6

*Modified from Bruchovsky, N. Comparison of the metabolites formed in the rat prostate following the in vivo administration of seven natural androgens. *Endocrinology*. 89:1212, 1222, 1971, and from Walsh, P. C. Physiologic basis for hormonal therapy in carcinoma of the prostate. *Urol Clin North Am.* 1:125-40, 1974.

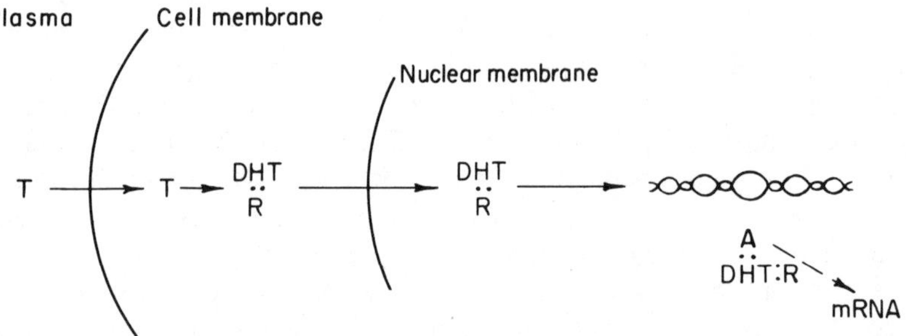

Figure 1. Testosterone (T) crosses plasma membrane by simple diffusion and is converted to dihydrotestosterone (DHT). DHT combines with the cytoplasmic receptor (R) to form the dihydrotestosterone-receptor complex. This complex is transferred to the nucleus where it combines with acceptors (A) located on the chromatin. These events stimulate the synthesis of messenger RNA (mRNA) and then protein synthesis.

(From Walsh, P. C. Physiologic basis for hormonal therapy in carcinoma of the prostate. *Urol Clin North Am.* 1:125-40, 1974.)

The principal circulating androgens secreted by the testes of adult males are testosterone and androstenedione whereas androgens synthesized by the adrenal are androstenedione and dehydroepiandrosterone. The enzymatic pathways for synthesis of these androgens from a common precursor, cholesterol, are depicted in Figure 2, and the production rates, plasma levels, and relative potencies in Table 2. Five major enzymes are involved in androgen synthesis, which preferentially follows the Δ^4 pathway. It should be noted that 95% of circulating plasma testosterone originates from the testis and, therefore, bilateral orchiectomy removes the major source of androgen production. Approximately 4% of plasma testosterone and 2% of androstenedione are converted by 5-α reduction into dihydrotestosterone.[6] Minute quantities of dihydrotestosterone are also formed by direct glandular secretion.

Over 95% of testosterone and dihydrotestosterone is bound with

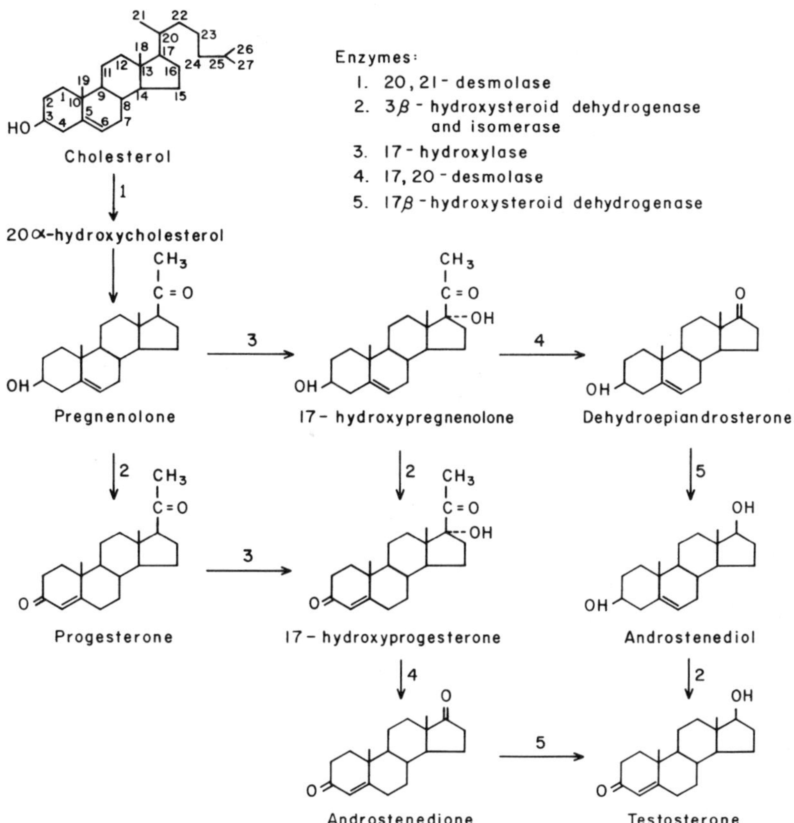

Figure 2. Pathways for synthesis of testosterone in testes. The preferred pathway in men is the Δ^4 pathway.

(From Walsh, P. C. Physiologic basis for hormonal therapy in carcinoma of the prostate. *Urol Clin North Am.* 1:125-40, 1974.)

Table 2
The Major Circulating Androgens in Man

Hormone	Source	Production Rate (MG PER D)	Plasma Level (NG PER 100 ML)	Relative Potency
Testosterone	Testis	7.0	559 ± 151	100
Dihydrotestosterone	Peripheral tissues	0.3	50 ± 14	268
Androstenedione	Adrenal	3.0	114 ± 21	39
Dehydroepiandrosterone	Adrenal	29.0	553 ± 178	15

Modified from Walsh, P.C. Physiologic basis for hormonal therapy in carcinoma of the prostate. *Urol Clin North Am.* 1:125–40, 1974.

high affinity to a β-globulin present in the plasma, testosterone-estradiol-binding globulin (TeBG; sex hormone-binding globulin; SHBG), and with lower affinity to plasma albumin. The concentration of TeBG in serum is increased by the administration of estrogens.[8-10] It is believed that the free moiety of testosterone is the functionally important one at the cellular level. Adrenal androgens lack the 17-β hydroxyl group and thus are bound almost exclusively to albumin.[11] Corticotropin (ACTH) regulates the synthesis of adrenal androgens.

Testosterone is produced by the Leydig cells of testes under the influence of pituitary luteinizing hormone (LH). Testicular cells other than Leydig cells can synthesize testosterone from a steroid such as progesterone, but production of pregnenolone from cholesterol (step 1 in Figure 2) cannot occur outside the Leydig cells.[12] Testosterone is secreted into the interstitial fluid from which it is either taken up by the seminiferous tubules and transported to the epididymis or channeled through pericellular membrane to spermatic venous blood.[13] The retention of androgen within the seminiferous tubules may be related to the presence of a specific androgen-binding protein (ABP). Transport to the venous system is incompletely understood, but it is known that testosterone binds to cortisol-binding globulin, albumin, and TeBG in the blood stream. Testosterone is converted peripherally by 5-α reduction to dihydrotestosterone or by aromatization to estradiol. Plasma testosterone levels remain relatively constant between the ages of 20 and 60 years after which a steady decrease occurs in most males.[14] This is associated with an increase in circulating TeBG levels so that free testosterone levels are depressed even further. In addition to this there is a similar reduction in plasma dihydrotestosterone levels. In contrast, the levels of plasma estradiol increase with age so that the overall alteration of the testosterone:estradiol ratio becomes significant.[15,16]

Circulating androgens are metabolized in the liver to 17-ketosteroids, conjugated with glucuronic and sulfuric acid, and excreted in the urine. In contrast to estrogens, only small amounts of androgen are excreted through the bile or feces. About 30% of urinary 17-ketosteroids is of testicular origin, whereas 70% is of adrenal origin. Because of the interreaction between these metabolites it is impossible to determine which steroids in the urine are of testicular and which of adrenal origin. Hence measurement of urinary 17-ketosteroids is not a reliable index of androgen function.[17]

PHYSIOLOGIC RATIONALE FOR HORMONAL THERAPY

The principal goal of hormonal therapy in treatment of prostatic cancer is suppression of androgenic stimuli to the prostate. This can be achieved through four mechanisms: 1) ablation of androgen sources, 2) suppression of pituitary gonadotropin release, 3) inhibition of androgen synthesis, and 4) interference with androgen action at target tissues.[18]

Ablation of Androgen Sources

Orchiectomy Bilateral orchiectomy causes a prompt decline in plasma testosterone levels from 500 ng/100 ml to 50 ng/100 ml.[19,20] Early studies by Scott and Vermeulen demonstrated that although urinary 17-ketosteroids fell rapidly after castration, this was followed by a secondary increase up to the pretreatment level in 9 of 10 patients.[21] Since then it has become apparent that elevations of urinary 17-ketosteroids can occur secondary to pain, anxiety, and stress and that, therefore, elevation of urinary 17-ketosteroids in castrated patients represents a nonspecific response to a situation of stress.[22] Determination of plasma testosterone levels is a much more reliable index of androgen function, and several clinical studies have shown that plasma testosterone is uniformly suppressed for up to two years following orchiectomy.[19,20,23,24] Furthermore, Walsh and Siiteri have measured plasma testosterone levels in castrated males with reactivation of prostatic cancer and demonstrated no secondary elevation of plasma testosterone in these patients.[7]

Adrenalectomy and Hypophysectomy Because 95% of circulating androgen is of testicular origin and thus removed by orchiectomy, and as no increase in adrenal androgens has been demonstrated with relapsing prostatic carcinoma, the role of adrenal or pituitary ablation in an attempt to lower extra-testicular androgen stimulation of the prostate is nebulous.[7] Furthermore, it is well-known that the adult prepubertal castrate has a small atrophic prostate with no secretion. Because the levels of adrenal and pituitary hormones in these subjects are similar to levels in the castrated patient with prostatic carcinoma, it is logical to conclude that the pituitary and the adrenal are of doubtful significance in stimulating prostatic growth in the absence of testes. Despite this lack of firm biochemical and morphologic support, ablation of the adrenal and the hypophysis has been accompanied by a 40% to 70% subjective improvement in the clinical condition.[25] In addition to removing the secretion of ACTH, hypophysectomy also causes a decrease in secretion of prolactin. Although prolactin has been reported to increase accumulation and utilization of androgen in the prostate, it is inactive in the absence of androgen.[26] In clinical studies on patients with carcinoma of the prostate, Bhanalaph, Varkarakis and Murphy were unable to detect any further fall in plasma testosterone following adrenalectomy.[27] However, in a previously reported study, Reynoso and Murphy demonstrated that adrenalectomy produced an increase in pituitary gonadotropin release.[28] This indicates that adrenalectomy may decease the feedback inhibition of LH and FSH release, and that failure to demonstrate suppression of plasma testosterone levels may be due to lack of sensitivity of the assay at levels of plasma testosterone of less than 50 ng/100 ml.

Suppression of Pituitary Gonadotropin Release

Treatment with Estrogens It is generally accepted that in the noncastrated male estrogens act primarily by suppressing release of LH from the pituitary and thus decreasing endogenous production of testosterone. Assuming this to be the case, it is possible to monitor the adequacy of estrogen treatment in prostatic cancer by measuring plasma testosterone levels. Studies by Kent and his coworkers and by Houghton, Turner, and Cooper have demonstrated that doses of 1.0 mg or less of diethylstilbestrol (DES) did not cause uniform suppression of plasma testosterone to castrate levels.[9,29] However, doses of 3.0 mg and more produced a uniform and prolonged suppression.[19,20] Increasing the dose of DES to 30 mg/day did not cause a further suppression of plasma testosterone.[30] As estrogen administration also causes an increase in testosterone-estradiol-binding globulin the levels of free testosterone may be significantly lower than values for total hormone.[8-10] Based on these data the optimal dosage of DES for treatment of prostatic cancer appears to be 3.0 mg per day. Although this is the case, clinical studies have demonstrated that 1.0 mg of DES is as effective as 5.0 mg in preventing deaths from prostatic cancer and progression of Stage C disease to Stage D disease.[31] No clinical studies have compared the 1.0 mg dose to the 3.0 mg dose. This variation between the clinical effectiveness of the administered dose of DES and its ability to lower plasma testosterone suggests that to achieve maximal regression of metastatic prostatic carcinoma it may not be necessary to lower plasma testosterone levels to the castrate range.

Although suppression of pituitary gonadotropin release is their primary mode of action in the intact subject, in the castrated animal estrogens have both stimulating and inhibiting effects on the prostate. In the castrated rat and the orchiectomized dog estrogens act synergistically with androgens in stimulating prostate growth.[32-34] Recent experimental work has demonstrated the presence of specific macromolecular proteins that bind estradiol with great affinity in the human prostate.[35,36] In addition estrogens promote the release of prolactin from the hypophysis. These data appear to suggest a direct stimulatory role for estrogens on the prostate.

Utilizing the canine prostatic fistula model, Huggins and Clark demonstrated in 1940 that overdosage with estrogens caused a complete cessation of prostatic secretion.[37] This was associated, however, with an increase in weight of the prostate gland and with histologic evidence of squamous metaplasia of the prostatic ducts, suggesting a causal role for ductal obstruction in preventing prostatic secretion. When estrogens were given in smaller doses such that the level of prostatic secretion was maintained at a low but constant level, these changes were not seen and the prostate gland remained involuted. They concluded that in the intact dog "the prostate decreases in size when estrogen is injected in amounts to depress prostatic secretion profoundly. . . . The shrinkage is related to depression of male hormone production. . . . Overdosage of estrogen (in the castrated dog maintained with exogenous androgen)* causes the prostate gland of dogs to enlarge."[37]

More recently it has been shown that estradiol inhibits the 3-β hydroxy steroid dehydrogenase and isomerase enzyme complex, thus blocking synthesis of testosterone from precursors.[38,39] In addition, estrogens can inhibit both DNA polymerase and 5-α reductase activity, suggesting a direct nuclear site of inhibition.[40,41] However, these latter two phenomena have been demonstrated only in vitro using doses of estrogen that far exceed levels that can be achieved in man. Finally, recent experiments have demonstrated that estrogens inhibit the conversion of testosterone to dihydrotestosterone by minces of human benign prostatic hyperplasia.[42] Taking all the conflicting evidence into consideration, it appears that the primary effect of estrogens in the clinical setting of prostatic carcinoma is to decrease testicular androgen synthesis by inhibiting pituitary gonadotropin release. With the low doses of DES utilized clinically, any direct effect on the prostate gland, whether excitatory or inhibitory, remains conjectural.

Chlorotrianisene (TACE) TACE is a synthetic estrogen that was manufactured in an attempt to produce an agent that would provide the clinical benefits of DES without its feminizing side effects. The drug was adopted because it failed to increase the size of the adrenal gland in rats, a known effect of estrogen administration to rodents, and because it

---

*Statement in parentheses is ours.

causes less gynecomastia.[43] Chlorotrianisene has been used for over 20 years and is assumed to act by suppression of LH release from the pituitary. Several investigators have demonstrated clinical remission of prostatic cancer in patients treated with TACE, but these remissions have been generally subjective, poorly documented, and in patients in whom other endocrine manipulations such as orchiectomy have been concomitantly performed.[44-47] In addition O'Connor and Sokol demonstrated that a significant proportion of patients on TACE benefited from subsequent castration. More recently Baker et al. have demonstrated that in daily doses of 24 mg TACE has no effect on plasma LH and FSH, although depressing plasma testosterone by 40% to 60%.[8] This latter effect could not be confirmed by Shearer et al., who demonstrated normal plasma testosterone levels and normal spermatogenesis in three patients with prostatic cancer treated with TACE.[20] These data strongly suggest that TACE is a weak estrogen which is why it fails to produce adrenal hyperplasia in the rodent. Therefore at the present time the role of chlorotrianisene in the treatment of prostatic cancer appears ill-defined.

Premarin Premarin is a conjugated natural estrogen that has been used in an effort to reduce cardiovascular and feminizing side effects of stilbestrol. Shearer et al. demonstrated that Premarin in doses of 2.5 mg orally tid was as effective as 3 mg of DES in reducing plasma testosterone, but was ineffective in doses of 1.25 mg tid.[20] In preliminary studies, Premarin in doses of 1.25 mg daily for a month followed thereafter by 2.5 mg daily has been as effective as 1 mg of DES in causing clinical regression of prostatic cancer.[48,49]

Progestational Agents Progestins affect the integrity of the prostatic epithelium by inhibiting gonadotropin secretion, by inhibiting androgen synthesis in the testis and by competing for binding of dihydrotestosterone by prostatic nuclei.[18] Trunell et al. reported on 19 patients with previously untreated or relapsing prostatic cancer to whom they administered progesterone.[50] Approximately 90% of the untreated group and 70% of the relapsing group obtained clinical benefit from progesterone treatment. In a recent study Blackard reported no increased benefit from Provera in a daily dose of 30 mg, either alone or in combination with diethylstilbestrol, over 1 mg of diethylstilbestrol alone.[47] Based on these data, and because progestational agents have been demonstrated to have synergistic effects when administered with androgens in certain experimental systems,[51] these agents are not in wide usage currently.

Ethinyl Estradiol (Estinyl) This synthetic estrogen has been used in several clinical trials in patients with prostatic cancer.[25] In doses of 0.05 mg twice daily ethinyl estradiol causes a reduction of plasma testosterone similar to that caused by 3 mg of diethylstilbestrol.[20] The clinical response rate and the incidence of side effects are comparable to stilbestrol.

Diethylstilbestrol Diphosphate (Stilphostrol, Honvan) When given orally this drug is hydrolyzed in the stomach and acts in a manner similar to DES. It is hypothesized that on intravenous administration it is concentrated in the prostatic cells and acts as a cytotoxic agent, although this has never been proven.[52] Fergusson demonstrated that following the administration of radioactive Stilphostrol to patients with prostatic carcinoma, no radioactivity was recovered from biopsies of the prostate gland.[53] The drug was metabolized in the liver and excreted in feces and urine. It is thus apparent that any salutory effect that the drug exerts is based on a central estrogenic effect rather than a local cytotoxic effect. The main advantage of this agent is that it is water soluble and can be given intravenously in high doses. Therapy consists of 0.5 to 2.0 g given intravenously in 250 to 500 ml of 5% dextrose over a period of one to four hours, or an oral dose of 100 mg taken three times a day. On oral administration, it has been demonstrated to depress plasma testosterone to castrate levels.[20] In a small series Band et al. demonstrated remission of disease in three of 15 patients who had relapsed three to four years following orchiectomy.[54] The remissions were characterized by increased motor function, healing of bony metastases, decrease in prostatic size, and relief of pain. Although Hawtrey et al. demonstrated considerable relief of pain and improved activity in a small number of patients with paraparesis secondary to carcinoma who were given Stilphostrol, conventional hormonal therapy was utilized concomitantly in all, and decompression laminectomy in most, of these patients.[55]

Polyestradiol Phosphate (Estradurin) Estradurin is a long-acting estrogen administered in 80 to 200 mg doses once a month. It acts primarily by pituitary inhibition, and the response rate and side effects are similar to those with diethylstilbestrol.

Inhibition of Androgen Synthesis

In this group are included agents that inhibit one of the enzymes involved in synthesis of testosterone from cholesterol (Table 3). Although most of these agents are not available for widespread clinical use preliminary trials in patients with relapsing carcinoma of the prostate have suggested encouraging results.[7,56-58]

Aminoglutethimide acts early in the synthesis chain to prevent conversion of cholesterol to pregnenolone by inhibiting the 20-21 desmolase enzyme.[18] This results in inhibition of all adrenal steroidogenesis, including androgens. Due to lack of feedback suppression large amounts of ACTH are secreted, and this may ultimately overcome the drug-induced blockade unless replacement doses of glucocorticoids are given.[56] Spironolactone acts further down the pathway and selectively inhibits

Table 3
Inhibitors of Androgen Synthesis

Agent	Enzymatic Reaction
Aminoglutethimide	20,21-desmolase
Spironolactone Cyproterone acetate	17,20-desmolase
Cyanoketone Cyproterone acetate Estradiol—17β Hydroxymethylene Medrogestone	3β-hydroxysteroid dehydrogenase and isomerase

From Walsh, P. C. Physiologic basis for hormonal therapy in carcinoma of the prostate. *Urol Clin North Am.* 1:125-40, 1974.

synthesis of androgens. When spironolactone was administered at doses of 400 mg per day to healthy male volunteers, a significant rise in progesterone and 17-α hydroxy progesterone was documented.[59] Although no fall in plasma testosterone levels was demonstrated, a transient increase in gonadotropin levels was detected. This indicates that failure to demonstrate a decrease in plasma testosterone may have been due to low doses of spironolactone used (when compared to animal experiments) or that in the presence of an intact pituitary gonadal axis, the rise in LH may restore plasma testosterone to normal levels.

Medrogestone is a third steroid that acts by inhibiting testosterone biosynthesis. Although medrogestone causes involution of the prostate in the intact rat, it is not able to block DNA synthesis induced by exogenous testosterone administered to the castrated rat.[60]

Cyproterone acetate, although possessing some ability to inhibit steroidogenesis, acts primarily as an antiandrogen in blocking androgen uptake by the cell. A number of other agents (estradiol, cyanoketone, hydroxymethylene) have been shown to act by inhibiting the 3-β hydroxy steroid dehydrogenase-isomerase complex.

Two of these agents have been tested clinically in patients with metastatic carcinoma of the prostate in relapse following orchiectomy. Robinson, Shearer and Fergusson obtained palliation in 50%, and Sanford et al. in three of seven patients treated with aminoglutethimide.[56,61] Complete adrenal suppression was demonstrated in all patients in the latter series, indicating that aminoglutethimide effectively performs a medical adrenalectomy. Walsh and Siiteri demonstrated that spironolactone induced a 50% drop in plasma androstenedione and dehydroepiandrosterone levels in all patients, and a limited clinical remission in three of seven patients with relapsing metastatic prostatic cancer.[7] However, because it is doubtful that androgens of adrenal origin play any significant role in stimulating the prostate, it is unlikely that this approach will produce any significant remission of metastatic disease in patients with reactivation of disease after an initial response to orchiectomy or DES.

Interference with Androgen Action at Target Tissues

Antiandrogens are agents that produce their effect by direct competition with androgens at the target organ. All compounds studied to date act by inhibiting the nuclear uptake of dihydrotestosterone. In experimental systems antiandrogens inhibit the testosterone-induced synthesis of DNA.[62] Several antiandrogens have been studied in detail and their structure and relative potency are shown in Figure 3. Cyproterone acetate is the agent that has been investigated most extensively. It is a progestational agent that is well-absorbed following oral administration and

ANTIANDROGEN	*STRUCTURAL FORMULA*	*RELATIVE POTENCY*
Cyproterone acetate	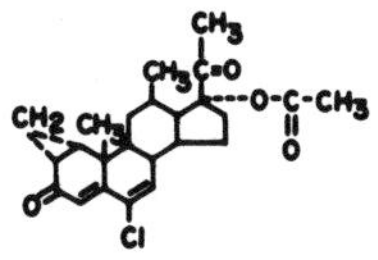	100
Flutamide (Sch 13521)	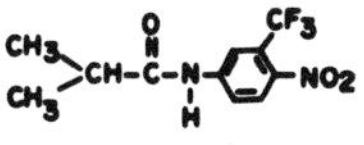	100-140
Cyproterone	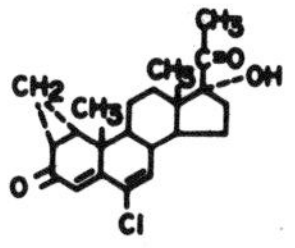	30
MK 316	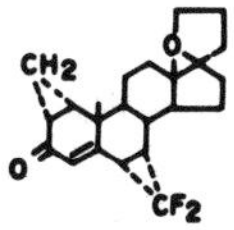	20
Chlormadinone acetate	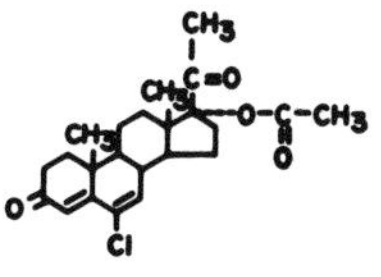	10
R 2956	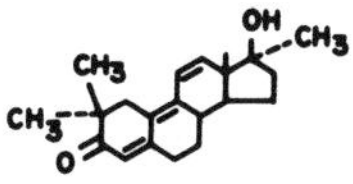	10
Medrogestone	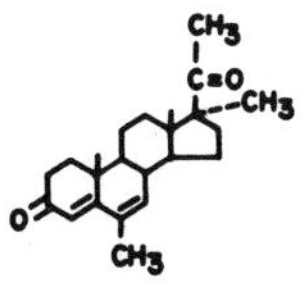	2

Figure 3. Relative potency of antiandrogens to inhibit uptake of exogenous androgen by ventral prostate of castrated rat.

acts by inhibiting gonadotropin release, by interfering with testicular androgen synthesis, and by inhibiting formation of the dihydrotestosterone-receptor complex in prostatic nuclei.[63,64] In clinical trials Wein and Murphy demonstrated clinical remission in 60% of 26 patients with advanced prostatic cancer treated with 200 mg doses of cyproterone acetate.[58] Smith, Walsh and Goodwin utilizing 300 mg of cyproterone acetate in 28 patients refractory to estrogen therapy and orchiectomy, were able to achieve relief of pain for a duration of one to 36 months in 12 patients.[57] Although the latter group did not detect any estrogenic side effects due to the drug, 15 of 55 patients in the former study developed some of the stigmata of estrogen treatment.

Flutamide (Sch 13521) is a nonprogestational, nonsteroidal antiandrogen that neither inhibits gonadotropin release nor suppresses plasma testosterone. It has been shown to cause involution of the seminal vesicle and ventral prostate in the intact rat. Flutamide inhibits transfer of labeled androgen from the cytosol to the nucleus and also inhibits testosterone-induced DNA synthesis by prostatic nuclei.[65] In doses of 750 to 1500 mg daily it caused decrease of pain, relief of obstruction, and decrease of prostatic size in seven of 18 patients with carcinoma of the prostate, most of whom had prior endocrine therapy in some form.[66]

Recent studies from the Memorial Hospital demonstrated clinical response in six of 26 patients with metastatic cancer refractory to conventional hormonal therapy and in 19 of 21 patients in whom the drug was used as a primary agent.[67,68] However, these responses have been transient and the incidence of estrogenic side effects was no less than in patients treated with DES. Of interest is the fact that when Flutamide was used as a primary form of hormonal therapy, all nine patients who were sexually potent prior to treatment remained so on the drug.[68,69] This appears to be superior to the 42% incidence of potency following orchiectomy and estrogens.[70]

CLINICAL STUDIES OF ENDOCRINE THERAPY

In their classical treatise Huggins and Hodges reported on the effects of estrogen administration and orchiectomy on eight patients with metastatic prostatic cancer.[1] Following treatment, in five to nine days a marked regression of the tumor associated with a striking decrease in serum acid phosphatase was noted. Subsequent administration of testosterone produced an elevation of serum acid phosphatase back into the abnormal ranges. They concluded that "prostatic cancer is influenced by androgenic activity in the body . . . (and) disseminated cancer of the prostate is inhibited by eliminating androgens through castration or neutralization of their activity by estrogen injection." Following this report utilization of endocrine therapy became widespread and often indiscriminate. It was used in all stages of disease, and the dose of estrogen ranged from one to 500 mg per day.

In an attempt to solve "the problems concerning the selection of the form of endocrine modification most efficacious for the particular needs of the patient . . . (and to determine) the most opportune time to institute therapy and the choice of secondary therapy once relapse had occurred," a cooperative study was established, the results of which were reported in 1950 by Nesbit and Baum.[71] They published a five-year follow-up of 263 patients with and 324 patients without metastases from prostatic cancer at the time of admission to the study, and compared the results to a previous report by Nesbit and Plumb.[72] Treatment of patients was by orchiectomy alone, estrogen alone (the equivalent of 1 to 5 mg of diethylstilbestrol orally each day) or a combination of the two. They concluded that endocrine therapy in any form improved survival rates whether or not metastases were present. In patients with metastases orchiectomy was more effective than estrogen administration, and the combination of the two offered no benefit over orchiectomy alone.

The study reported by Nesbit and Baum had one major weakness in that there were no concurrent controls.[71] The "controls" represented patients treated in the pre-antibiotic era between the years 1925 and 1940 when perhaps the expected survival rates in the age-matched general population were low. Indeed, in an analysis of patients with prostatic cancer treated by transurethral resection alone in the pre-endocrine era, Pool and Thompson reported a five-year survival of 14% in patients treated in the period between 1926 and 1936, and 27% for the period between 1937 and 1941.[73] This indicated that death rates from cancer of the prostate were falling even prior to the advent of endocrine therapy. If this latter group treated by Pool and Thompson is utilized as the control for Nesbit and Baum's study, the dramatic improvement in survival with endocrine therapy disappears.[70,72]

The conclusions of this study remained unchallenged until the results of the Veterans Administration studies were published. The Veterans Administration Cooperative Urological Research Group (VACURG) was organized in 1960 for the purpose of studying the treatment of various urological disorders and especially carcinoma of the prostate by means of large scale, randomized, prospective clinical trial.[74] Three studies have been initiated so far: study 1, begun in 1960; study 2, in 1967; and study 3, in 1969. In study 1 all patients with Stage A or Stage B disease underwent radical prostatectomy; half, chosen by statistical randomization, were given supplementary estrogens (DES 5 mg daily). For Stages C and D, patients were randomized to either placebo, 5.0 mg of DES daily, orchiectomy plus placebo, or orchiectomy plus 5.0 mg of DES daily. *In any group, if the patient did poorly, the treatment was changed, but the results were included in the original group.* The results of this study indicated that in patients with Stage A and Stage B disease supplementary estrogen not only failed to improve the length of survival, but also that patients receiving estrogens actually showed poorer survival rates than patients who did not receive them (Figure 4). Survival rates were significantly lower in Stage C patients receiving orchiectomy and estrogen than in the other three treatment groups. No significant survival differences were detected in Stage D patients.[74]

When survival data were analyzed according to the causes of death, it became obvious that patients in the estrogen-treated groups had lower death rates from cancer of the prostate and higher death rates from other causes, mainly cardiovascular (myocardial infarctions, cerebrovascular

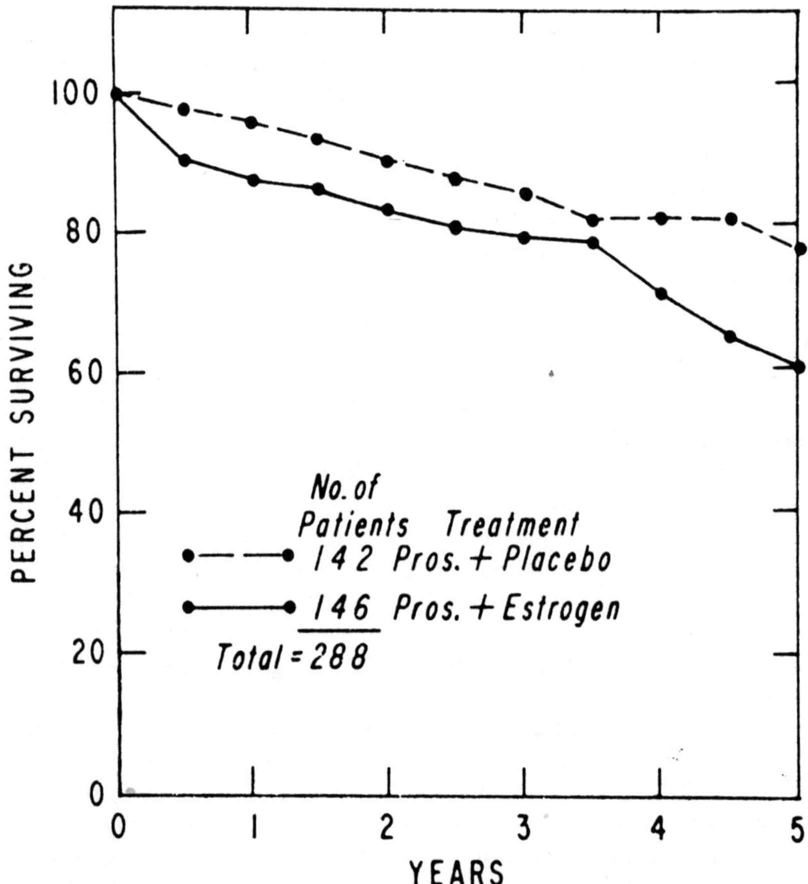

Figure 4. Survival rates of Stage A and B patients by treatment assigned, as of 15 August 1966.

(From VACURG. Treatment and survival of patients with cancer of the prostate. *Surg Gynecol Obstet.* 124:1012, 1967.)

accidents, congestive heart failure, atherosclerotic heart disease, pulmonary embolism) (Table 4). The greatest risk of cardiovascular death was in the first year of estrogen administration. The fact that estrogens lower the death rate from prostatic cancer does not indicate that they form the preferred mode of hormonal therapy. Because estrogens cause a true increase of noncancer mortality, what "estrogen treatment gains from the cancer, it more than loses to other causes of death."[75] It is possible that if these people had lived long enough they would have succumbed to their cancer.

Table 4
Deaths by Stage, Treatment, and Cause: Prostate Study 1

Stage	A		B	
Treatment*	Px + P	Px + E	Px + P	Px + E
Number of patients	60	60	85	94
Cancer of prostate	3	2	8	2
Cardiovascular	20	25	25	32
Other causes	7	10	9	12
Total deaths	30	37	42	46

Stage	C				D			
Treatment*	P	E	O + P	O + E	P	E	O + P	O + E
Number of patients	262	265	266	257	223	211	203	216
Cancer of prostate	46	18	35	25	105	82	97	82
Cardiovascular	88	112	96	108	55	76	56	59
Other causes	43	50	54	48	29	23	29	40
Total deaths	177	180	184	181	189	181	182	181

*Px = radical prostatectomy
P = placebo
E = 5.0 mg diethylstilbestrol daily
O = orchiectomy
From Byar, D. P. The VACURGs studies of cancer of the prostate. *Cancer.* 32:1127, 1973.

When the data were analyzed as to the relief of symptoms obtained from endocrine therapy (in contrast to an increase in survival) it became obvious that estrogen administration offered no benefits to patients with Stage A and Stage B disease. Analysis of the data at six months (to eliminate bias due to a change in treatment) showed that those patients treated with endocrine therapy were less likely to have an enlarged and hard prostate gland or elevated acid phosphatases. However, no significant differences were demonstrated in the appearance of osseous metastases, involvement of the central nervous system, or subjective responses such as decrease in pain, weight gain, or increased activity.

Several criticisms have been raised about study 1. First, about 40%

of patients seen were excluded from the study for various reasons. Second, the number of patients in each group at risk for the given time period was not presented. Finally, patients could be changed from one mode of treatment to another whenever the investigator felt that a change in treatment was necessary for the welfare of the patient. Approximately 20% of patients were switched from one treatment form to another at some point in the study, and in most cases the change was from placebo to some form of endocrine therapy. About 70% of Stage C and 100% of Stage D patients were ultimately changed from placebo to some other form of treatment.[76] Despite this, all results were tabulated on the basis of the initial form of therapy. This may have skewed the results favorably with respect to the placebo group. Therefore, this study does not compare the results of hormone treatment to no-hormone treatment as is often stated, but in fact compares early hormonal therapy to hormonal therapy that is delayed until onset of symptoms. Unless this fact is understood, the true impact of the results is misinterpreted. In the ultimate analysis what the VACURG study does show is that delayed hormonal therapy is as beneficial as early hormonal therapy in affecting survival from metastatic prostatic carcinoma. As the main role of hormonal therapy is symptomatic palliation, treatment should be withheld until patients become symptomatic.

The first VACURG study raised the possibility that lower doses of estrogen may control the cancer and at the same time cause less cardiovascular death. Study 2 was started in 1967 in order to explore this possibility. Patients with either Stage A or Stage B cancer were randomized either to prostatectomy or placebo, and patients with Stage C or Stage D disease were randomized to either placebo or diethylstilbestrol in daily doses of 0.2, 1.0, or 5.0 mg. Early results in patients with Stage A and Stage B disease seem to demonstrate no differences between either group, although detailed statistical analysis has not been performed.[31] In patients treated with DES the 1.0 mg dose was associated with fewer cardiovascular deaths than the 5.0 mg dose, and was as effective as the 5.0 mg dose in reducing deaths due to carcinoma of the prostate. Survival rates were poorest in Stage D patients on placebo treatment, perhaps because participating physicians were less likely to take patients off study. When the rates at which Stage C patients converted to Stage D were studied, it was found that the rate of progression was remarkably slow for the two higher doses of estrogen (Figure 5). In spite of this overall survival rates were not dissimilar among the various groups in Stage C patients. These data further reinforce the conclusion that delaying endocrine therapy does not affect patient survival. It may be hypothesized that Stage D patients in this study perhaps form the only group in which a comparison between endocrine therapy and no-endocrine therapy can be drawn, as patients on placebo were usually not switched to endocrine therapy. If the poorer survival for Stage D patients on placebo is borne out on further analysis of the data, it may be inferred that endocrine therapy may indeed increase survival rates from prostatic carcinoma.

The third VACURG study was started in 1969. Treatment for Stages A and B were the same as in study 2 (prostatectomy vs placebo), but patients in Stage C and Stage D were randomized either to 1.0 mg of

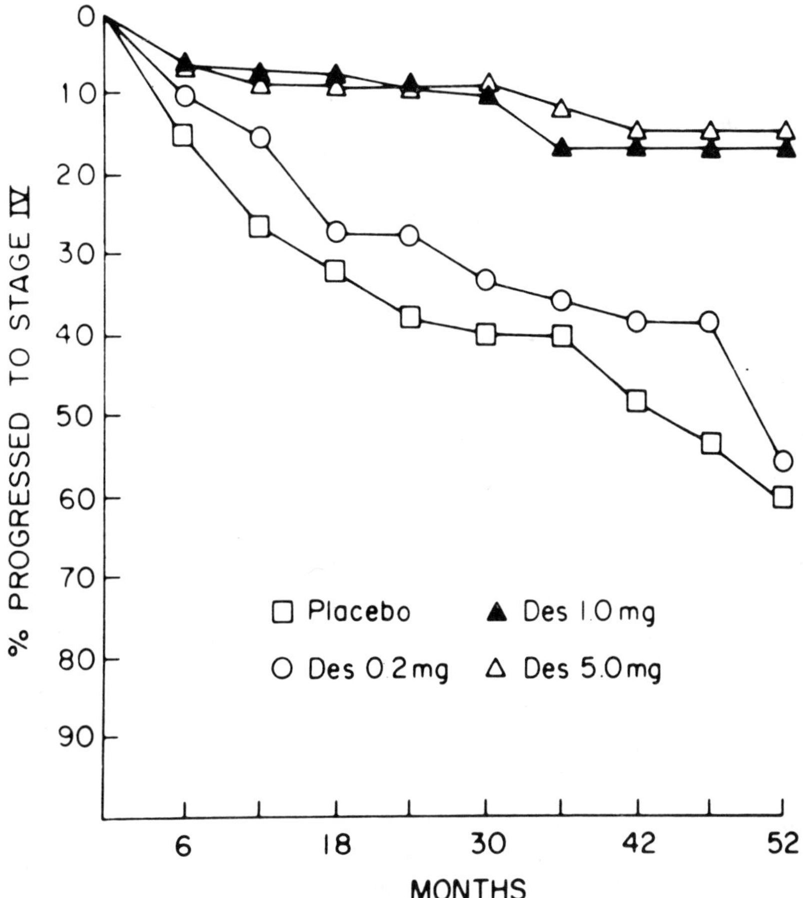

Figure 5. Percent of Stage C patients in study 2 who progressed to Stage D (see text) as a function of time.

(From Byar, D. P. The VACURG studies of cancer of the prostate. *Cancer.* 32:1129, 1973.)

DES daily, 1.25 mg of Premarin daily for one month followed by 2.5 mg daily, 3.0 mg of Provera daily, or 30 mg of Provera plus 1 mg of DES daily. Preliminary results indicate that none of these regimens is superior to DES alone in terms of survival.[49,50]

Although the VACURG studies have provided important insight into the endocrine treatment of prostatic cancer, they raise several important questions. Should estrogen therapy be used at all, except in patients who are unwilling to submit to orchiectomy? As the overall survival curves are similar in all treatment groups, it is difficult to champion any particular form of endocrine therapy. However, poor patient compliance in taking medicines over a prolonged period of time and increased risk of cardiovascular deaths in the first year of estrogen therapy, especially in patients over 75 years of age, argue in favor of orchiectomy as the preferred mode of treatment in patients with metastatic carcinoma of prostate.[77,78] In addition, the first VACURG study demonstrated significantly poorer survivals in Stage C patients treated with orchiectomy combined with estrogens. In another publication Brendler and Prout reporting on the results of the Cooperative Study Group in Prostatic Cancer (which evaluated the role of placebo versus DES in patients refractory to castration), revealed that at four weeks no statistically significant difference in progression of the disease could be detected between either group.[79] Although some authors[80] have reported increased survival rates in patients treated with orchiectomy plus DES, based on the data mentioned above and the fact that estrogens act synergistically with androgens in promoting prostatic growth in the castrated rat and orchiectomized dog, we usually do not use estrogen therapy in castrated patients.

Another unanswered question concerns the preferred dose of DES in patients who refuse orchiectomy. The VACURG data indicate that 1.0 mg of DES reduces cancer death while not increasing cardiovascular deaths. However, several investigators have demonstrated that plasma testosterone levels are not uniformly depressed with 1.0 mg of DES whereas a dose of 3.0 mg produced uniform suppression.[20,29] Therefore, it can be argued that on a purely theoretical basis the optimal daily dose of DES is 3 mg. However, because no clinical data on the incidence of cardiovascular deaths with the 3-mg dose are available, and as the clinical response rate with the 1 mg dose may be as good as with the higher dose (although this has not been tested), the exact dose of DES that should be used is still a matter of controversy.

Finally, the question arises as to the timing of endocrine therapy. The second VACURG study shows that Stage C patients treated with endocrine therapy at the time of diagnosis show a significantly lower rate of progression of disease. However, the fact that overall survival rates were not affected by treatment indicates that these patients do poorly once the disease starts to progress. In addition, the first VACURG study showed that early endocrine therapy did not delay onset of osseous metastases or neurologic symptoms. It is thus our policy to withhold endocrine therapy until symptoms warrant it.

Treatment of Vesical Outlet and Ureteral Obstruction

Although some authorities recommend transurethral resection for vesical obstruction due to prostatic cancer,[25] it has been our experience that this procedure may be associated with increased morbidity in these patients. In many cases prostatic cancer invades the membranous urethra and distorts the normal anatomy, rendering transurethral resection imprecise in this situation. In an analysis of our last hundred transurethral resections for both benign and neoplastic conditions of the prostate gland, urinary incontinence resulted in only four patients with carcinoma of the prostate and in no patient with benign hyperplasia (R.M.E. Engel, personal communication, 1975). In addition there is the theoretical risk of venous tumor dissemination in these patients. Therefore, in patients with urinary retention we are inclined to perform bilateral orchiectomy and delay removal of the indwelling Foley catheter until obstruction has resolved. Occasionally this may take several weeks. We resort to transurethral resection of the prostate gland only if the obstruction fails to resolve with this plan of treatment.

Recent reports have demonstrated occasional prolonged survival in patients with prostatic cancer, pelvic metastases, and ureteral obstruction.[81,82] In addition, Michigan and Catalona have assessed the response of ureteral obstruction to endocrine therapy in these patients.[83] They showed that 88% responded to orchiectomy (as demonstrated by a reduction in hydronephrosis) and that this response rate was not enhanced by the concomitant administration of DES. The average survival in the responders was 37 months and the one-year survival over 90%. Radiation therapy caused a decrease of hydronephrosis in two of eight patients who had 'escaped' on endocrine therapy. Based on these data we favor aggressive treatment in these patients. We utilize bilateral orchiectomy in those who have not already had it, and pelvic radiation in those who have. Supravesical diversion is utilized as necessary by means of nephrostomy or in situ ureterostomy.

Treatment of Relapse after Hormonal Therapy

The prognosis of patients who have reactivation of prostatic cancer on hormonal therapy remains dismal and therapeutic measures serve only to ameliorate symptoms. Because no single method has proven superior to the others this group of patients has been treated with a heterogeneity of methods not characteristic of any other group. In an attempt to define the role of chemotherapy in patients with relapsing cancer a cooperative study involving six institutions was set up in 1973 (the National Prostatic Cancer Project). In a preliminary report of the project, Scott et al. stated that of 125 patients entered in the study 58% were dead with an average survival time of 26 weeks.[52] Althugh the study is still far from complete, initial results seem to indicate that chemotherapy may increase average survival.[84] Currently the study is also evaluating the role of chemotherapy as a primary treatment modality in metastatic prostatic carcinoma. Because the results with additional hormonal therapy (adrenalectomy, hypophysectomy) are so poor in patients with reactivation of disease, we are currently treating all patients in relapse with chemotherapy.

GUIDELINES TO TREATMENT OF METASTATIC PROSTATIC CARCINOMA

Based on the rationale outlined in this discussion, the following principles are followed in treatment of metastatic prostatic carcinoma at the Brady Urological Institute:

1) Hormonal therapy is withheld until symptoms arise.
2) The preferred form of hormonal therapy is bilateral orchiectomy. Estrogens are not administered to these patients. DES in daily doses of 3 mg is utilized in those patients who refuse orchiectomy.
3) Vesical outlet obstruction secondary to prostatic carcinoma is treated primarily with endocrine therapy in preference to transurethral resection.
4) Ureteral obstruction in locally invasive prostatic carcinoma is attacked aggressively.
5) Because pituitary and adrenal hormones have not been demonstrated to play a significant role in stimulating prostatic carcinoma in the absence of the testes, relapse following orchiectomy is treated with chemotherapy under the dictates of the National Prostatic Cancer Project.

CONCLUSION

Although more than 30 years have elapsed since the monumental discoveries of Huggins and his coworkers, an effective method for prolonging survival in patients with metastatic prostatic carcinoma has not yet been elucidated. A significant drawback in our comprehension of the disease has been the inability to predict the biological behavior of the tumor in an individual patient. While some patients with prostatic cancer survive for long periods of time without any apparent ill effects from the disease, others succumb to the tumor within the space of a few weeks. Furthermore, of all patients with prostatic adenocarcinoma, only 60% to 70% will respond to hormonal therapy, and in those responding the duration of response varies from individual to individual. In several experimentally induced tumor systems as well as in human breast cancer a clear correlation has been demonstrated between hormonal responsiveness and receptor content.[85-89] Because it has been difficult to identify the androgen receptor in the cytosol of human prostatic tissue such a correlation has not yet been demonstrated in prostatic cancer.[90] However, recent investigations utilizing the potent synthetic androgen, methyltrienolone (R1881), appear to indicate that the receptor can be readily identified in the nuclei of prostatic cells.[91] If these preliminary results are confirmed by subsequent investigation, the physician may have a sensitive tool to predict hormonal response of the individual tumor. Quantitation of the androgen receptor may provide an indication of the duration of response to therapy or may identify those patients in relapse who will benefit by further endocrine manipulation. The discovery that normal prostatic tissues can be converted into neoplastic tissues by viruses in certain experimental systems, the discovery and characterization of spontaneous prostatic adenocarcinomas in the rat, and the suggestion that human prostatic carcinomas bear specific cell surface antigens that are capable of eliciting immunologic responses in the host, all portend an exciting era of new knowledge.[92-97] It can be predicted safely that the understanding and the management of prostatic cancer will be revolutionized in the near future when these investigative efforts are nurtured to fruition.

REFERENCES

1. Huggins, C., and Hodges, C. V. Studies on prostatic cancer 1. The effect of castration, of estrogen and of androgen injection on serum phosphatases in metastatic carcinoma of the prostate. *Cancer Res.* 1:293-7, 1941.

2. Huggins, C., Stevens, R. E., and Hodges, C. V. Studies on prostatic cancer. II. The effects of castration on advanced carcinoma of the prostate gland. *Arch Surg.* 43:209-23, 1941.

3. Bruchovsky, N., and Wilson, J. D. The conversion of testosterone to 5α-androstan-17β-ol-3-one by rat prostate in vivo and in vitro. *J Biol Chem.* 243:2012-21, 1968.

4. Anderson, K. M., and Liao, S. Selective retention of dihydrotestosterone by prostatic nuclei. *Nature.* 219:277-8, 1968.

5. Bruchovsky, N. Comparison of the metabolites formed in the rat prostate following the in vitro administration of seven natural androgens. *Endocrinology.* 89:1212-22, 1971.

6. Wilson, J. D. Metabolism of testicular androgens. Edited by D. W. Hamilton and R. O. Greep. In *Handbook of Physiology,* Section 7, Endocrinology. Vol. V. Male Reproductive System. Baltimore: The Williams and Wilkins Co., 1975, 491-508.

7. Walsh, P. C., and Siiteri, P. K. Suppression of plasma androgens by spironolactone in castrated men with carcinoma of the prostate. *J Urol.* 114:254-5, 1975.

8. Baker, H.W.G., Burger, H. G., deKretser, D. M. et al. Effects of synthetic oral oestrogens in normal men and patients with prostatic carcinoma: lack of gonadotropin suppression by chlorotrianisene. *Clin Endocrinol.* (Oxford) 2:297-306, 1973.

9. Houghton, A. L., Turner, R., and Cooper, E. H. Sex hormone-binding globulin in carcinoma of the prostate. *Brit J Urol.* 49:227-32, 1977.

10. Kato, T., and Horton, R. Studies of testosterone-binding globulin. *J Clin Endocrinol Metab.* 28:1160-8, 1968.

11. King, R.J.B., and Mainwaring, W.I.P. *Steroid-cell Interactions.* London: Butterworth, 1974.

12. Eik-Nes, K. Biosynthesis and secretion of testicular steroids. Edited by D. W. Hamilton and R. O. Greep. In *Handbook of Physiology,* Section 7. Endocrinology, Vol. V. Male Reproductive System. Baltimore: The Williams and Wilkins Co., 1975, 95-116.

13. Hanssen, V., Ritzen, E. M., French, F. S. et al. Androgen transport and receptor mechanisms in testis and epididymis. Edited by D. W. Hamilton and R. O. Greep. In *Handbook of Physiology.* Section 7. Endocrinology Vol. V. Male Reproductive System. Baltimore: The Williams and Wilkins Co., 1975, 173-202.

14. Vermeulen, A. Testicular hormonal secretion and ageing in males. Edited by J. T. Grayhack, J. D. Wilson, and M. J. Scherbenske. In *Benign Prostatic Hyperplasia.* NIAMDD Workshop Proceedings Feb. 20-21, 1975. pp 177-82, Government Printing Office DHEW publication number (NIH) 76, 1976.

15. Pirke, K. M., and Doerr, P. Age-related changes in free plasma testosterone, dihydrotestosterone, and oestradiol. *Acta Endocrinol.* 80:171-8, 1975.

16. Rubens, R., Dhont, M., and Vermeulen, A. Further studies on Leydig cell function with age. *J Clin Endocrinol Metab.* 39:40-5, 1974.

17. Paulsen, C. A. The testis. Edited by R. H. Williams. In *Textbook of Endocrinology.* 5th Ed. Philadelphia: W. B. Saunders, 1974.

18. Walsh, P. C. Physiologic basis for hormonal therapy in carcinoma of the prostate. *Urol Clin North Am.* 2:125-40, 1975.

19. Robinson, M.R.G., and Thomas, B. S. Effect of hormonal therapy on plasma testosterone levels in prostatic carcinoma. *Br Med J.* 4:391-4, 1971.

20. Shearer, R. J., Hendry, W. F., Sommerville, I. F. et al. Plasma testosterone: an accurate monitor of hormone treatment in prostate cancer. *Br J Urol.* 45:668-77, 1973.

21. Scott, W. W., and Vermeulen, C. Studies on prostatic cancer. V. Excretion of 17-ketosteroids, estrogens and gonadotropins before and after castration. *J Clin Endocrinol Metab.* 2:450-6, 1942.

22. Gallagher, T. F., Whitmore, W. F., Zumolf, B. et al. Studies in prostate cancer before and after orchiectomy. Edited by E. P. Vollmer, Jr. In *Workshop on the Biology of the Prostate and Related Tissues. Natl Cancer Inst. Monograph* 12:131-8, 1963.

23. Mackler, M. A., Liberti, J. P., Smith, M.J.V. et al. The effect of orchiectomy and various doses of stilbestrol on plasma testosterone levels in patients with carcinoma of the prostate. *Invest Urol.* 9:423-5, 1972.

24. Young, H. H., II, and Kent, J. R. Plasma testosterone levels in patients with prostatic carcinoma before and after treatment. *J Urol.* 99:788-92, 1968.

25. Resnick, M. I., and Grayhack, J. T. Treatment of stage IV carcinoma of the prostate. *Urol Clin North Am.* 2:141-61, 1975.

26. Grayhack, J. T. Pituitary factors influencing growth of the prostate. Edited by E. P. Vollmer, Jr. In *Workshop on the Biology of the Prostate and Related Tissues. Natl. Cancer Inst. Monograph* 12:131-8, 1963.

27. Bhanalaph, T., Varkarakis, M. S., and Murphy, G. P. Current status of bilateral adrenalectomy for advanced prostatic carcinoma. *Ann Surg.* 179:17-23, 1974.

28. Reynoso, G., and Murphy, G. P. Adrenalectomy and hypophysectomy in advanced prostatic carcinoma. *Cancer.* 29:941-5, 1972.

29. Kent, J. R., Bischoff, A. J., Arduino, L. J. et al. Estrogen dosage and suppression of testosterone levels in patients with prostatic carcinoma. *J Urol.* 109:858-60, 1973.

30. Adler, A., Burger, H., Davis, J. et al. Carcinoma of the prostate: response of plasma luteinizing hormone and testosterone to oestrogen therapy. *Br Med J.* 1:28-30, 1968.

31. Byar, D. P. The veterans administration cooperative urological research group's studies of cancer of the prostate. *Cancer.* 32:1126-30, 1973.

32. Huggins, C. Discussion of paper by D. Price. Edited by E. P. Vollmer. In *Workshop on the Biology of the Prostate and Related Tissues. Natl Cancer Inst. Monograph* 12:27, 1963.

33. Tesar, C., and Scott, W. W. A search for inhibitors of prostatic growth stimulators. *Invest Urol.* 1:482-98, 1964.

34. Walsh, P. C. and Wilson, J. D. The induction of prostatic hypertrophy in the dog with androstanediol. *J Clin Invest.* 57:1093-7, 1976.

35. Armstrong, E. G., and Bashirelahi, N. A specific binding protein for 17-β-estradiol in retired breeder rat ventral prostate. *Biochem Biophys Res Commun.* 61:628-34, 1974.

36. Hawkins, E. F., Nijs, M., and Brassinne, C. Steroid receptors in the human prostate. 2. Some properties of the estrophilic molecule of benign prostatic hypertorphy. *Biochem Biophys Res Commun.* 70:854-61, 1976.

37. Huggins, C., and Clark, P. J. Quantitative studies of prostatic secretion. II. The effect of castration and of estrogen injection on the normal and on the hyperplastic prostatic glands of dogs. *J Exp Med.* 72:747-62, 1940.

38. Goldman, A. S. Further studies of steroidal inhibitors of Δ^5-3^β-hydroxysteroid dehydrogenase and Δ^5-3^β-ketosteroid isomerase in pseudomonas testosteroni and in bovine adrenals. *J Clin Endocrinol Metab.* 28:1539-46, 1968.

39. Yanaihara, T., and Troen, P. Studies of the human testis. III. Effect of estrogen on testosterone formation in human testis in vitro. *J Clin Endocrinol Metab.* 34:968-73, 1972.

40. Harper, M. E., Fahmy, A. R., Pierrepoint, C. G. et al. The effect of some stilbestrol compounds on DNA polymerase from human prostatic tissues. *Steroids.* 15:89-103, 1970.

41. Shimazaki, J., Horaguchi, T., and Ohki, Y. Properties of testosterone

5α-reductase of purified nuclear fraction from ventral prostate of rats. *Endocrinol Jpn.* 18:179-87, 1971.

42. Farnsworth, W. E. A direct effect of estrogens on prostatic metabolism of testosterone. *Invest Urol.* 6:423-7, 1969.

43. Thompson, C. R., and Werner, H. W. Studies on estrogen tri-p-anisylchloroethylene. *Proc Soc Exp Biol Med.* 77:494-7, 1951.

44. Bennett, A. H., Dowd, J. B., and Harrison, J. H. Estrogen and survival data in carcinoma of the prostate. *Surg Gynecol Obstet.* 130:505-8, 1970.

45. Carroll, G., and Brennan, R. V. TACE in the treatment of carcinoma of the prostate: an 80 months survey. *J Urol.* 80:155-7, 1958.

46. O'Connor, V. J., and Sokol, J. K. Secondary regression in carcinoma of the prostate after orchiectomy. Presented at the annual meeting of the American Urological Association, 1959.

47. Smith, P. G., Rush, T. W., and Evans, A. T. Preliminary report on the clinical use of TACE (chlorotrianisene) in the treatment of prostatic carcinoma. *J Urol.* 65:886-91, 1951.

48. Blackard, C. E. The veterans administration cooperative urological research group's studies of carcinoma of the prostate: a review. *Cancer Chemother Rep.* 59:225-227, 1975.

49. Byar, D. VACURG studies on prostatic cancer and its treatment. Edited by M. Tannenbaum In *Urologic Pathology: The Prostate,* Philadelphia: Lea and Febiger, 1977.

50. Trunnell, J. B., Duffy, B. J., Marshall, V. F. et al. Use of progesterone in treatment of cancer of prostate. *J Clin Endocrinol Metab.* 11:663-76, 1951.

51. Mowscowicz, I., Bieber, D. E., Chung, K. W. et al. Synandrogenic and antiandrogenic effects of progestins: comparison with nonprogestational antiandrogens. *Endocrinology.* 95:1589-99, 1974.

52. Scott, W. W., Johnson, D. E., Schmidt, J. D. et al. Chemotherapy of advanced prostatic carcinoma with cyclophosphamide or 5-fluorouracil: results of first national randomized study. *J Urol.* 114:909-11, 1975.

53. Fergusson, J. D. Endocrine-control therapy in prostatic cancer. *Br J Urol.* 30:397-406, 1958.

54. Band, P. R., Banerjee, T. K., Patwardhan, V. C. et al. High-dose diethylstilbestrol diphosphate therapy of prostatic cancer after failure of standard doses of estrogens. *Can Med Assoc J.* 109:697-9, 1973.

55. Hawtrey, C. E., Welch, M. J., Jr., Schmidt, J. D. et al. Paraplegia and paraparesis due to prostatic cancer: use of intravenous diethylstilbestrol diphosphate. *Urology.* 4:431-4, 1974.

56. Sanford, E. J., Drago, J. R., Rohner, T. J., Jr. et al. Aminoglutethimide medical adrenalectomy for advanced prostatic carcinoma. *J Urol.* 115:170-4, 1976.

57. Smith, R. B., Walsh, P. C., and Goodwin, W. E. Cyproterone acetate in the treatment of advanced carcinoma of the prostate. *J Urol.* 110:106-8, 1973.

58. Wein, J. W., and Murphy, J. J. Experience in the treatment of prostatic carcinoma with syproterone acetate. *J Urol.* 109:68-70, 1973.

59. Stripp, B., Taylor, A. A., Bartter, F. C. et al. Effect of spironolactone on sex hormones in man. *J Clin Endocrinol Metab.* 41:777-81, 1975.

60. Sufrin, G., and Coffey, D. S. Differences in the mechanism of action of medrogestone and cyproterone acetate. *Invest Urol.* 13:1-9, 1975.

61. Sufrin, G., and Coffey, D. S. A new model for studying the effects of drugs on prostatic growth. 1. Antiandrogens and DNA synthesis. *Invest Urol.* 11:45-54, 1973.

62. Robinson, M.R.G., Shearer, R. J., and Fergusson, J. D. Adrenal suppression in the treatment of carcinoma of the prostate. *Br J Urol.* 46:555-9, 1974.

63. Fang, S., and Liao, S. Antagonistic action of antiandrogens on the formation of a specific dihydrotestosterone-receptor protein complex in rat ventral prostate. *Mol Pharmacol.* 5:428-31, 1969.

64. Walsh, P. C., and Korenman, S. G. Mechanism of androgenic action effect of specific intracellular inhibitors. *J Urol.* 105:850-1, 1971.

65. Sufrin, G., and Coffey, D. S. Flutamide: mechanism of action of a new non-steroidal antiandrogen. *Invest Urol.* 13:429-34, 1976.

66. Stoliar, B., and Albert, D. J. Sch 13521 in the treatment of advanced carcinoma of the prostate. *J Urol.* 111:803-7, 1974.

67. Sogani, P. C., Ray, B., and Whitmore, W. F., Jr. Advanced prostatic carcinoma: Flutamide therapy after conventional endocrine treatment. *Urology.* 6:164-6, 1975.

68. Sogani, P. C., and Whitmore, W. F., Jr. Experience with flutamide in previously untreated patients with advanced prostatic cancer. *J Urol.* (In press)

69. Irvin, R. J., and Prout, G. R. A new antiprostatic agent treatment of prostatic carcinoma. *Surg Forum.* 24:536-7, 1973.

70. Ellis, W. J., and Grayhack, J. T. Sexual function in aging males after orchiectomy and estrogen therapy. *J Urol.* 90:895-9, 1963.

71. Nesbit, R. M., and Baum, W. C. Endocrine control of prostatic carcinoma: clinical and statistical survey of 1818 cases. *JAMA.* 143:1317-20, 1950.

72. Nesbit, R. M., and Plumb, R. T. Prostatic carcinoma: a follow-up on 795 patients treated prior to the endocrine era and comparison of survival rates between these and patients treated by endocrine therapy. *Surgery.* 20:263-72, 1946.

73. Pool, T. L., and Thompson, G. J. Conservative treatment of carcinoma of the prostate. *JAMA.* 160:833-7, 1956.

74. Byar, D. P. Treatment of prostatic cancer: studies by the veterans administration cooperative urological research group. *Bull NY Acad Med.* 48:751-66, 1972.

75. Veterans administration cooperative urological research group. Treatment and survival of patients with cancer of the prostate. *Surg Gynecol Ostet.* 124:1011-17, 1967.

76. Blackard, C. E., Byar, D. P., Jordan, W. P., Jr. et al. Orchiectomy for advanced carcinoma—a reevaluation. *Urology.* 1:553-60, 1973.

77. Rosenstock, I. Patients' compliance with health regimens. *JAMA.* 234:402-3, 1975.

78. Bayard, S., Greenberg, R., Showalter, D. et al. Comparisons of treatments for prostatic cancer using an exponential-type life model relating survival to concomitant information. *Cancer Chemother Rep.* 58:845-59, 1974.

79. Brendler, H., and Prout, G. R., Jr. A cooperative group study of prostate cancer: stilbestrol versus placebo in advanced progressive disease. *Cancer Chemother Rep.* 16:323-7, 1962.

80. De Vere White, R., Paulson, D. F., and Glenn, J. D. The clinical spectrum of prostatic cancer. *J Urol.* 117:323-7, 1977.

81. Brin, E. N., Schiff, M., Jr., and Weiss, R. M. Palliative urinary diversion for pelvic malignancy. *J Urol.* 113:619-22, 1975.

82. Khan, A. U. and Utz, D. C. Clinical management of carcinoma of the prostate associated with bilateral ureteral obstruction. *J Urol.* 113:816-19, 1975.

83. Michigan, S., and Catalona, W. J. Ureteral obstruction from prostatic carcinoma: response to endocrine and radiation therapy. *J Urol.,* 1977. (In press)

84. Murphy, G. P., Gibbons, R. P., Johnson, D. E. et al. Comparison of estramustine phosphate and streptozotocin in patients with advanced prostatic carcinoma who have had extensive radiation. *J Urol.* 118:288-91, 1977.

85. Bruchovsky, N., and Meakin, J. W. The metabolism and binding of

testosterone in androgen-dependent and autonomous transplantable mouse mammary tumors. *Cancer Res.* 33:1689-95, 1973.

86. Jensen, E. V., and DeSombre, E. F. Mechanism of action of the female sex hormones. *Ann Rev Biochem.* 41:203-30, 1972.

87. McGuire, W. L., and Julian, J. A. Comparison of macromolecular binding of estradiol in hormone-dependent and hormone-independent rat mammary carcinoma. *Cancer Res.* 31:1440-5, 1971.

88. Jensen, E. V., Block, G. E., Smith, S. et al. Edited by T. L. Dao. In *Estrogen Target Tissues and Neoplasia.* Chicago: University of Chicago Press, 1972, pp 23-57.

89. McGuire, W. L. Estrogen receptors in human breast cancer. *J Clin Invest.* 52:73-7, 1973.

90. Menon, M., Tananis, C. E., McLoughlin, M. G. et al. Androgen receptors in human prostatic tissue: a review. *Cancer Treat Rep.* 61:265-71, 1977.

91. Menon, M., Tananis, C. E., Hicks, L. L. et al. Characterization of the binding of a potent synthetic androgen, methyltrienolone (R1881) to human tissues. *J Clin Invest.* 1978. (In press)

92. Paulson, D. F., Rabson, A. F., and Fraley, E. E. Viral neoplastic transformation of hamster prostatic tissue in vitro. *Science.* 159:200-1, 1968.

93. Dunning, W. F. Prostatic cancer in the rat. Edited by E. P. Vollmer. In *Workshop on the Biology of the Prostate and Related Tissues. Natl. Cancer Inst. Monograph* 12:351-70, 1963.

94. Smolev, J. K., Heston, W.D.W., Scott, W. W. et al. Characterization of the Dunning R3327H prostatic adenocarcinoma: an appropriate animal model for prostatic cancer. *Cancer Treat Rep.* 61:273-87, 1977.

95. Brannen, G. E., Gomolka, D. M., and Coffey, D. S. Specificity of cell membrane antigens in prostatic cancer. *Cancer Chemother Rep.* 59:127-38, 1975.

96. Bubenik, J., Pearlmann, P., Helmstein, S. et al. Immune response to urinary bladder tumors in man. *Int J Cancer.* 5:39-44, 1970.

97. Catalona, W. J., and Scott, W. W. Carcinoma of the prostate. Edited by J. H. Harrison, R. F. Gittes, A. Perlmutter et al. In *Campbell's Urology.* Philadelphia: W. B. Saunders Co. (In press)

Drug Development for Carcinoma of the Prostate

12

Arnold Mittelman

The basis of drug development for the treatment of prostatic carcinoma has been the hormonal relationship between prostate, testes, and anterior pituitary gland. Classic studies demonstrated the dependence of the structure and function of the dog prostate upon androgens derived from the testes.[1,2] Rational application of these findings to the therapy of prostatic carcinoma is still of major importance. Our increasing knowledge of the relationship between the various steroid structures and the prostate cell, normal or malignant, provides a broadened basis of therapeutic drug development. Findings of specific receptor sites in prostatic cells for androgens and estrogens have major therapeutic implications.[3,4]

Unique biochemical processes within the prostate gland have been extremely useful in diagnosis. Elevated specific prostatic acid phosphatase in blood has long been used as an index of activity of prostatic carcinoma. Acid phosphatase and other prostatic enzymes such as 5-α reductase and arginase may provide pathways for agents that modulate or inhibit these enzymatic steps.

The natural history of prostatic carcinoma, its predominant patterns of spread, and organ involvement will exert considerable influence on the future development of hormonal and nonhormonal chemotherapeutic agents for advanced prostatic carcinoma. A realistic approach to therapy of carcinoma of the prostate lies in the dominant form of this disease. Detection of early, surgically curable carcinoma of the prostate is uncommon. It must also be realized that extensive blastic skeletal metastases are characteristic of advanced disease. Obstructive urinary symptoms and chronic urinary tract infections are also hallmarks of this condition.[5] These two factors alone emphasize the need for non-myelosuppressive chemotherapeutic agents.

ANTIANDROGENS

This term is used in a general sense and is applicable to any substance that interferes with or suppresses the action of androgens upon prostatic tissue. Historically estrogenic substances were first used in this context. The observations of Huggins et al. pointed to the use of estrogens as useful therapeutic agents for prostatic carcinoma.[2] A number of these substances had been isolated and identified during the late 1930s.

Naturally occurring estrogens such as estrone and estradiol (Figure 1) were subsequently available for use; and synthesis and biologic activity of nonsteroidal estrogen occurred at about the same time. Diethylstilbestrol (Figure 2) is the most effective representative of the stilbene derivatives. It is a cheap, stable, orally effective estrogen, and is probably the most widely used substance for the therapy of prostatic carcinoma. An intravenous preparation, diethylstilbestrol diphosphate (Stilphostral), (Figure 3) was synthesized in 1946. It was hoped that intravenous phosphate would permit a higher concentration of diethylstilbestrol to enter the prostatic cancer cells. There are clinical data suggesting that some patients who no longer respond to oral diethylstilbestrol may be benefited by the diphosphoric ester.[6,7] Controlled clinical trials have not been made.

Another estrogenic variant, polyestradiol phosphate (Estradurin) (1955) (Figure 4) is a water soluble polymerization product wherein sev-

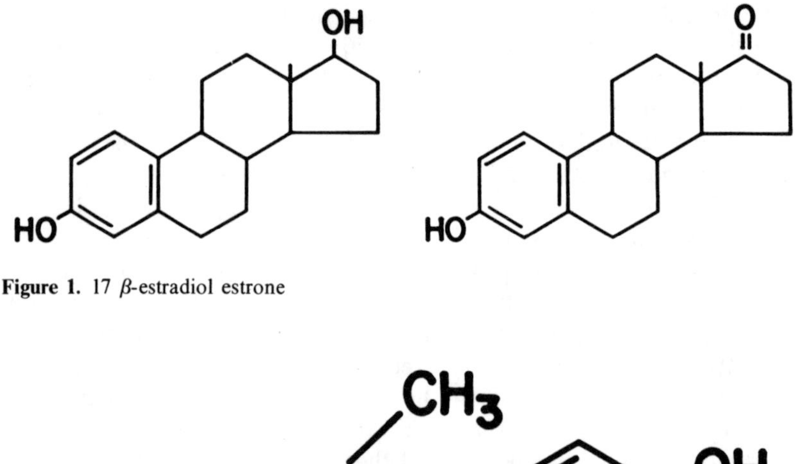

Figure 1. 17 β-estradiol estrone

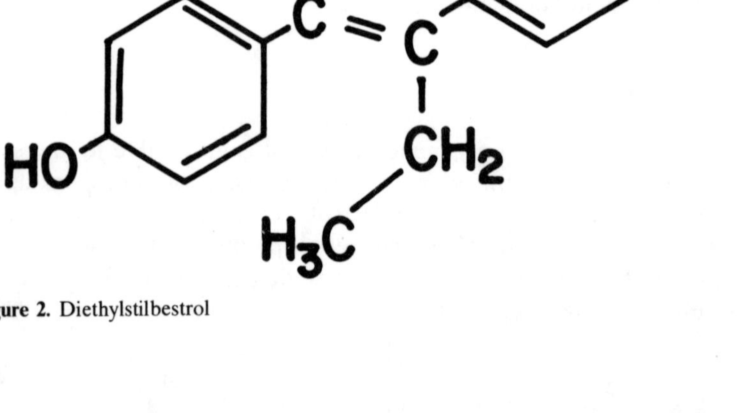

Figure 2. Diethylstilbestrol

eral estradiol molecules are firmly united with phosphate bonds. Sustained release of estradiol with stable blood and tissue levels may be obtained after intramuscular injection. This type of compound was primarily devised for patients who had an intolerance to oral estrogen preparations. Therapeutic superiority of such a compound when compared to diethylstilbestrol has not been established.[8] The mechanism of action of such a polymer is not clear. Jonsson reported a variable effect upon urinary 17-ketosteroids when Estradurin is given intramuscularly.[9] These workers could not correlate clinical benefit with reduction of urinary 17-ketosteroid excretion.

All of the estrogenic compounds described have significant side effects that may interfere with their continued clinical use. Salt and water retention, gynecomastia, and occasional hepatic toxicity characterize all these agents to a greater or lesser degree. The ideal hormonal agent for prostatic carcinoma would be one that possesses significant antitumor effect but would have no other biologic effects associated with steroid structure. Recently Scott et al. reviewed the possible usefulness of a number of

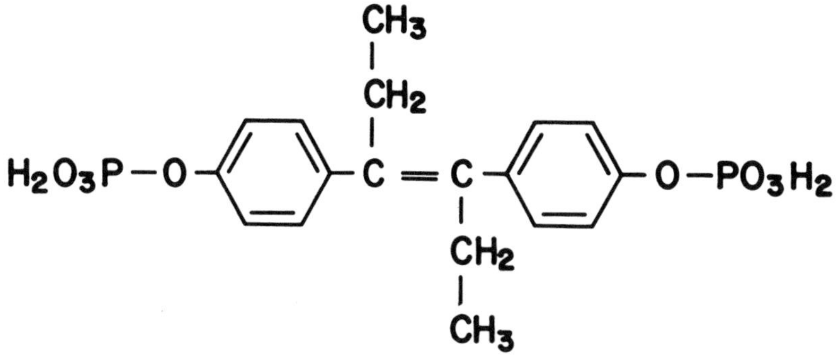

CH_3, CH_2, H_2O_3P-O, $C = C$, $O-PO_3H_2$, CH_2, CH_3

Figure 3. Diethylstilbestrol diphosphate

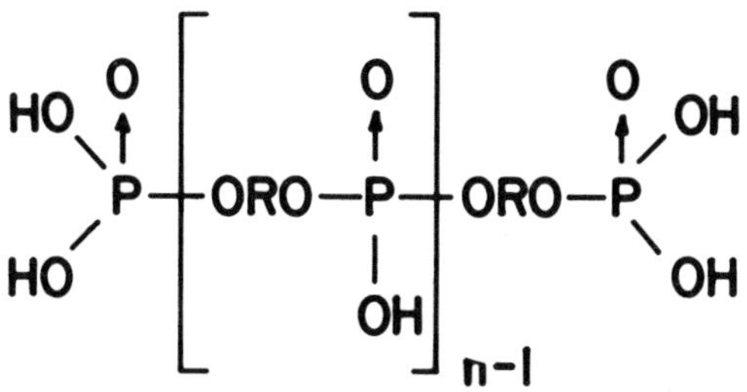

HO, O, HO, P, ORO—P, O, OH, ORO—P, O, OH, OH, n-1

(—ORO—is the estradiol radical and n is about 80)

Figure 4. Polyestradiol phosphate (Estradurin)

modified C_{21} steroids (Figures 5-8) derived from progesterone.[10]

Cyproterone acetate (SH 714) (Figure 5) has had extensive study in animal systems and has had clinical trials in Europe and the United States.[11-13] Experimental evidence indicates that this compound exerts its antiandrogenic effect by competitive antagonism with androgens at

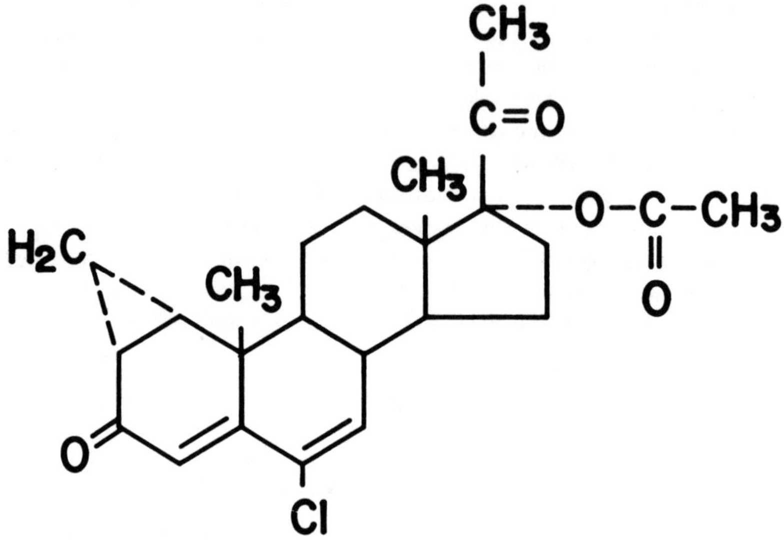

Figure 5. Structural formula of cyproterone acetate

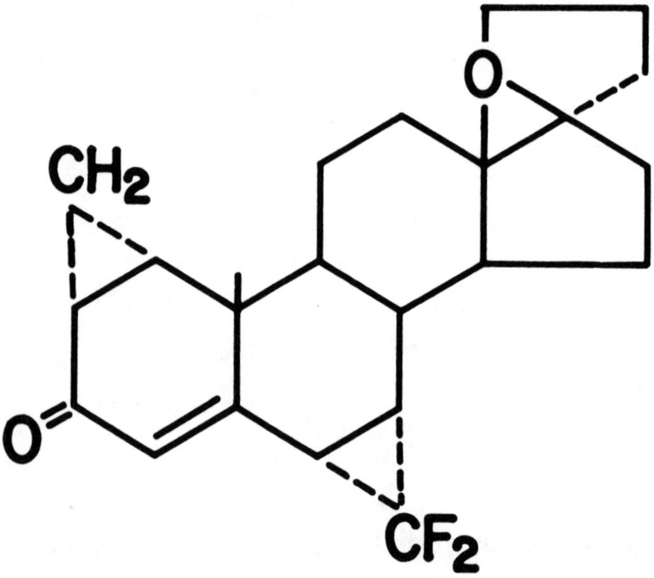

Figure 6. MK 316

the receptor sites of target organs such as the prostate gland.[14] This steroid does not seem to have estrogenic or corticoid effects although such have been reported to occur. Its physiologic activity is predominantly progestational. This compound has been reported to induce objective and subjective improvement in patients with advanced carcinoma of the prostate.[12,13] Previously untreated patients with advanced Stage D carcinoma of the prostate seem to respond more often than patients who have had previous endocrine therapy. Comparative clinical trials have not as

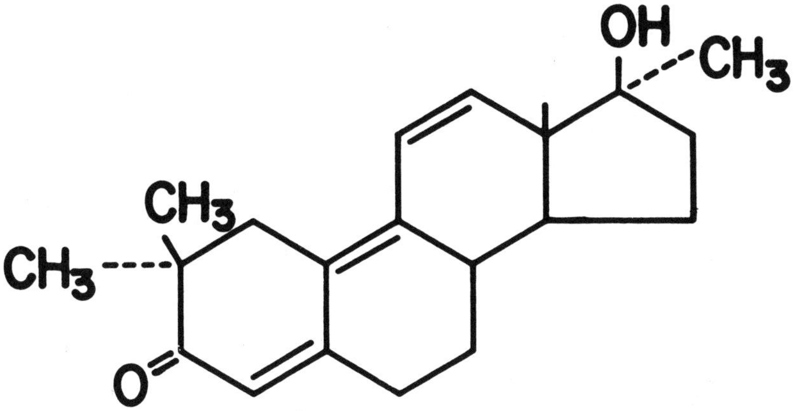

OH
CH3
CH3
CH3
O

Figure 7. R-2956

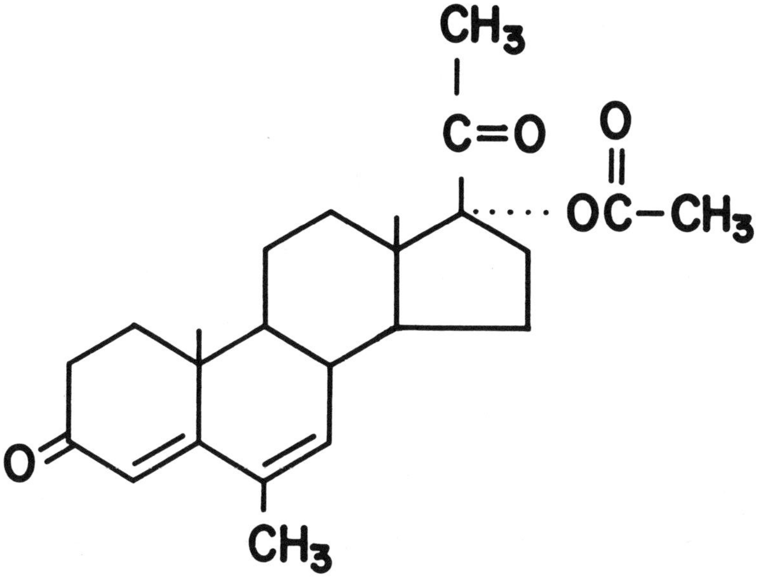

CH3
C=O
O
OC—CH3
O
CH3

Figure 8. Megesterol acetate (17 α-acetoxy-6-methyl-pregna-4,6-diene-3,20 dione)

yet been reported. Compounds V, VI, VII have similar biologic effects in animal systems but have not had clinical trials.[10] Another progesterone derivative, megesterol acetate (Figure 8), has been reported to be useful in the treatment of advanced carcinoma of the prostate.[15] The author indicated that this compound is not associated with estrogenic or androgenic effects. No retention of salt and water was observed in previously untreated patients with advanced carcinoma of the prostate.

A nonsteroidal compound, Flutamide (Figure 9), has been reported to have significant antiandrogen activity on male accessory sex organs.[16] Liao et al. indicated that Flutamide exerts its biologic activity by suppressing the retention of a specific 5-α-dihydrotestosterone receptor complex in the nucleus of the rat prostate.[14] Antineoplastic activity has been reported for this compound in patients with advanced carcinoma of the prostate.[17,18] Whether the mechanism of action is the same in man as it is in the rodent prostate is open to speculation.

Chlorotrianisene (TACE) (Figure 10), has long been used in carcinoma of the prostate for patients who are intolerant to diethylstilbestrol or are no longer responding. The compound is weakly estrogenic and has

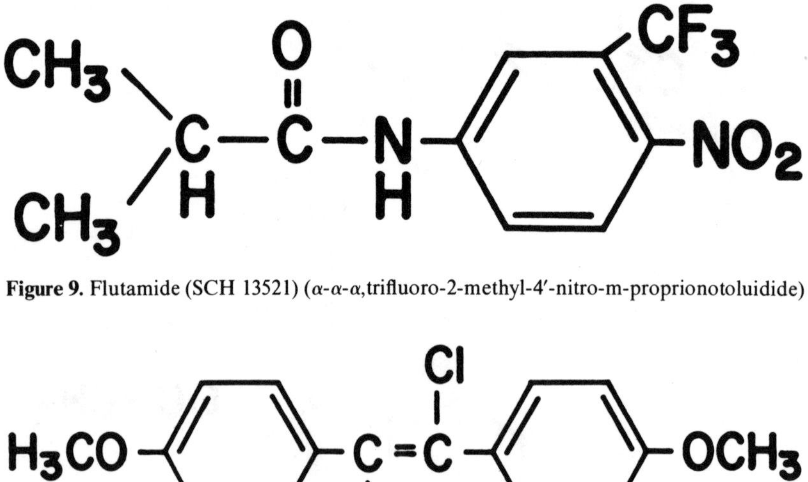

Figure 9. Flutamide (SCH 13521) (α-α-α,trifluoro-2-methyl-4′-nitro-m-proprionotoluidide)

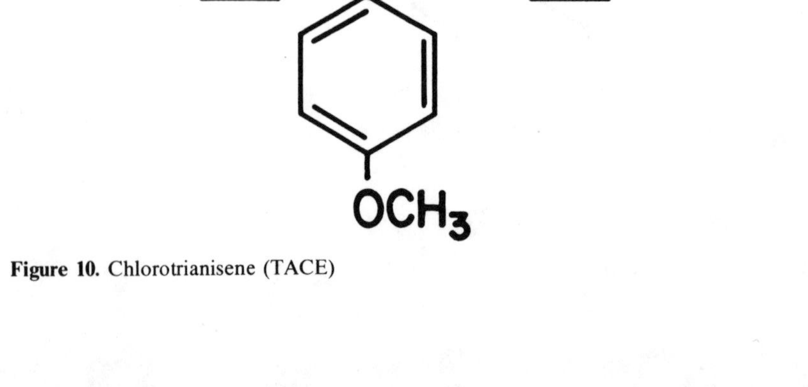

Figure 10. Chlorotrianisene (TACE)

been reported not to lower plasma testosterone. Its antineoplastic action may be due to a direct effect upon the prostatic neoplasm. The mechanism of action may be similar to that of Flutamide.

An examination of the structure of all nonsteroidal compounds that have antiandrogen properties reveals some common features. All have at least one phenolic ring with substituted alphatic groups of varying lengths.

MOLECULAR CHEMOTHERAPY

Combining our empirical knowledge and new concepts derived from molecular biology we may begin to speak of a molecular chemotherapy. Molecular biology has made significant contributions to our understanding of the mechanism of hormone action. The discovery of specific receptor sites in target tissues and an understanding of their cell interactions has particular significance for drug development in such hormonally linked tumors as prostate and breast.

The rather specific enzyme content of the prostate gland also offers potential pathways for development of antineoplastic drug therapy.

THE CARRIER CONCEPT

The therapeutic efficacy of many of our currently available cytotoxic agents is limited primarily by their lack of specificity. It would be of obvious advantage to be able to deliver agents selectively to the tumor and have their cytotoxicity expressed as an intracellular phenomenon. In a recent review Konyves et al. have described the development of chemotherapeutic agents utilizing carrier moieties.[19,20] Amino acids, carbohydrates, synthetic estrogens, and steroids have been attached to alkylating groups.[21-23] Figure 11 indicates the general formulation. The Leo Group (Konyves, Fex, and Hogberg) observed that toxicity was greatly diminished and tumor specificity enhanced when R (group) was a steroid of C_{19} or C_{21} structure. Based upon this observation a series of compounds were synthesized. One such compound (Estra 1, 3,5(10)-trien-3,17 β-diol,3N-bis (2-chlorethyl)-carbamate 17 β-dehydrogen phosphate) called estramustine phosphate or Estracyt has been used in the treatment of carcinoma of the prostate (Figure 12). It has been shown to be effective in the treatment of advanced hormonally resistant carcinoma of the prostate.[24] There are also reports of its possible effectiveness in 'early' untreated Stage D disease. This compound has little hematologic toxicity. Sandberg's group has shown that human prostatic tissue is capable of spliting Estracyt into its components. No other tissue tested could do this.[25]

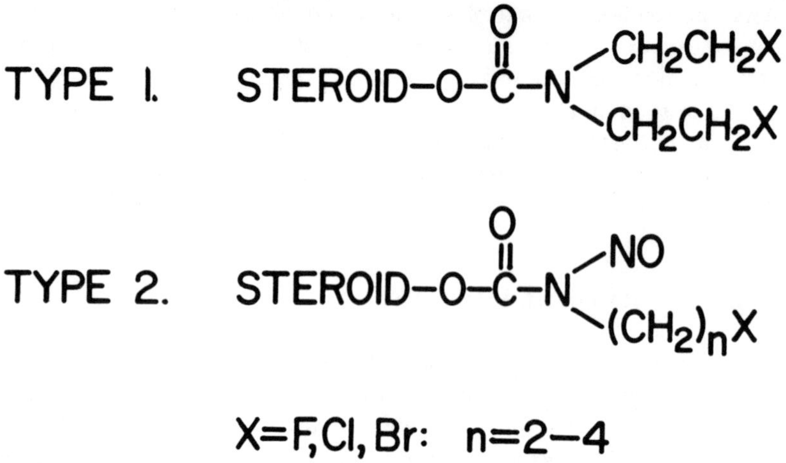

$$\text{TYPE 1.}\quad \text{STEROID–O–}\overset{\text{O}}{\overset{\|}{\text{C}}}\text{–N}\begin{matrix}\diagup CH_2CH_2X \\ \diagdown CH_2CH_2X\end{matrix}$$

$$\text{TYPE 2.}\quad \text{STEROID–O–}\overset{\text{O}}{\overset{\|}{\text{C}}}\text{–N}\begin{matrix}\diagup NO \\ \diagdown (CH_2)_nX\end{matrix}$$

$$X = F, Cl, Br:\quad n = 2–4$$

Figure 11. Estracyt [Estradiol-3-N-bis (2-chloroethyl) carbamate-17-phosphate]

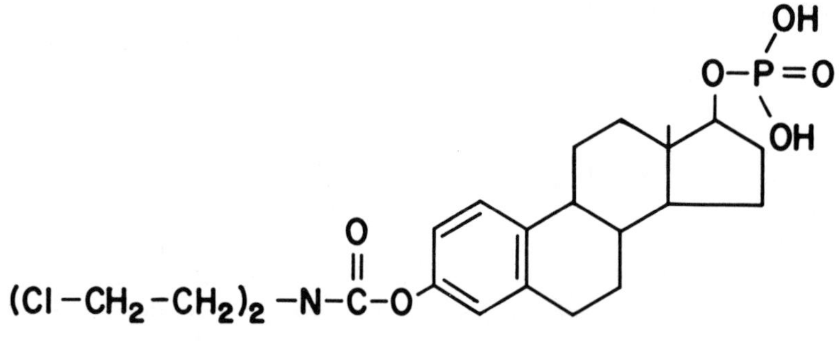

$$(Cl-CH_2-CH_2)_2-N-\overset{\text{O}}{\overset{\|}{\text{C}}}-O-\text{[steroid]}-O-P(=O)(OH)_2$$

Figure 12. General structure for substituted steroids

The carbamate group may also be used to link other types of cytotoxic agents than the nor-nitrogen mustards. Hogberg et al. have proposed the substitution of a nitroso group to replace one of the two chloroethyl groups of the bis (2-chloroethyl) carbamate moiety (Figure 13).[26] Several promising compounds have emerged from this program. Among them is a 19-nortestosterone derivative that has excellent antitumor activity but no hematologic toxicity (Figure 14). Bloch et al. have approached the development of steroidal conjugate in another manner (personal communication, 1977). Bifunctional carboxilic acids such as succinic acid are proposed bridges which would link the carrier moiety to the cytotoxic agent. Esterification of steroids with succinic acid has been described.[27] Bloch proposes the formulation of various steroid esters with antimetabolites, alkylating agents, and such intercoacting agents as adriamycin and daunorubicin. Although these compounds would have obvious relevance to endocrine-affected neoplasms, they certainly could be used in other tumor types. The presence of steroid receptors on nonendocrine-related tumors cells is a more widespread phenomenon than previously appreciated.[28]

There are other forms of carrier compounds that could be developed. A variety of antitumor agents may be conjugated to porphyrins.[29] Dougherty has shown that specially prepared hemotoporphyrins localized preferentially in a wide variety of rodent and human neoplasms.[3]

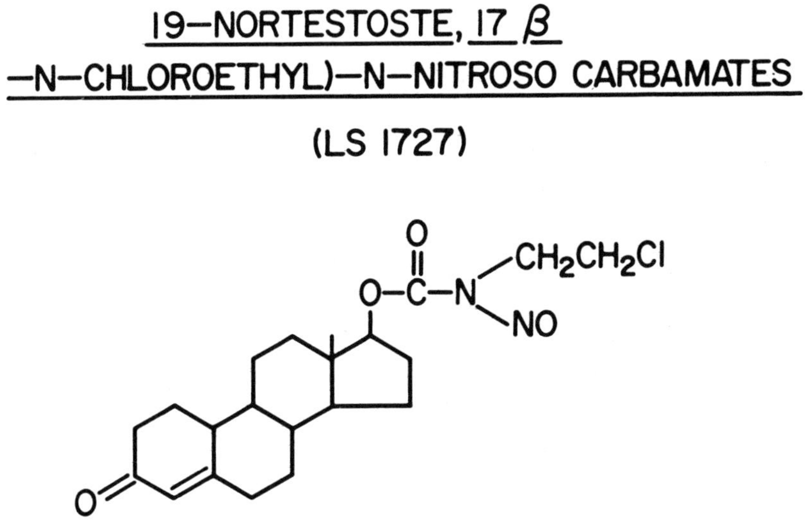

19–NORTESTOSTE, 17 β –N–CHLOROETHYL)–N–NITROSO CARBAMATES

(LS 1727)

Figure 13. 19-nortestoste, 17 β-N-chloroethyl-N-nitroso carbamates (LS 1727)

CARBAMYL PHOSPHATE

L–Aspartate

N–(Phosphonacetyl)– L–Aspartate

Carbamyl–L–Aspartate

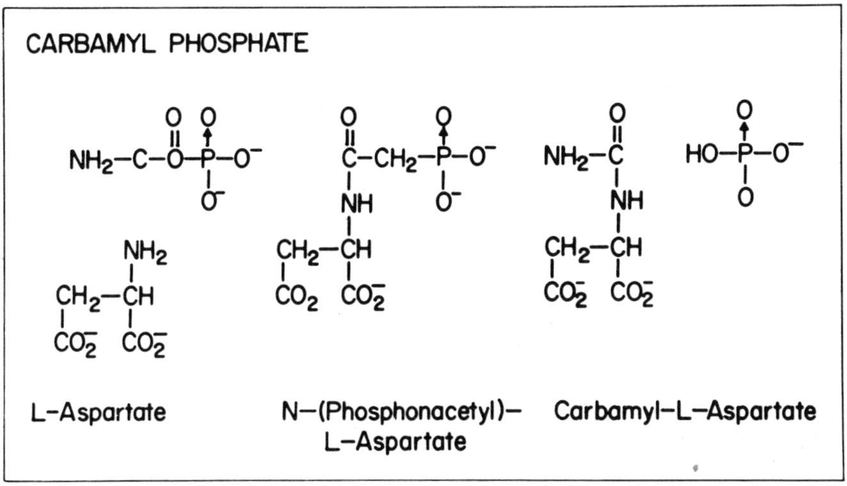

Figure 14. Transition state analogue of L-asparate transcarbamylase

Activation of singlet oxygen by light energy transmitted to the porphysin-containing tumor results in cell destruction.[29] The clinical usefulness of this process was recently demonstrated by Kaufman.[30]

TRANSITION STATE ANALOGS

The presence of enzymes of a certain specificity in human prostatic tissue offers the possibility of synthesizing specific inhibitors of these enzymes. Recently Collins and Starke have pointed out the high specificity that transition state enzyme analogs may obtain.[31] It has been postulated that enzymes must bind most tightly to the 'activated' form of their substrates which resemble the transition state of the reaction being catalyzed. A given transition state analog would bind much more tightly to a given enzyme than the true substrates. Kim and Starke have illustrated this with the transition state analog for aspartate transcarbamylase, N-(phosphonacetyl) L-aspartate.[32]

Transition state analogs could be developed for such prostatic tissue enzymes as acid phosphatase, arginase, 5α-reductase.

CONVENTIONAL CHEMOTHERAPEUTIC AGENTS

Within the past four years various reports have appeared concerning the efficacy of such agents as 5-FU, Cytoxan, and Adriamycin for advanced prostatic carcinoma. Several of these studies have been prospective randomized trials. Among the most noteworthy are those studies performed by the National Prostatic Cancer Project Treatment Group. This group has shown that 5-FU and Cytoxan have exceedingly modest objective effects upon advanced hormonally resistant carcinoma of the prostate with a clear enhancement of survival in the chemotherapy group when compared to controls.[33] The use of platinum, Adriamycin, and methotrexate have all been reported. As yet, these therapies cannot be evaluated.[34,35]

Although these comments are not meant to be a complete review of chemotherapy of advanced carcinoma of the prostate, they do indicate lack of dramatic response to current conventional chemotherapy.

REFERENCES

1. Huggins, C., and Clark, P. J. Quantitative studies on prostatic secretion. II. The effect of castration and of estrogen injection on normal and on hyperplastic prostate glands of dogs. *J Exp Med.* 72:747, 1940.

2. Huggins, C., Stevens, R. E., Hodges, C. V. Studies on prostatic cancer. II. The effect of castration on clinical patients with carcinoma of the prostate. *Arch Surg.* 43:209, 1941.

3. Sufrin, G., Kirdani, R. Y., Sandberg, A. et al. Estrogen binding and estrogen receptors in the prostate. *Surg Forum.* 26:584-6, 1975.

4. Tveter, K. J., Unhjem, O., Attramadal, A. et al. Androgenic receptors in rat and human prostate. *Advances in the Biosciences.* Schering Workshop on Steroid Hormone 'Receptor'. Berlin, December 7-9, 1970.

5. Murphy, G. P., Saroff, J., Joiner, J. et al. Prostatic carcinoma: treated at a catagorical center 1960-1969. *NY State J Med.* Sept 1975, pp 1663-9.

6. Band, R. P., Baneree, T. K., and Patwordhan-Eid, T. C. High-dose diethylstilbestrol diphosphate therapy of prostatic cancer after failure of standard doses of estrogen. *Can Med Assoc J.* 109:697-9, 1973.

7. Rohlf, P. L., and Flocks, R. H. Stilphostrol therapy in 100 cases of prostatic carcinoma. *J Iowa Med Soc.* 59:1096-8, 1969.

8. Goodhope, C. D. Polyestradiol phosphate for carcinoma of the prostate: a clinical study. *J Urol.* 77:312-14, 1957.

9. Jonsson, G. Treatment of prostatic carcinoma with polyestradiol phosphate combined with ethinylestradiol. *Scand J Urol Nephrol.* 5:97-102, 1971.

10. Scott, W. W. Rationale and results of primary endocrine therapy in patients with prostatic cancer. *Proc Natl Conf Urologic Cancer.* Washington: March 29-31, 1973, pp 1119-25.

11. Neumann, F. Use of cyproterone acetate in animal clinical trials: hormones and antagonists. *Gynecol Invest.* 2:150-79, 1972.

12. Scott, W. W. Cyproterone acetate treatment of disseminated prostatic cancer and benign nodular hyperplasia. Raspe and Brosig, eds. *International Symposium on the Treatment of Carcinoma of the Prostate, Berlin 1969.* Vol. I. Oxford: Pergamon Press, 1971, pp 161-3.

13. Wein, A. J., and Murphy, J. J. Experience in the treatment of prostatic carcinoma with cyproterone acetate. *J Urol.* 109:68-70, 1973.

14. Liao, S., Howell, D. K., Chang, T. M. Action of a nonsteroidal antiandrogen Flutamide on the receptor binding and nuclear retention of 5-dihydrotestosterone in rat ventral prostate. *Endrocrinology.* 94:1205-8, 1974.

15. Johnson, D. E., Daesler, K. E., and Ayala, A. G. Megestral acetate for treatment of advanced carcinoma of the prostate. *J Surg Oncol.* 7:9-15, 1975.

16. Neri, R. O., and Monahan, M. Effects of a novel nonsteroidal antiandrogen on canine prostatic hyperplasia. *Invest Urol.* 10:123-6, 1972.

17. Prout, G. R., Jr., Irwin, R. J., Klimau, B. et al. Prostatic cancer and SCH 13521. II. Histological alterations and the pituitary gonadal axis. *J Urol.* 113:834, 1975.

18. Stoliar, B., and Albert, D. J. SCH 13521 in the treatment of advanced carcinoma of the prostate. *J Urol.* 111:803-7, 1974.

19. Mittelman, A., Shukla, S. K., Welvaart, K. et al. Oral estramustine phosphate (NSC-18199) in the treatment of advanced (Stage D) carcinoma of the prostate. *Cancer Chemother Rep.* 59:219-23, 1975.

20. Alfthan, D. S., and Rush, I. L. Estracyt in advanced prostatic carcinoma. *Ann Chir Gynaecol.* 56:234, 1969.

21. Jonsson, G., Hogberg, K. B. Treatment of advanced prostatic carcinoma with estracyt: a preliminary report. *Scand J Urol Nephrol.* 5:103, 1971.

22. Kirdani, R. Y., Mittelman, A., Murphy, G. P. et al. Studies on phenolic steroids in human subjects. XIV. Fate of a nitrogen mustard of estradiol 17B. *J Clin Endocrinol Metab.* 41:305-18, 1975.

23. Seligman, A., Steinberger, N. J., Paul, B. D. et al. Design of pindle poison activated specifically by prostatic acid phosphatase (PAP) and new methods

for PAP cytochemistry. *Cancer Chemother Rep.* 59:233-42, 1975.

24. Tritsch, G. L., Shukla, S. K., Mittelman, A. et al. Estracyt (NSC-89199) as a substrate for phosphatases in human serum. *Invest Urol.* 12:38-9, 1974.

25. Kadohama, N., Kirdani, R. Y., Murphy, G. P. et al. Estramustine phosphate: metabolic aspects related to its action in prostatic carcinoma. *J Urol.* 119:Feb. 1977.

26. Hogberg, B., Fex, H., Konyves, I. et al. (A. B. Leo, Sweden) 1973, U.S. Pat. No. 3, 963, 707, 1973.

27. Jackson, A. G., Kenner, B. W., Moore, G. A. et al. *Tetrahedron Lett.* 40:3627 (1976).

28. Jenson, E. V., and DeSombre, E. R. Steroid hormone receptors in breast cancer. Edited by Jorge R. Pasqualine. In *Receptors and Mechanism of Action of Steroid Hormones.* New York: Marcel Dekker, Publisher, 1977, pp 569-601.

29. Grindey, G. B., Fill, R., Weishaup, K. R. and Bayle, D. G. Photoradiation Therapy II. Cure of animals tumors with hematoporphysin and light. *J Nat Cancer Inst.* 1:115-21, 1975.

30. Kaufman, J., Dougherty, T., Goldfarb, A., et al. Photoradiation therapy of malignant tumors. *ASCO Proceedings.* May, 1977.

31. Collins, K. D., and Stark, G. R. Aspartate transcarbomylase, interaction with the transition state analogue N-(phosphonacetyl)-L-aspartate. *J Biol Chem.* 246:6599-605, 1971.

32. Swyryd, E. A., Seaver, S. S., and Stark, G. R. (Phosphonacetyl)-L-aspartate, a patent transition state analog inhibitor of aspartate transcarbomylase. Blocks proliferation of mammalian cells in culture. *J Biol Chem.* 21:6945-50, 1974.

33. Scott, W. W., Johnson, D. E., Schmidt, J. E. et al. Chemotherapy of advanced prostatic carcinoma with cyclophosphamide or 5-fluorouracil. Results of first national randomized study. *J Urol.* 114:909-11, 1975.

34. Eagan, R. T., Utz, D. C., Myers, R.M.P. et al. Comparison of adriamycin (NSC 123127) and the combination of 5-fluorouracil (NSC 19893) and cyclophosphamide (NSC 27271) in advanced prostatic cancer: a preliminary report. *Cancer Chemother Rep.* 59:203-7, 1975.

35. Merrin, C. Treatment of advanced carcinoma of the prostate (Stage D) with infusion of cis diamino dichloro platinum (CDDP) and mannitol. Meeting Abstract *Proc Am Assoc Cancer Res.* 18:100, 1977.

Management of Disseminated Prostatic Carcinoma

13

Gerald P. Murphy

Disseminated prostatic cancer has been essentially and primarily managed by palliation with endocrine therapy. The rationale, basis, and epidemiologic factors associated with this reality have been previously reviewed in this book. In sequential therapeutic considerations it has long been held that advanced prostatic cancer in the majority of patients evolves at a regular and somewhat slow pace from a focal lesion to arrive ultimately at the widespread, disseminated state. This impression is not realistic in terms of the available data we have collected in our area of the United States, or from comparison with other studies that have been described in the literature.[1-3] Review of autopsy and full clinical follow-up data confirm the distressing fact that a substantial and significant percentage of patients present with widespread and disseminated disease when first seen. This is not due to a deficit in availability of clinical, diagnostic, and therapeutic resources, but constitutes a rather realistic statement that prostatic cancer may not always present as a localizing, slowly progressive disease. Moreover, there is an impression that a number of these individuals do not respond for very long or to a very extensive degree to the conventional forms of hormonal therapy. For this reason additional hormonal manipulations for the management of reactivated prostatic cancer have been attempted in the past.[4] Adrenalectomy and hypophysectomy, or their combination, have been carefully evaluated and found to have some limited effect. However, when compared with other forms of nonhormonal chemotherapy, sufficient long-term responses can be achieved with chemotherapy and have been found to be superior to bilateral adrenalectomy or hypophysectomy.[5] Understandably there must exist a concern for the toxic effects of systemic chemotherapy and for appropriate selection in those patients who can best benefit. The National Prostatic Cancer Project and investigators at Roswell Park Memorial Institute starting in 1972 have considered a number of these parameters in an attempt to determine those patients who could best be treated. Prior radiation therapy does limit the number of available cytotoxic agents that can be safely used in some patients.[6] However, there are other agents that do not have cytotoxic effects which can be used safely. Reliable and predictable criteria regarding assessment of the primary tumor, the disseminated disease, and its histologic appearance have been studied by this national group and found to be useful.[7] Their first result confirms that chemotherapy using cyclophosphamide or 5-fluorouracil can be effective even in this advanced stage of the disease.[8] It should be recognized in dealing with an advanced disseminated disease that there must be limited hope for improved survival or complete resolution. Despite this there have been some rather persistent and remarkable responses including disappearance of osteoblastic metastases in prostatic carcinoma following treatment with agents such as Estracyt.[9]

Because of the ability to treat patients with prostatic cancer for longer periods of time and perhaps more intensively with nonhormonal cytostatic agents, assessment of disease extent has been a matter of increased concern both in terms of prognosis as well as determining response rates for soft tissue lesions heretofore not frequently considered, and for cancers located in sites such as the central nervous system that have not been a matter of previous therapeutic concern.[10,11] A variety of efforts has been successfully employed to assess the overall patient status using additional biologic markers in advanced disease states.[12,13] These methods have also been further improved by additional refinements in prostatic acid phosphatase assay as well as in the isoenzymes of alkaline phosphatase. Both of these latter tests have been successfully employed and are being currently field-tested by the National Prostatic Cancer Project.

Some previous reports have recounted the clinical experience and usefulness of various types of treatments of advanced prostate cancer with chemotherapy. They are as effective today as they have been previously described.[14] However, this is a continuing field, since additional results from ongoing studies previously underway, as well as the evaluation of other new agents, requires our responsive position to reassess this area frequently. For example, when an advanced cancer state improves with treatment, adjuvant therapy is considered at an earlier phase. As a result various chemotherapeutic agents are currently being introduced at the time of surgery or radiotherapy for localized or less extensive prostatic cancer. These studies will require some time before definitive answers are available but the results can be awaited with anticipation.

We have pointed out that relatively little emphasis had been placed on chemotherapy of prostatic cancer until the last few years.[15] Factors which in our opinion are responsible for the very gradual inroads into this modality of antitumor therapy include 1) the increased incidence of prostatic cancer in older men who often succumb to other chronic illnesses, 2) the frequent dramatic responses seen with orchiectomy or oral estrogen therapy, 3) urologists' unwillingness to embark on a new dimension in cancer treatment, and 4) the relative infancy of the field of cancer chemotherapy in general.

In spite of the high incidence of prostatic cancer, adequate drug testing in this disease has been woefully neglected. Only about 10% of currently available antitumor drugs have been adequately tested in prostatic cancer. This figure compares with 90% of currently available drugs which have been tested against colon and lung cancer, and 34% against testicular cancer. Such little experience with chemotherapy in prostatic cancer is regrettable, since chemotherapy in some cases may be the only modality of unquestioned effectiveness in killing tumor cells anywhere in the body.

Until recently, clinical use of chemotherapy in prostatic cancer had been restricted to sporadic and anecdotal case reports and a few uncontrolled series. Current investigations into the merits of chemotherapy include the efforts of several well-organized cooperative studies, such as the National Prostatic Cancer Project (a National Cancer Institute Organ Site Program, Division of Cancer Research Resources and Centers, grant-supported program of research). I will refer to the various groups and their drug protocols throughout this chapter. Much of the material presented will necessarily be prospective since the field of chemotherapy in prostatic cancer is so new and ever-changing.

NATIONAL PROSTATIC CANCER PROJECT

Recognizing that a randomized trial of the chemotherapy of advanced (Stage D, relapsing, hormonal-resistant) prostatic cancer had never been conducted, the National Prostatic Cancer Project (NPCP) of the United States in 1973 began such an objective comparison using 5-FU or Cytoxan compared with a wide variety of other conventionally available nonchemotherapeutic agents. The results to date are most encouraging.[16]

This group of investigators currently consists of those listed at the end of this chapter, and the specific initial protocol (protocol 100) is presented in Figure 1. Specific criteria for careful patient selection have been maintained (Table 1). Objective and subjective criteria of remission during or after therapy have also been tested and found most satisfactory (Lists 1 and 2).

The response to initial and crossover therapy for these patients is shown in List 3 and Figure 2. As of April 1976 there was a longer duration of response (stable and/or partial regression) in patients during the initially randomized chemotherapies than during crossover or standard therapy. A proportionately larger number of patients obtained more clinical benefit on Cytoxan than on standard therapy ($P<0.02$). There was also a proportionately larger number of patients who responded to 5-FU than to standard therapy but the difference was not statistically

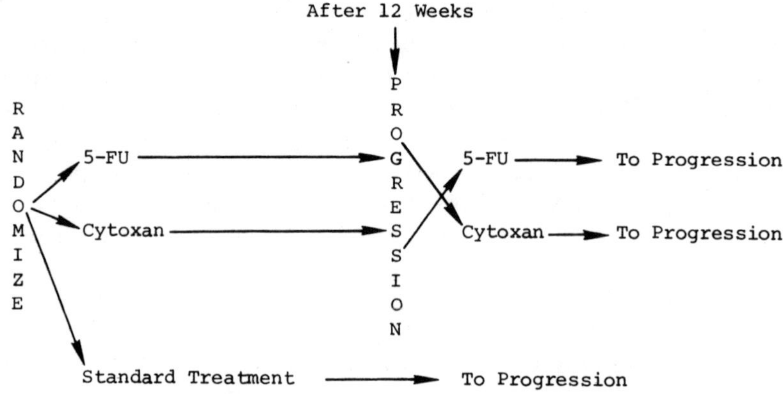

Figure 1. Protocol 100—First Protocol of the National Prostatic Cancer Project (1973). Treatment schema: 5-FU, 600 mg/M² IV per week vs Cytoxan, 1 g/M² IV per 3 weeks vs standard treatment. A crossover between chemotherapies will be done at progression unless death intervenes.

Table 1
Objective Response to Treatment After at Least Three Weeks on Study*

Treatment	Stable	Partial Regression	Progression	Total
Initial				
5-FU	8	4	21	33
Cytoxan	16	3	22	41
Standard	7	0	29	36
Total	31	7	72	110
Crossover to				
5-FU	6	0	14	20
Cytoxan	4	1	14	19
Total	10	1	28	39

*National Prostatic Cancer Project Protocol 100, observations as of April 1, 1976.
Significant difference ($P<0.02$) between response on initial randomization to Cytoxan and standard treatments.

significant ($P>0.05$). None of the patients randomized to standard therapy exhibited a partial regression of disease in comparison to seven who responded to the chemotherapies. For patients crossed from Cytoxan to 5-FU, disease of six became stable. Crossover therapy from 5-FU to Cytoxan resulted in stabilization of disease for four patients, and one obtained a partial regression (Table 1, Figure 2). There was a significant difference ($P<0.05$) for patients whose disease was stabilized on the initial and/or crossover chemotherapies in comparison to the results obtained for patients on standard therapy.

Twenty-two of the original evaluable patients are still alive. These are distributed among the responses as follows: 5-FU patients: stable (5/8), partial regression (2/4), progression (1/21); Cytoxan patients:

List 1
National Prostatic Cancer Project
Chemotherapy Protocol 100–Criteria for
Patient Selection

A. Historically confirmed metastatic prostatic carcinoma in relapse on endocrine therapy.
B. Less than 2000 rads pelvic irradiation.
C. No prior cytotoxic chemotherapy.
D. No other primary neoplasm.
E. Expected survival more than 90 days.
F. WBC greater than 4000/cu mm.
G. Platelet count greater than 100,000/cu mm.

List 2
Protocol 100–Evaluation of Therapy
Partial Objective Regression

A. A 50% reduction in measurable or palpable soft tissue tumor mass when present.
B. Return of an elevated acid phosphatase to normal.
C. The recalcification of some osteolytic lesions if present.

List 3
Protocol 100–Evaluation of Therapy
Objective Progression
(or also relapse after adequate therapy)

Any of the following criteria:
A. Significant deterioration in symptoms, decrease in weight, or decrease in performance status.
B. Appearance of new areas of malignant disease.
C. Increase in any previously measurable lesion (soft tissue and lung, excluding bone) by more than 50% in two perpendicular diameters.
D. An increase in acid or alkaline phosphatase *alone* is not to be considered an indication of progression. These should be used in conjunction with other criteria.

stable (6/16), partial regression (1/3), progression (2/22); standard therapy: stable (1/7), progression (4/27).

All patients whose disease continued to progress on initial randomization to the three arms of the study survived for an approximate mean

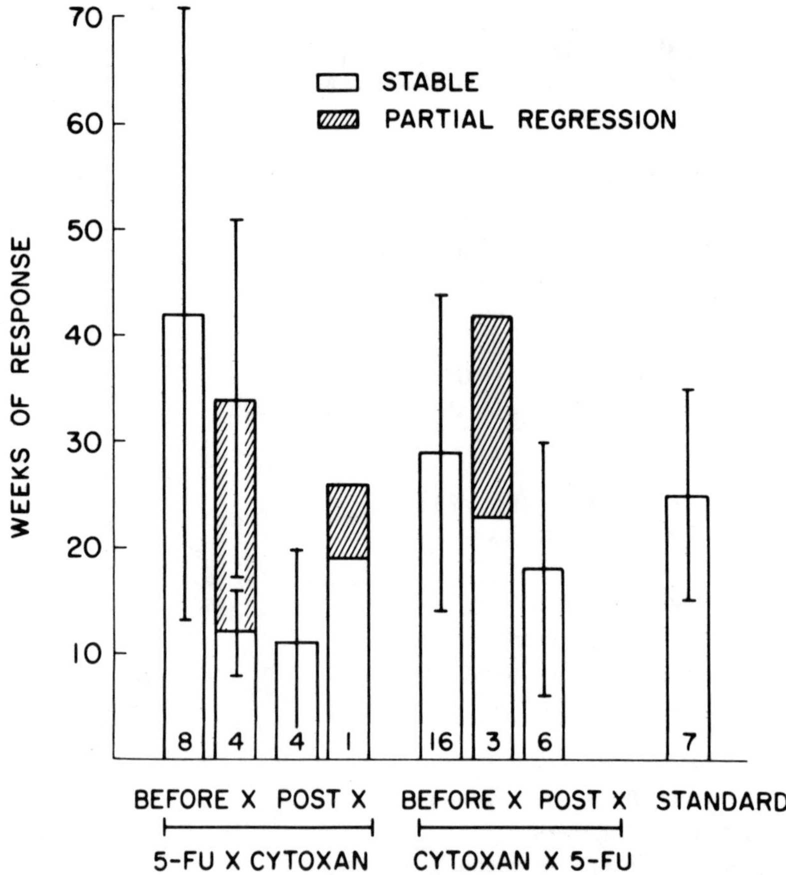

Figure 2. Duration of Response—Protocol 100, results as of April 1, 1976. The columns denote weeks of response by mean and one standard deviation. Numbers of patients receiving treatment are indicated within the columns. On crossover therapy (Post X) patients treated with 5-fluorouracil received Cytoxan and Cytoxan-treated patients received 5-FU. The benefit of chemotherapy is readily seen.

duration of 36 to 37 weeks. The duration of survival for patients who responded to chemotherapy (stable plus partial regression) was comparatively longer for 5-FU-treated patients ($P<0.01$) and Cytoxan-treated patients ($P<0.05$) than for patients in progression under these treatments. Patient survival for those responding (stable and partial regression) to chemotherapy in general was longer than for patients responding (stable) on standard therapy.

Since survival is dependent on total therapy, we compared those patients whose disease progressed before or after crossover therapy with those whose disease intially progressed and then responded (stable and progression) to therapy, or who initially responded and then failed to respond to crossover therapy. The duration of survival progressively increased as follows: responders before and/or after crossover therapy lived longer than those patients whose disease progressed throughout the study. The survival of those patients whose disease progressed before and after crossover therapy was significantly poorer than for the group of patients whose disease responded initially and then progressed on crossover therapy ($P<0.05$) and the group whose disease responded to both chemotherapeutic agents ($P<0.01$). For either group of patients who responded, survival was longer than for patients whose disease was stable on standard therapy.

This represents a continued in-depth evaluation of survival for a randomized national trial for chemotherapy of advanced prostatic cancer. The first protocol has been very successful in this regard. The results are encouraging in that they support the objectivity of the significant response data and the beneficial objective and subjective results obtained from the use of the first two chemotherapeutic agents evaluated, Cytoxan and 5-FU, in the treatment of relapsing advanced prostatic carcinoma.

OTHER PROTOCOLS

Some patients who have previously received >2,000 rads radiotherapy to the pelvis were found intolerant of bone marrow-depressant cytotoxic agents such as Cytoxan or 5-fluorouracil. Accordingly, Protocol 200 (Figure 3) was introduced. Patient entry for this protocol began July 1, 1974 and was completed April 2, 1976. During this 21-month period of patient accrual, 125 patients were entered into the study. Only two protocol violations occurred; one was a patient entered without previous irradiation treatment, and the other a patient whose life expectancy was less than 90 days.

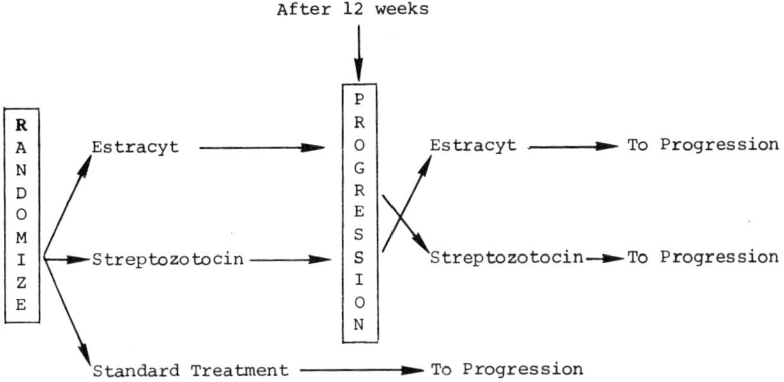

Figure 3. Protocol 200—Treatment schema: Estracyt, 600 mg/M² orally daily in 3 divided doses vs streptozotocin 500 mg/M² IV daily for 5 days every 6 weeks vs standard treatment. A crossover will be done at progression between chemotherapies unless death intervenes.

Analysis of the prognostic factors on entrance into the study revealed no significant differences for each arm of the study with regard to 1) age distribution, 2) initial performance status, 3) elevation of acid phosphatase determination, 4) serum hemoglobin level, and 5) presence of chronic disease. These findings suggested that no single treatment arm received more than its share of patients with favorable or unfavorable prognoses.

As mentioned in the second nationally randomized cooperative chemotherapy trial of the National Prostatic Cancer Project, 125 patients with histologically confirmed progressing, advanced carcinoma of the prostate (clinical Stage D) who had had prior pelvic irradiation of at least 2,000 rads received as initial therapy one of two non-myelosuppressive agents, estramustine phosphate or streptozotocin, for comparison with patients randomized to receive standard treatment. Patients whose disease was progressive after 12 weeks on chemotherapy were crossed over to receive the alternative therapeutic agent. Response to treatment was evaluated in 105 patients on the basis of previously established and defined criteria.

All known prognostic factors were comparable among the three treatment arms. The objective response rates to therapy were 19% in the standard arm (stable only), 30% in the estramustine phosphate arm (stable and partial regression), and 32% in the streptozotocin arm (stable only). Thus far, four patients who crossed to estramustine phosphate and two patients who crossed to streptozotocin responded to therapy. In a number of response parameters estramustine phosphate had an advantage over the other two treatment arms. Nausea and vomiting were the predominant toxicities for patients in all treatment arms. Average survival time is longer for patients receiving the chemotherapies. Estramustine phosphate seems to be the superior drug, and both chemotherapies are superior to standard treatment. A significant number of patients are still being treated actively, and their responses will affect the final conclusions only more favorably.[17]

The patients in this study were compared to the previous chemotherapy study (Protocol 100) conducted by the National Prostatic Cancer Project for such factors as age on entrance to study, initial performance status, initial serum acid phosphatase, hemoglobin levels on study, number of orchiectomized patients, and the presence of chronic diseases. All but two of the comparisons were nonsignificant. Patients entered on Protocol 100 were 2.4 years older than those on the present protocol and had a significantly better initial performance status than patients in the present study. Although patients in both studies had tumors in progression in clinical Stage D and had failed on conventional therapy, patients in the present study were regarded as more difficult to treat since prior radiotherapy to the pelvis ruled out the use of myelosuppressive antineoplastic agents, and because of the initial poor performance status of these patients. Although estramustine phosphate had a definite advantage over streptozotocin in terms of partial responses and other response parameters, it is gratifying and encouraging that any measure of response could be obtained with either agent in these patients who were at the time those for whom so little in the way of treatment could be offered. The increased duration of survival in this and the previous study supports the objectivity of the response data and the beneficial effects of chemotherapy.

There was a higher percentage of poorly differentiated and a lower incidence of medium differentiated tumors in this group of clinical Stage D patients than was found in a retrospective review of Stage D patients at Roswell Park Memorial Institute.[3] Although prior studies have demonstrated a relationship between survival and primary tumor grade and between primary tumor grade and response to hormonal treatment, this was not evaluated further in the present study.[18,19] In an evaluation of patients on Protocol 100 it was reported that histologic pattern alone may not identify which individual pattern may respond favorably to treatment since additional factors may be operative.[7]

Eighty-two percent of the patients in this study entered with an elevated serum acid phosphatase level in comparison with the 74% who were on Protocol 100.[20] Survival was significantly shorter for those patients who entered the study with an elevated acid phosphatase, but this in itself may not be used as a predictor of response. Acid phosphatase, as it relates to prognosis and the monitoring of treatment response, requires further analysis, particularly with the advent of newly developed specific immunologic assays.[21,22]

The option of using chemotherapy as a modality of treatment for some patients is now being recognized. Additional single agents, combinations, and adjuvant chemotherapy will be evaluated by our group in the treatment of the advanced as well as earlier stages of prostatic adenocarcinoma.

In another new Protocol 300 (Figure 4) those patients who have not received extensive irradiation to the pelvis (more than 2,000 rads) are currently being randomized to receive procarbazine, DTIC, or Cytoxan. The status of the 86 patients accrued from April 1, 1975 through May 28, 1977 is available. Forty-nine patients have been on study for more than three weeks, eight patients were off study within three weeks, and 29 patients were recently entered on study. The objective responses were based on the 49 patients listed on study after at least three weeks of treatment. The response rates for cyclophosphamide, DTIC, and procarbazine, considering both stable patients as well as partial regressions as response, are 27%, 48%, and 29%, respectively.

There are other agents in addition to Estracyt that have shown promise in other Phase I and Phase II trials. We have also recently reported some additional progress, particularly in those patients receiving

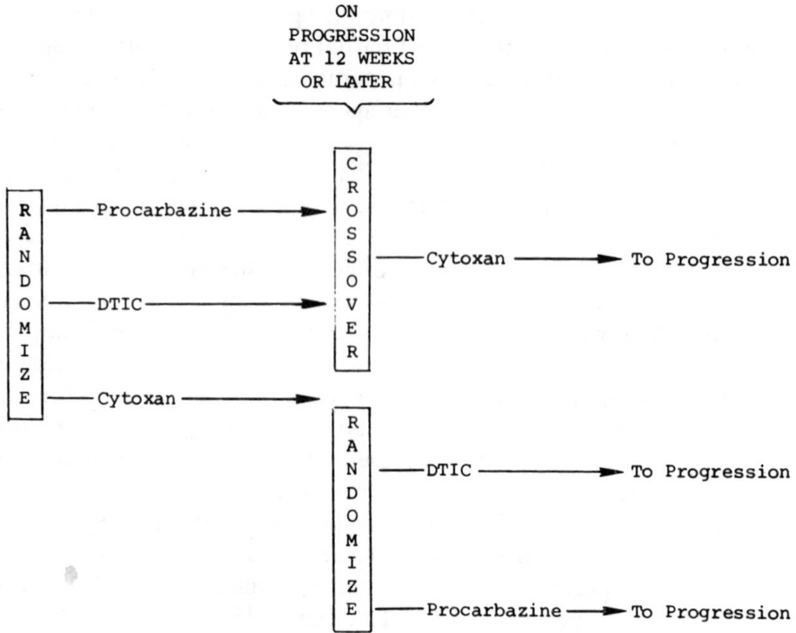

Figure 4. Protocol 300—Treatment schema: DTIC, 200 mg/M² IV days 1-5, 21 days rest, then repeat cycle vs Procarbazine, 100 mg/M² orally daily days 1-22, 3 weeks rest; Rx days 44-65, 3 weeks rest, etc. vs Cytoxan, 1 g/M² IV every 3 weeks. A crossover will be done at progression unless death intervenes.

long-term Estracyt. Seven of these patients (four Stage D and three Stage C) who have received continuous Estracyt for more than one year are being observed. These patients receiving long-term therapy are particularly important in consideration of drug effect and lack of toxicity. The seven patients receiving long-term Estracyt are described in Table 2. All patients had advanced symptomatic disease with an average of 2.5 years from diagnosis to protocol (range six months to seven years). Five of these seven patients have progressed on estrogen therapy. Four had Stage D and three Stage C, according to Whitmore's staging system (Stage C—extensive carcinoma without metastasis and induration extending beyond the capsule of the prostate; Stage D—metastatic cancer, eg, bones or soft tissue).[23] The response and side effects in the seven patients are summarized in Table 3.

Estracyt, a chemical combination of nitrogen mustard and estradiol, has been found effective in advanced prostatic carcinoma in patients whose conditions are refractory to estrogens.[24-29] The average duration of response was at least one year in other early reports.[25,27] The toxic side effects of this agent are related to the steroid moiety of Estracyt, with none of the patients demonstrating hematologic depression. This has been reported previously.[24,27,30] One of these seven patients had gastrointestinal toxicity which appeared one year after starting therapy and was not relieved by decreasing the dose (Table 2).

Gynecomastia occurred in two of seven patients in our experience. However, the feminizing side effects were less prominent with Estracyt than with diethylstilbestrol in doses of more than 1 mg/day. One patient with previously diagnosed congestive heart failure developed pedal edema. This was easily controlled by diuretics. No severe toxicity appeared with prolonged Estracyt therapy (Table 3). Estracyt appears to be a safe and effective treatment for patients with prostatic carcinoma who have failed to respond to conventional therapy. On the basis of these long-term responses, it may also have a role in the treatment of earlier stages of prostatic cancer.

In addition to studies of Estracyt, we have also studied combination therapy with a new agent, prednimustine (Stereocyt, Leo 1031). Prednimustine is an ester of chlorambucil and prednisone with a high therapeutic index in animal studies, low toxicity for normal stem cells, and effectiveness in limited trials in various human tumors.[29,31-36] Between July 1975 and April 1976, 21 patients with symptomatic Stage D prostatic carcinoma were treated with the combination of estramustine and prednimustine. The doses of estramustine and prednimustine were 600 $mg/M^2/day$ and 15 $mg/M^2/day$, respectively, and were given daily in divided oral doses. The dosage was adjusted according to toxicity. The pretreatment data on the 21 patients are shown in Table 4. Their mean age was 66. All had prior estrogen therapy, 12/21 (57%) had orchiectomy, 11/21 (52%) radiation therapy, and 6/21 (28%) had previous chemotherapy. The mean duration from initial diagnosis to protocol therapy was 3½ years. The criteria for objective and subjective response were those defined by the National Prostatic Cancer Project.

The response of the patients is shown in Table 5. Five patients had an objective response lasting between four to six months; three of these patients are still in remission. Four additional patients had a subjective response consisting of complete disappearance of bone pain, improvement in sense of well-being, appetite, and weight gain. A majority of responding patients demonstrated some improvement within the first month of therapy. Seven patients were stable for two to six months, and two of them have relapsed after four to six months of therapy.

The percentages of responses in this study (24% objective and 43% subjective) show the potential usefulness of this combination in the treatment of patients with advanced prostatic cancer. All patients had progressive metastatic disease after failure on hormonal treatment, and in most of the cases also on radiation therapy or chemotherapy. Despite their advanced stages, they demonstrated a relatively high response rate without significant toxicity. Previous study with chemotherapy on patients failing on hormonal therapy have demonstrated less than a 10% objective response.[37]

The use of the steroid structure as a carrier for alkylating agents,

Table 2
Characteristics of Long Survivors on Estracyt Therapy

				Previous Therapy				
Case No.	Age	Stage*	Grade†	Type‡	Duration of Response (yrs.)	Time to Estracyt from Initial Diagnosis (yrs.)	Stage* at Start of Estracyt	Reason for Start on Estracyt
1	69	B	WD	E	2	2½	C	Urinary obstruction
2	82	C	PD	E	1½	1½	D	Bone pain
3	59	C	WD	Rad	3	7	D	Bone pain
				E	None			
4	75	C	MD	Rad	½	½	C	Perineal pain
5	53	D	PD-MD	E	2	2	D	Bone pain
6	76	D	PD-MD	O+E	2	2	D	Bone pain
7	68	C	WD	–	–	1½	C	Urinary obstruction

*According to classification of Whitmore[24]

† WD—well differentiated; MD—moderately differentiated; PD—poorly differentiated

‡ E—estrogens; Rad—radiation; O—orchiectomy

Table 3
Response and Side Effects from Estracyt Therapy

		Response		Side Effects		
No.	Duration of Estracyt Therapy (Months)	Subjective	Objective	Mild	Moderate	Severe
1	37+	+	Stable	—	—	—
2	36+	+	Elevated acid and alkaline phosphatase returned to normal (Figure 1)	—	—	—
3	28 (31+)*	+	(Stable)*	(Edema)	—	—
4	26+	+	Decrease in size of prostate and return of abnormal cystogram to normal	(Gynecomastia)	—	—
5	6 (14+)*	+	(Stable)*	—	—	—
6	12	+	Disappearance of blastic metastases (Figures 2-5)	—	(Nausea, vomiting)	—
7	12+	+	Stable	(Gynecomastia)	—	—

*In parentheses: Combined Estracyt and Leo 1031 therapy
Criteria for objective and subjective responses are those established by the National Prostatic Cancer Project

Table 4
Characteristics of Patients on Start of Therapy

	No.	Mean	Range
No. Patients	21		
Age (years)		66	54-85
Previous therapy			
Estrogen	21		
Orchiectomy	12		
Radiation	11		
Chemotherapy	6		
Years from diagnosis		3.5	0.5-10

Table 5
Response to Prednimustine and Estramustine in Advanced Prostatic Carcinoma

	No. Patients	Percentage
Objective response*	5	24
Subjective response*	4	19
Total response	9	43
Stable disease	7	33
Progression	5	24
Total	21	100

*National Prostatic Cancer Project criteria[30]

which increases their specificity and decreases their toxicity, has been proposed by Konyves and Liljekvist.[31] Kirdani et al. showed a specific action of estramustine on canine and rat prostates, which is probably a combined effect of the estrogen and the nitrogen mustard moieties of the drug.[38] Tritsch et al. also showed a marked affinity of prostatic acid phosphatase for the phosphate group of estramustine.[39]

Prednimustine, on the other hand, does not show a special affinity to the prostate, but it has a better therapeutic index than each of its constituents in animal tumors.[31] It has been found effective in a variety of solid tumors as well as in patients with lymphoma who have relapsed on chlorambucil and prednisone.[33,35] Our preliminary results indicate that prednimustine as a nonspecific alkylating agent may increase the responses obtained by the specific drug estramustine in advanced prostatic cancer.

The results thus described from studies at our own institution or the National Prostatic Cancer Project strongly suggest that chemotherapy can be of significant therapeutic benefit in relapsing advanced prostatic cancer in man. Our National Prostatic Cancer Project studies naturally are now evolving toward the careful use of chemotherapy at earlier clinical stages of this disease in the reasonable expectation that such intervention if carefully done, could result in even greater clinical benefit than that seen in the advanced and sometimes terminal stages.

Thus, a new Protocol (500) (Figure 5) has been recently instituted. This ongoing study will treat newly diagnosed clinical Stage D patients who have not had prior hormonal therapy. The results from this randomized trial could be of major significance. In addition, Protocol 600 (Figure 6) has been instituted. The purpose of investigators in this study is to determine the efficacy of the addition of chemotherapy (Estracyt or Cytoxan) to estrogen therapy as a means of controlling Stage D prostatic

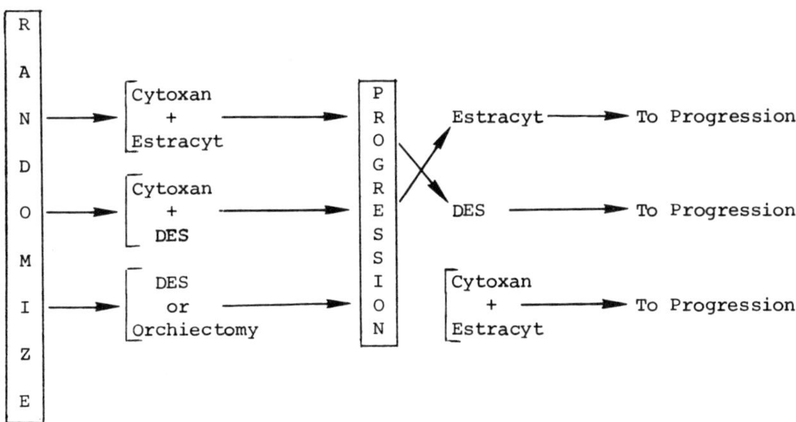

Figure 5. Protocol 500—Treatment schema: Cytoxan, 1 g/M^2 IV every 3 weeks plus Estracyt, 600 mg/M^2 orally daily in 3 divided doses vs Cytoxan 1 g/M^2 IV every 3 weeks plus diethylstilbestrol, 1 mg tid orally vs diethylstilbestrol, 1 mg tid orally, or orchiectomy.

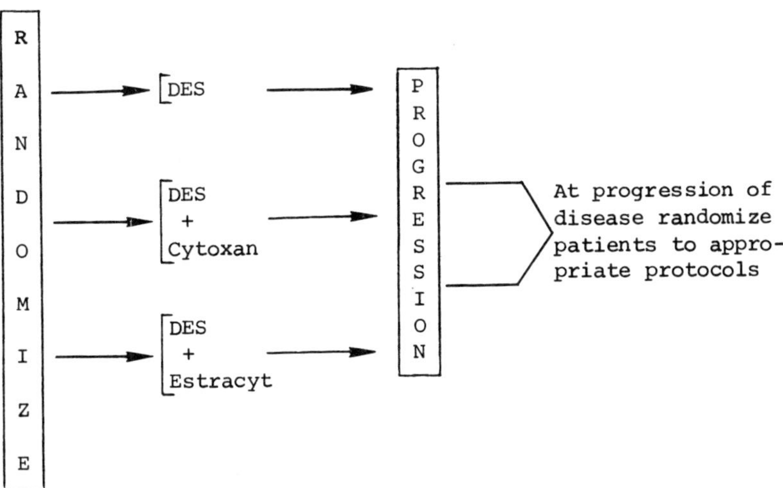

Figure 6. Protocol 600—Treatment schema: Diethylstilbestrol, 1 mg tid orally vs diethylstilbestrol, 1 mg tid orally plus Cytoxan, 1 g/M^2 IV every 3 weeks vs diethylstilbestrol, 1 mg tid orally plus Estracyt, 600 mg/M^2 orally daily in 3 divided doses.

carcinoma. The study will determine the success of therapy in part by the prevention of recurrence, duration of stability, and/or absence of progression.

In additional studies we have found that Leo 1031 alone is also effective in patients with advanced, hormone-resistant prostatic cancer.[40] Twenty-three patients with advanced, hormone-resistant prostatic cancer were treated with daily oral prednimustine, which is a combination of prednisolone and chlorambucil. Eight patients (35%) responded subjectively with disappearance of skeletal pain and improvement in appetite, weight, and sense of well-being. Three patients had objective evidence of tumor regression, ie, recalcification of lytic bone lesions, shrinkage of enlarged prostates, and return of acid phosphatase to normal. Clinical toxicity was moderate, and only occasional myelosuppression was encountered.

The ease of administration and predictable toxicity of prednimustine make it a potentially useful agent alone or in combination, for advanced prostatic cancer.[40]

There have been additional studies by others using other single agents in advanced prostatic cancer. Hydroxyurea has been reported to have some effect although Melphalan has not.[41,42] These agents and others are under ongoing, adjuvant, therapeutic review by additional study groups.

Adjuvant immunotherapy characterized by BCG has been attempted in prostatic cancer.[43] We have not found it to be of substantial or sustained benefit in that form, and the experience of others seems to confirm this viewpoint.[44] In the future, less toxic agents may be considered for management of the patient with advanced, disseminated prostatic cancer.

Additional earlier adjuvant therapeutic studies will without doubt show increased survival rates and increased numbers of patients with full resolution of disease, based upon these results that have been carefully reviewed in patients with advanced hormonal resistance to prostate cancer.

We feel that it is necessary to continue the evaluation of the activity of single agents in order to arrive ultimately at combinations which may be demonstrably effective in the treatment of all stages of prostatic cancer. Therefore, in May 1977 we initiated Protocol 700, shown in Figure 7, for treatment of progressing patients with distant metastatic disease who have not had prior extensive pelvic irradiation. The chemotherapeutic agents to be compared are hydroxyurea vs MeCCNU vs Cytoxan. Similarly, for those patients who had prior extensive pelvic irradiation, Protocol 800, shown in Figure 8, was initiated in June of 1977 and will compare Estracyt vs vincristine vs Estracyt plus vincristine.

While we continue to evaluate the activity of single agents in those patients with progressing disease, adjuvant chemotherapy is planned for clinical Stages B, C, and D-1 patients.

SUMMARY

Advanced, disseminated, hormone-resistant prostatic cancer represents a substantial percentage of our patient population to date. Despite

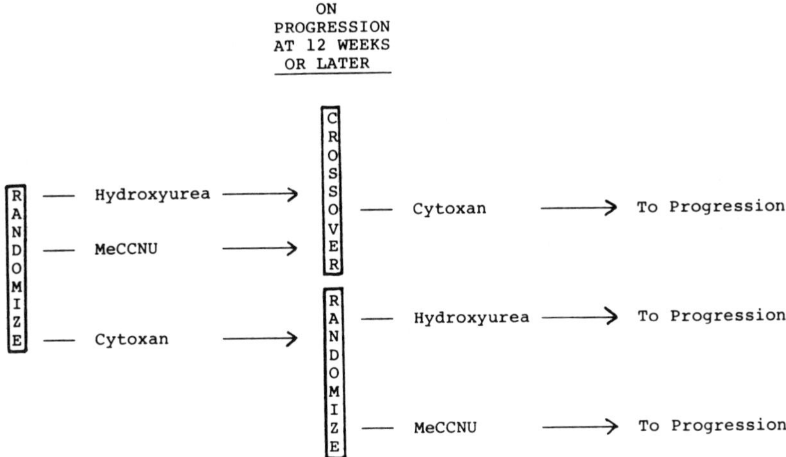

Figure 7. Protocol 700—Treatment schema: Hydroxyurea, 3 g/M² p.o. every 3 days in 3 divided doses vs MeCCNU, 175 mg/M² p.o. every 6 weeks vs Cytoxan, 1 g/M² IV every 3 weeks.

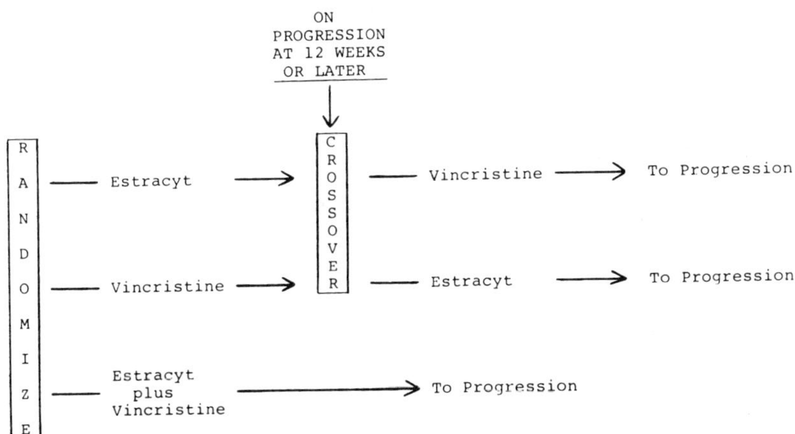

Figure 8. Protocol 800—Treatment schema: Estracyt, 600 mg/M² p.o. daily in 3 divided doses, vincristine, 1 mg/M² IV once every 2 weeks *or* Estracyt, 600 mg/M² p.o. daily in 3 divided doses *plus* vincristine, 1 mg/M² IV once every 2 weeks.

advances and techniques in diagnosis and screening, we are faced with a disease that frequently is diagnosed in the advanced stage. For some time, sequential randomized studies of the effectiveness of nonhormonal chemotherapeutic agents has been wanting. The National Prostatic Cancer Project has over 800 patients that have been evaluated in such trials. Additional Phase I and Phase II studies have been done at individual institutions. Based on these results, urologists today are able to offer patients with this phase of the disease effective cytotoxic agents which have minimal toxicity and can produce remission and even improve survival. The agents must be used discriminately because those patients with extensive prior radiotherapy and compromised bone marrow reserve must receive certain agents that do not have additional toxicity. Regardless of that fact, patients with both radiated and nonradiated primary prostatic tumors who had hormonal therapy and are in relapse can now be offered useful and effective agents. Earlier treatment, both in the advanced stage of the disease and at an early surgical and radiotherapeutic primary treatment stage, is underway and hopefully will provide a better outlook for patients with prostatic cancer.

National Prostatic Cancer Project
Chemotherapy:
Participating Treatment Centers
(October 1977)

Gerald P. Murphy, M.D., Project Director
Roswell Park Memorial Institute
Buffalo, New York.

Robert P. Gibbons, M.D.
Virginia Mason Research Center
Seattle, Washington.

George R. Prout, M.D.
Massachusetts General Hospital
Boston, Massachusetts.

William W. Scott, M.D., Treatment Chairman
Johns Hopkins Hospital
Baltimore, Maryland.

Douglas E. Johnson, M.D.
M. D. Anderson Hospital and Tumor Institute
Houston, Texas.

Stefan Loening, M.D.
University of Iowa Hospitals and Clinics
Iowa City, Iowa.

Clair Cox, M.D., Chairman, Department of Urology
University of Tennessee Medical College
Memphis, Tennessee.

Joseph D. Schmidt, M.D.
University Hospitals
University of California at San Diego
San Diego, California.

REFERENCES

1. Murphy, G. P., Joiner, J. R., and Saroff, J. Prostatic cancer. Evolution of treatment at a comprehensive cancer center (1970-1974). *Urology.* 8:357-62, 1976.

2. Murphy, G. P., Joiner, J. R., Vana, J. et al. Treatment of prostatic carcinoma in Western New York. *NY State J Med.* 76:869-73, 1976.

3. Murphy, G. P., Saroff, J., Joiner, J. et al. Prostatic carcinoma. Treated at categorical center, 1960-1969. *NY State J Med.* 75:1663-9, 1975.

4. Murphy, G. P. Management of reactivated prostatic cancer. Edited by P. L. Munson, J. Glover, E. Diczfalusy et al. In *Vitamins and Hormones. Advances in Research and Applications. International Symposium on Endocrine Control of the Prostate.* Vol. 33. New York: Academic Press, December 1975, 399-415.

5. Welvaart, K., Merrin, C. E., Mittelman, A. et al. Stage D prostatic carcinoma. Survival rate in relapsed patients following new forms of palliation. *Urology.* 4:283-6, 1974.

6. Schmidt, J. D., Johnson, D. E., Scott, W. W. et al. Chemotherapy of advanced prostatic cancer. Evaluation of response parameters. *Urology.* 7:602-10, 1976.

7. Gibbons, R. P., Scott, W. W., Johnson, D. E. et al. Prostatic carcinoma: relationship between primary tumor, histologic grade, and response to chemotherapy. *Urology.* 8:222-6, 1976.

8. Scott, W. W., Johnson, D. E., Schmidt, J. D. et al. Chemotherapy of advanced prostatic carcinoma with cyclophosphamide or 5-fluorouracil: results of first national randomized study. *J Urol.* 114:909-11, 1975.

9. Catane, R., Kaufman, J., Mittelman, A. et al. Disappearance of osteoblastic metastases in prostatic carcinoma following estramustine therapy. *JAMA.* 237:2471, 1977.

10. Varkarakis, M. J., Winterberger, A. R., Gaeta, J. et al. Lung metastases in prostatic carcinoma. Clinical significance. *Urology.* 3:447-52, 1974.

11. Catane, R., Kaufman, J., West, C. et al. Brain metastasis from prostatic carcinoma. *Cancer.* 38:2583-7, 1976.

12. Chu, T. M., Shukla, S. K., Mittelman, A. et al. Comparative evaluation of serum acid phosphatase, urinary cholesterol, and androgens in diagnosis of prostatic cancer. *Urology.* 6:291-4, 1975.

13. Sandberg, A. A., Rosenthal, H., Mittelman, A. et al. Prostatic cancer. Transcortin levels during treatment with estramustine phosphate. *Urology.* 6:17-21, 1975.

14. Murphy, G. P., Saroff, J., Joiner, J. R. et al. Chemotherapy of advanced prostatic cancer by the National Prostatic Cancer Group. *Semin Oncol.* 3:103-6, 1976.

15. Murphy, G. P. Chemotherapy of advanced prostatic cancer. *Rev Surg.* 34:75-87, 1977.

16. Scott, W. W., Gibbons, R. P., Johnson, D. E. et al. Comparison of 5-fluorouracil (NSC-19893) and cyclophosphamide (NSC-26271) in patients with advanced carcinoma of the prostate. *Cancer Chemother Rep.* 59:195-201, 1975.

17. Murphy, G. P., Gibbons, R. P., Johnson, D. E. et al. A comparison of estramustine phosphate and streptozotocin in patients with advanced prostatic carcinoma who have had extensive irradiation. *J Urol.* 118:288-91, 1977.

18. Pool, T. L., and Thompson, G. J. Conservative treatment of carcinoma of the prostate. *JAMA.* 160:833-7, 1956.

19. Schirmer, H.K.A., Murphy, G. P., and Scott, W. W. Hormonal therapy of prostatic cancer: a correlation between histologic differentiation of prostatic cancer and the clinical course of the disease. *Urol Digest.* 4:15-19, 1965.

20. Johnson, D. E., Chu, T. M., Scott, W. W. et al. Current clinical significance of serum acid phosphatase levels in advanced prostatic carcinoma as studied by the National Prostatic Cancer Project. *Urology.* 8:123-6, 1976.

21. Choe, B. K., Pontes, E. J., McDonald, I. et al. Immunochemical studies of prostatic acid phosphatase. *Cancer Treat Rep.* 61:201-4, 1977.

22. Chu, T. M., Wang, M. C., Scott, W. W. et al. Immunochemical detection of serum prostatic acid phosphatase methodology and clinical evaluation. *Invest Urol.* 15:319-23, 1978.

23. Whitmore, W. F. The rationale and results of ablative surgery for prostatic cancer. *Cancer.* 16:1119-32, 1963.

24. Jonsson, G., and Hogberg, B. Treatment of advanced prostatic carcinoma with Estracyt. A preliminary report. *Scand J Urol Nephrol.* 5:103-7, 1971.

25. Lindberg, B. Treatment of rapidly progressing prostatic carcinoma with Estracyt. *J Urol.* 108:303-6, 1972.

26. Mayer, E. J. Orale Estracyt—behandlung beim prostatakarzinom. *Ther Umsch.* 32:114-19, 1975.

27. Mittelman, A., Shukla, S. K., and Murphy, G. P. Extended therapy of stage D carcinoma of the prostate with oral estramustine phosphate. *J Urol.* 115:409-12, 1976.

28. Nilsson, T., and Jonsson, G. Clinical results with estramustine phosphate (NSC-89199): a comparison of the intravenous and oral preparations. *Cancer Chemother Rep.* 59:229-32, 1975.

29. Konyves, I., Nordenskjöld, B., Plym-Forshell, G. et al. Preliminary clinical and absorption studies with prednimustine in patients with mammary carcinoma. *Eur J Cancer.* 11:841-4, 1975.

30. Mittelman, A., Shukla, S. K., Welvaart, K. et al. Oral estramustine phosphate (NSC-89199) in the treatment of advanced (Stage D) carcinoma of the prostate. *Cancer Chemother Rep.* 59:219-23, 1975.

31. Konyves, I. and Liljekvist, J. The steroid molecule as a carrier of cytotoxic groups. In *Advances in Tumour Prevention, Detection, and Characterization.* Proceedings of the Sixth International Symposium on the Biological Charcterization of Human Tumours, Copenhagen, May 13-16, 1975. New York: American Elsevier Publishing Company, 3:98-105, 1976.

32. Evenaar, A. H., Wins, E.H.R., and van Putten, L. M. Letter to the editor. Cell-killing effectiveness of an alkylating steroid (Leo 1031). *Eur J Cancer.* 9:773-4, 1973.

33. Aungst, C. W., Mittelman, A., and Murphy, G. P. Treatment of chronic lymphocytic leukemia and lymphosarcoma with a new chlorambucil ester of prednisolone (Leo 1031) (NSC-134087). *J Surg Oncol.* 7:457-60, 1975.

34. Brandt, L., Konyves, I., and Möller, T. R. Therapeutic effect of Leo 1031, an alkylating corticosteroid ester, in lymphoproliferative disorders. I. Chronic lymphocytic leukaemia. *Acta Med Scand.* 197:317-22, 1975.

35. Kaufman, J. H., Hanjura, G. L., Mittelman, A. et al. Study of Leo 1031 (NSC-134087) in lymphocytic lymphoma and chronic lymphocytic leukemia. *Cancer Treat Rep.* 60:277-9, 1976.

36. Möller, T. R., Brandt, L., Konyves, I. et al. Therapeutic effect of Leo 1031, an alkylating corticosteroid ester, in lymphoproliferative disorders. II. Lymphocytic Lymphoma. *Acta Med Scand.* 197:323-7, 1975.

37. Scott, W. W., Johnson, D. E., Schmidt, J. D. et al. Chemotherapy of advanced prostatic carcinoma with cyclophosphamide or 5-fluorouracil: results of first national randomized study. *J Urol.* 114:909-11, 1975.

38. Kirdani, R. Y., Müntzing, J., Varkarakis, M. J. et al. Studies on the antiprostatic action of Estracyt, a nitrogen mustard of estradiol. *Cancer Res.* 34:1031-7, 1974.

39. Tritsch, G. L., Shukla, S. K., Mittelman, A. et al. Estracyt (NSC-89199) as a substrate for phosphatases in human serum. *Invest Urol.* 12:38-9, 1974.

40. Catane, R., Kaufman, J. H., Madajewicz, S. et al. Prednimustine therapy for advanced prostatic cancer. *Br J Urol.* 50:29-32, 1978.

41. Lerner, H. J., and Malloy, T. R. Hydroxyurea in Stage D carcinoma of prostate. *Urology.* 10:35-8, 1977.

42. Houghton, A. L., Robinson, M.R.G., and Smith, P. H. Melphalan in advanced prostatic cancer: a pilot study. *Cancer Treat Rep.* 61:923-4, 1977.

43. Merrin, C., Han, T., Klein, E. et al. Immunotherapy of prostatic carcinoma with Bacillus *Calmette-Guerin. Cancer Chemother Rep.* 59:157-63, 1975.

44. Robinson, M.R.G., Rigby, C. C., Pugh, R.C.B. et al. Adjuvant immunotherapy with BCG in carcinoma of the prostate. *Br J Urol.* 49:221-6, 1977.

INDEX